Scars Tell Stories

*From a Cystic Fibrosis and
Heart-Double Lung Transplant Patient*

Dan Lagasse

USBN # 9798675102334 (paperback)

Published by
Kindle Direct Publishing
www.kdp.amazon.com

Cover graphics by Liz Murphy
miaeliidesigns@gmail.com

Contributions (pages 178-180 and 283-289)
by Doug Lagasse

Photographs (Cover and also page 284 and 289)
by Doug Lagasse

Scripture references are from the New International Version unless otherwise noted.

Printed in the United States of America

Dedication

To my daughters Shirena and Jessica,

Your trials in life will be different than mine.

I pray your faith will grow stronger through them.

Thanks

My greatest thanks go to my wife DeAnna, who has walked with me and remained devoted to me throughout my adult life. She knew I had cystic fibrosis when she married me, but couldn't fathom the ways it (and other illnesses) would impact our married life and lives of service. She is my champion and my hero. Her faithfulness and perseverance are testament to her love. She has, in a tangible way, given me life.

DeAnna also edited these stories, offered valuable insights and corrected my memory where it faltered. She has carried much of the unseen burden of my illnesses. She is the one who chose to marry a dying man because she loved me. She was the one who rose at four a.m. to give me therapy before she left each day to go to nursing school. She was the one who cooked special meals so I'd have energy and health. She slept in hospital cots beside me all over the world. She carried my suitcases and hauled the heavy groceries up the flights of steps to our apartment in Berlin. And she is the one who stayed alone in Iraq with two babies while I jetted off to Europe to get my lungs treated. When I became really ill she is the one who hoisted heavy oxygen tanks into the station wagon. She hauled the heavy wheel chair out of the car and pushed me to church each week. And she prayed in faith while I was slated to die. She is my hero.

I also thank my brother Doug, for being an awesome friend and for contributing his feedback, some photos, and a synopsis of his own transplant experience.

How many nurses deserve my thanks? How many doctors are due my gratitude? Anesthesiologists, respiratory therapists, pharmacists, and administrators. These medical staff work day in and day out without extra honor or pay. I owe them my deepest thanks. How many friends, only some of whom are mentioned in these true stories should be thanked? A person in need, as I often found myself, is dependent upon others, sometimes for really basic stuff. If you are one of the ones who has helped me (or has helped others like me) you deserve a huge thank you. Those good deeds have not gone unnoticed; they just aren't talked about. You are deserving of honor and praise for selflessness and kindness. No act of love, no matter how small, is ever wasted. Bless you.

Preface

Many really good lessons about living can be learned from stories. The whole point of this book is to retell stories from my crazy health journey and draw out the lessons learned in each instance. It is one thing to simply say I was hospitalized in nine countries; it is another to talk of being all alone and locked down in a psychiatric ward in London in perfectly good mental health. What can you learn from that? Plenty, as it turns out.

It is fairly obvious that everyone faces sickness in life. As a pastor I sat beside countless hospital beds while families tried to make sense of the suffering of a loved one. Was there meaning to it? Was there any purpose? Was God just being mean because we screwed up our lives? How come we suffer so much? We always want to know *why?*

I will say this regarding the purpose of suffering. Through it I have experienced the grace of God. I have been the recipient of his sustaining power and sometimes His healing hand. And I have grown to know Him more intimately as a result of the trials He saw fit to put me through. Therefore, I cannot help but put it down in writing so that your life might be impacted.

And that is why I tell you these stories.

CONTENTS

Chapter 1

Heart and Double-Lung Transplant

Bobby Robbins was prepared to open the sternum of the patient's chest. It was early on the morning of January 26, 1997. The man had been fully prepped. His skin was shaved, washed and then cleaned again with betadine. There was an IV to administer medications. The man was intubated to receive a steady flow of oxygen and he had an arterial line in place to monitor the O2 content of his blood. He was completely asleep. An automatic blood pressure cuff was attached to his left arm. And that was just the beginning of the preparations. He lay motionless on the gurney. The operating room was full of people, each with a key role to play in the day's surgery. The anesthesiologist was positioned at the patient's head, watching vital signs with diligence and monitoring each of the IV drugs.

The surgeon carefully worked the rotary saw, beginning what would eventually be a thirteen inch incision starting at the trachea and reaching almost to the belly button. Dr. Robbins was himself pretty weary after having just finished another rigorous surgery, but he was somewhat refreshed after having taken an eight hour break. Unexpectedly, Stanford Hospital had no less than three lung transplants take place on Super Bowl weekend in 1997. Doctor Bobbie had barely completed an eight hour surgery when a call came in that another set of organs had been donated in Modesto, California. Stanford had a patient on their list that badly needed them. The team wisely chose to wait to harvest the Modesto heart and double lungs, until Bobby had at least finished an eight hour break. Once harvested, the lungs would only be viable for four hours. On an early Sunday morning they were harvested in Modesto and flown over the Diablo Mountain Range to Stanford University Hospital in Palo Alto.

As scalpel and saw cut through flesh and cartilage, blood began to ooze, then flow, from the wound. *This is a lot of blood,"* Bobby thought. Assistants worked to staunch the flow with gauze, expecting the blood to eventually begin to clot. Some medication is typically given to a patient prior to surgery to slow clotting. But this patient's blood wasn't clotting at all. Parts of the blood are supposed to eventually thicken, forming a semi-solid mass.

Dr. Robbins had asked that blood products (packed red blood cells) and liters of blood be readied for transfusion. As the rib cage was pried apart and clamps set in place, the heart and lungs were exposed. Bobby realized he was in for a huge task. The heart looked healthy enough but the lungs were grey and stiff, not pink and spongy. This is often the case when the patient has had decades of lung infections. Of even greater concern was the lining of the lungs. They form an airtight sack so that the lungs can expand and contract within the lining. But this patient had had pneumonia many times. Each time scar tissue had formed that made the sack around the lungs adhere to the diseased lungs. The old lungs needed to come out, but the lining had to remain for the new lungs to function. The scars had to be cut - then repaired - over and over, before the old lungs could be removed. The patient would not survive unless that lining could sustain a vacuum around the new lungs.

After the heart bypass was in place Dr. Robbins carefully cut the trachea and connections between the heart and lungs. The patient's heart was in good condition and per his wishes would be donated to another patient. This had all been prearranged after many tests to determine the heart health. The heart was cooled and preserved and began its journey to southern California where a man with congenital heart disease was also waiting for a transplant to save his life.

An adult male body holds about 5.5 liters of blood. Bobby's patient was very thin and underweight. By the end of today's surgery, thirty-two liters of blood would be pumped into the patient to replace the blood that flowed out of every incision. That's almost six times the body's volume! The machine that suctioned the flow of blood could not keep up with the leakage from the many incisions. The operating table was soon red, as were sterile gloves, gowns and even the floor. As the anesthesiologist recalled some ten years later, "That was the bloodiest and messiest surgery I have seen in my entire career. I will never forget that!"

Dr. Bobby Robbins fought valiantly on. The new heart and lungs were in place but the bleeding was catastrophic. "Give it up, Bobby," his colleagues told him. "You've done everything you can." He persisted. Hour after hour had gone by as he struggled to stop the bleeding and help the new lungs begin to function. He sutured and cauterized continually. But the sack around the lungs were so full of blood and clots that the new lungs could not begin to expand. He knew he had to manually clear that space.

With the sternum stapled shut, he rolled the patient on his side, lifting the arm above the head. He would need to perform a thoracotomy. He cut a ten inch incision running between the ribs from the back of the patient around to the front, then pried the ribs apart to access the lung cavity. More suctioning and cleaning of the cavity ensued. The incision was stapled shut. Two 5/8 inch chest tubes were inserted through the patient's back to allow fluid to leave the right chest cavity. These had to be taped securely with high adhesive plastic tape to the skin, to prevent any air from escaping into the vacuum of the chest cavity.

With that side done Bobby knew he had to do the same on the other side. They carefully rolled the patient onto his other side. Another incision, more suctioning, two more tubes, and closing the wound with staples. Now it was just a matter of time to see if the patient survived. It had been a long long day. Ten and a half hours. He left the operating room and went into the adjacent room to clean up. It was time to give the family an update.

As Dr. Bobby Robbins entered the waiting room the patient's wife, parents, and a group of relatives and friends could see the news was not good. Bobby's face showed his exhaustion and weariness. He came straight to the point.

"It's been a very difficult surgery," he began, addressing the young wife. "Your husband has lost a lot of blood and it's been difficult to stop the bleeding and to allow the new lungs to begin to function. I'm sorry. We've done everything we can, but we're losing him." After answering a few questions he disappeared back down the hallway.

The family gathered around in the small waiting room. There were five people present. They got on their knees and they poured their hearts out to Jesus, asking for a miracle.

I am that patient. But this is not where the story begins…

Chapter 2

Heat Stroke

ystic fibrosis (CF) was first labeled as such in 1938 by Dorothy Anderson, a pathologist at the New York Babies Hospital. It was known as early as 1857 that babies whose brow "tasted of salt" would soon die. But no therapies existed for the mysterious illness. In the beginning of the nineteen hundreds the disease was associated with meconium-ileus, a bowel obstruction in babies. Eventually babies who survived this problem would develop serious lung illness, pancreas problems, and sinus issues. It was always terminal, a childhood killer.

None of the three boys born in our family (born in 1955, 1958 and 1960) had meconium-ileus, and if our brows tasted of salt it was never noted. We did receive the sweat chloride test (developed in 1953), which simplified the testing for cystic fibrosis. However, the tests were inconclusive. My older brother, David, age five, showed symptoms of coughing and a failure

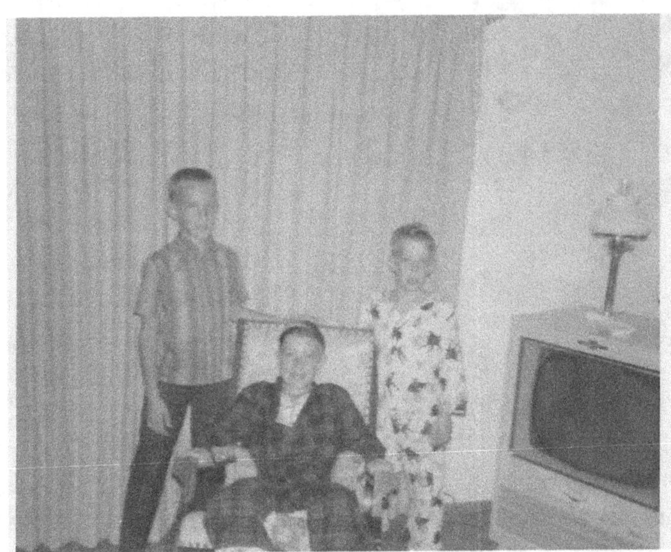

DAN, DAVID AND DOUG - WITH CHICKEN POX

to gain weight. It was assumed that his positive CF test was accurate. My younger brother Doug and I were active and healthy in appearance, although skinny. So the test results were inconclusive. Everyone hoped that we didn't have CF. David received rudimentary treatments when he was little, some that later proved to be detrimental to his health, like sleeping in a mist tent. It was supposed to loosen secretions in his lungs, but instead it caused mold to grow in his mattress and probably his lungs. His sheets and pillow were constantly wet and he was miserable throughout the night.

Illness did not hinder our family's activities. I remember having perfect attendance at school for many years. My mother, Carolyn, viewed sickness more like a mental state than a physical one, so we were pushed to our limits. There was no pandering for illness. "Pull up your boot straps," I heard more than once. And I didn't even wear boots.

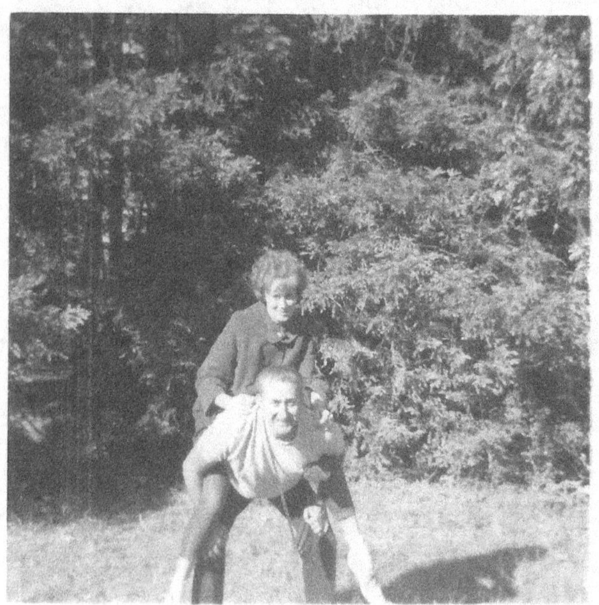

Mom and Dad liked camping, well, mostly dad. Mom agreed to it because finances were tight and, well, camping was cheap. At least it was a vacation for the family. We often joined other friends and headed for northern California where temperatures in the summer were usually a bit cooler than Santa Clara Valley. Plus the views were superior. Camping in California state parks was a child's dream. I grew up with fond memories of the California redwood forests. Rushing streams and canyons banked with bracken and sword ferns. The three of us boys spent hours running through the trees and hiding in fire blackened stumps and hollows.

In July of 1961 we piled into our powder blue fifty-seven Chevy Belair four-door and headed up Highway 101 towards Clear Lake. I was two years old. Clear Lake is the largest lake that is wholly in California and it has breathtaking views. We set up camp in the open, atop a hill with a nice view of the lake. Our family of five slept together in an ancient green army tent, which was designed for four. I think my dad obtained it after he served in the Korean conflict. It seemed to weigh a hundred pounds, and

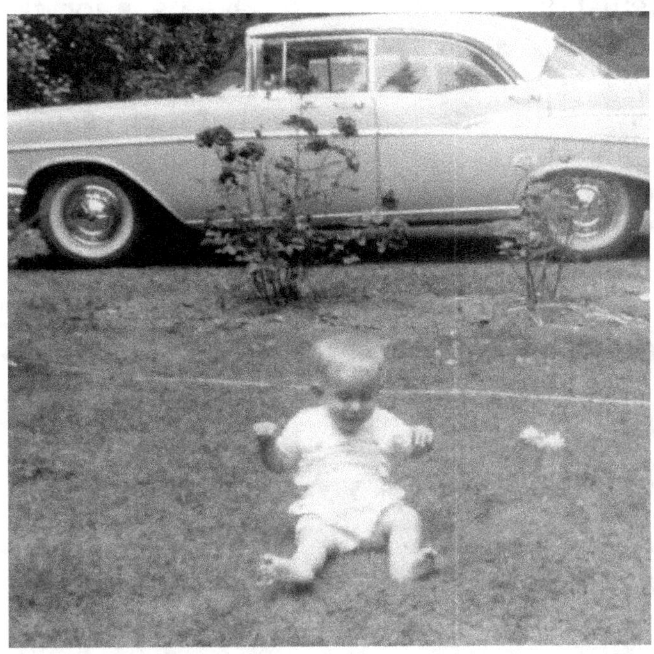

had a memorable musty odor. I remember the solitary window flap measured about twelve inches square. There was no circulation inside; and it was stifling hot in the campground near Clear Lake. One hundred and two degrees.

My mom Carolyn allowed me to run off my two-year old energy around the campground. Gathering sticks, throwing stones, chasing butterflies; I was a typical energetic child. Little Doug was being nursed in the shade of the tent. At least he was staying hydrated. I ran back and forth having a great time.

Then I collapsed in the dirt and went unconscious.

Emergency personnel eventually came and assessed I had heat exhaustion or heat stroke. I had been exposed to prolonged periods of activity in the extreme heat, without drinking. Dehydration led to my body's temperature control system to fail. Excessive salt loss accelerates dehydration as the electrolyte balance is thrown off. I had become confused and lost consciousness. My parents laid me in the shady area beneath the tent flap, removed my tee shirt and tried to cool my body off by dampening my skin with a moist towel.

I was rushed to the local hospital where doctors attempted to give me fluids. They were unable to find a vein in my arms, so an IV was started in my scalp, as an emergency measure to give my body some fluids and lower its core temperature.

When I was told this story - years after it happened - it made me think about the tremendous shock it must have been for my parents to have a son with a terminal illness - not to mention me almost dying at age two. Parents usually think about their children as the fruit of their lives, the continuation of a legacy and a chance to make a difference in the future world. Children are *not* supposed to die before their parents. Imagine the thought that perhaps *all* of your children will precede you in death. That was

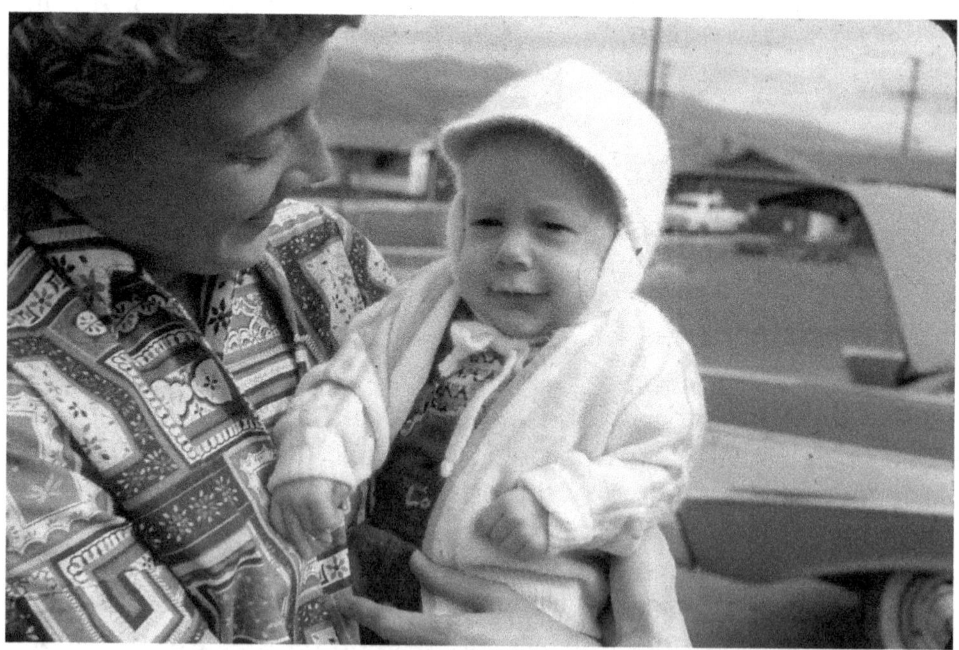

CAROLYN LAGASSE HOLDS HER THIRD SON DOUG

the future my parents thought likely. All three of their sons would eventually be confirmed to have the terminal illness cystic fibrosis. My younger brother Doug and I were officially diagnosed in our teen years, but that early test when we were young certainly made them suspicious that we all did indeed have CF.

Add to that the false guilt one could feel knowing that it was one's own genes that were passed on to create the double recessive-gene recipe for cystic fibrosis. Then there is the financial pressures of hospitalizations, the stress of handling insurance, the education process about a terminal illness, the travel to a myriad of doctors appointments, the social issues with friends and relatives, and the managing of daily therapies and treatments. It could easily become so overwhelming that a marriage disintegrates.

It took incredible strength for my parents Dave and Carolyn to not only care for and raise three children who all had cystic fibrosis, but also to remain married and continue to love one another. I do remember times when they would argue. A house is only so big and when mom and dad are unhappy everybody knows it. Mom would run around shutting the windows so neighbors couldn't hear them yelling. I tried to be the peacemaker in the home, but sometimes there was no peace to be had. *"How much did the stress of three sick sons contribute to their marital strife?"* I wonder. They remained committed to one another for their forty-eight years of marriage. Mom died of melanoma cancer when she was just sixty-six. I was forty at the time. Dad loved her to the end and grieved her loss for many years.

The familiar marriage vow contains the words, "For better or worse." Having three terminally ill sons could easily fall into the "worse" category. But they remained committed to one another. My father wrote down his definition of love: "Doing that which meets the basic needs of another." Clearly their love for one another defined our family and our outlook on life. Yes, we knew that 'God is Love.' 1 John 4:8 says, "Whoever does not love does not know God, because God is love."

But seeing it lived out day-to-day in the little things of life made all the difference. "If we have not love we are nothing," 1 Corinthians says. Selfless love became the foundation for my parents marriage, and for our family. This special love from God would sustain me through many a trial.

Chapter 3

Facing Death

I often awoke to the familiar sound of thumping. It was the half-cupped hands of my father striking the bony torso of my big brother David as he hung over the edge of his bed. And then there was the hacking, guttural, deep chested cough. He spit into a pale blue plastic kidney-shaped tray. And then after forty-five minutes of this, he got himself ready for school. Such were the sounds of his fragile life. They were also the sounds of an impending death.

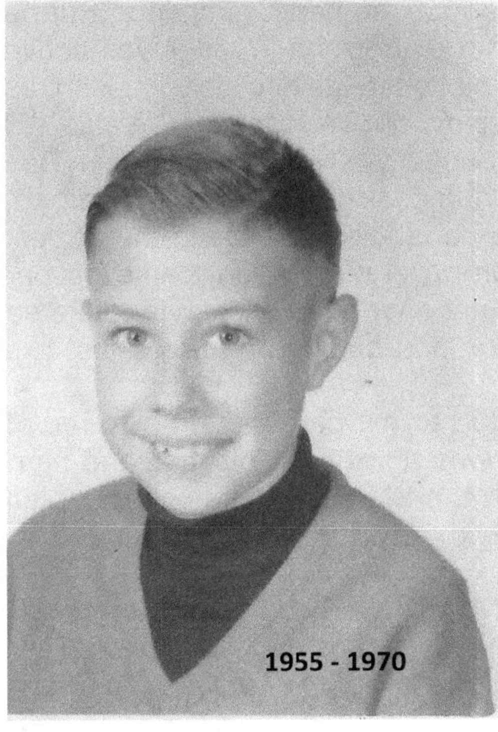

David was thin for his age, but he was energetic and smart. Very smart, if you trust those IQ tests. I remember when he created a home alarm system from his collection of electrical gadgets. He loved to create. He was thirteen; I was eleven. When our mother came home from grocery shopping at Gemco and she took her first step onto the flat pile rug at the lower steps in the house, the alarm's screaming whine startled her half to death. Appearing from his hiding place behind the door, David was ecstatic. Mom shouted in terror and dropped her bag of groceries. However, we were laughing loudly and jumping up and down.

Laughing makes one's lungs spasm. David launched into a lengthy cough, as his lungs tried hopelessly to clear his airways that were clogged with sticky mucus. This was typical for David early in life. Such realities must have been a cause of fear for my mom; perhaps that's why she gave us so many long lectures when we got into trouble. She was expressing her anxiety in the only way she could.

Twice a day my father would thump on David's chest and David would cough and try to clear his lungs. He had to lay in twelve different positions, at different angles on the bed, designed to drain different parts of the lungs. He diligently followed the medical regimen that the best lung doctors at Kaiser gave him. But he still ended up with recurring pneumonias. The antibiotics that were available were very few and other CF therapies untested.

However, his illness did not define his life. He did well in school, played the trombone, camped with the scouts, and marched with the high school band, even had a girlfriend. (But he didn't tell his younger brother much about her.) David was active as we all were. Doug and I enjoyed relatively good health as young kids with CF. We were skinny, but very active. We also did not let CF define us as individuals. We were involved in Boy Scouts, in our youth groups at church, and in bands. We camped, hiked, rode bikes, and made go-carts - like all kids in the sixties. When the wheels (repurposed from an old wagon) came off our cart or the brakes failed (it was just a wooden stick), we rocketed down our hilly street in Los Gatos and crashed. We bled just like every other kid on the block.

But our doctors had suggested to my parents that all three of their sons had cystic fibrosis. It was a terrifying disease and hard to even pronounce. One child at the Stanford Children's Hospital simplified it by pronouncing it, "sixty-five roses." That sounded so much nicer.

Having three boys with this illness was super rare; the odds were one in sixty-four, since neither parent had the illness. *Was this a case of a rotten role of the dice? Was it a curse? Or perhaps it was intended as a blessing?* I wondered. I am encouraged by the words of King David, a man who suffered greatly. About his body he says of the Lord, "For you created my inmost being; you knit me together in my mother's womb. I praise you because I am fearfully and wonderfully made; your works are wonderful, I know that full well."[1] It is reassuring to know I am not a mistake, and that even my body, with its failings, is wonderful.

One of the many hospitalizations David endured ended with an indelible memory. He was fifteen and in his freshmen year at Leigh High School. He was a patient at Kaiser in Santa Clara and both our parents were visiting him daily at the hospital. He'd been really sick with double pneumonia. The hospital wouldn't allow Doug nor me in to see him (the minimum visitor age was 14) but I had looked through the glass from the balcony at him and saw him in the hospital bed. One memorable night our parents left us home alone and went to visit David. At bedtime Doug and I went upstairs to the room we shared. Orange shag carpet and orange bedspreads. Yikes. We went to sleep.

I woke up suddenly at two a.m. In the depth of my heart I felt something really significant had occurred. I looked across at Doug in the semi-darkness; he was still fast asleep. I felt that something had changed in the world. It was perhaps my first experience with the mystical, the unexplainable. I didn't know what, but I knew that my life was somehow at that very moment dramatically different. I lay there awake for perhaps thirty minutes. Eventually I fell back asleep.

Our mom and dad came home from Kaiser at four a.m. They came into our bedroom, and turned on the light. This took us both by surprise. They sat down on the edges of our single beds. We could see a great sadness on their faces. The oddity of them waking us up in the middle of the night made us realize something significant had happened. They began by telling us that David had been fighting for every breath. "The doctors did everything they could, but...," their voices trailed off as they wept. We all cried till dawn.

---

[1] Psalm 139 1:13,14

I tear up now, even as I write this. There is some pain, some scars, that are so deep that they will for the rest of our lives be a source of grief. That is part of our humanity. But we are not without hope. My brother David knew he had a home in heaven, and we knew this too. He had placed his hope in the only one who ever rose from the dead and conquered death, Jesus. Again we are comforted by words from the apostle Paul, "For we believe that Jesus died and rose again, and so we believe that God will bring with Jesus those who have fallen asleep in him."[2]

Six boy scouts from Troop 363 carried David's coffin into the chapel at the First Baptist Church in San Jose. The entire fifty member troop filled several rows dressed in their uniforms. There were also teachers from Leigh High School, fellow students, members of the Leigh marching band, friends from church, neighbors from Danville Drive where we grew up, and of course family and relatives present, filling the room to capacity. David's short life had made an impact on many. His love for others, concern for the disadvantaged (he volunteered with Head Start), and his love for Jesus, was an example and encouragement to many. The scouts created an award in my brother's honor: "The David Lagasse Memorial Award." It is given to the scout each year who most demonstrates the ideals of scouting. A friend told me forty years later that he had received that award when he was in scouts, and it is his most cherished award he's received in life.

David's life was brief, but not without impact. Each of us has an important role to play in this world. "For we are God's handiwork, created in Christ Jesus to do good works, which God prepared in advance for us to do." [3] And David's work was finished.

---

[2] 1 Thessalonians 4:14

[3] Ephesians 2:10

Chapter 4

Getting Old is Hard

Getting old is hard for anybody. It is especially hard when you are a kid. My older brother David began getting sick when he was five. When you are five you are supposed to be climbing trees and playing good guy – bad guy, running around the yard with home-made pistols and rifles. David, on the other hand, was getting chest percussion therapy four times a day and coughing his head off. When our scout troop went on hikes he was last in line, huffing and puffing as he headed up the trail. He did his best at swimming, but had to be put in special P.E. while in Junior High. This is humiliating for a kid. He didn't want to be special. Nobody does.

One factor of getting old is the reduction of normal activities. It's the stuff everybody else can do. Taking long walks, climbing stairs, bathing oneself. Seniors experience this and realize what a bummer it is. Ever-so-slowly *age* crawls up on you. Things are taken away from your active life one by one. Your ability to see deteriorates. Your bones creak. Your joints hurt. You prefer sitting to walking. You'd rather play card games in the lodge then go downhill skiing. Your depth perception is shot and you face losing your driver's license. Just like that. Your mobility is taken from you and you are dependent on others. We all hate this loss of independence.

It is especially tough when this happens to a kid, or a young adult. Doug and I didn't show any CF symptoms (i.e. coughing thick mucus) so we thought we were normal healthy kids. In fact I didn't get really sick until I was fourteen. I had been on a week-long bus tour with the choir from my church. A lot of the kids had gotten sick. When I continued to have a fever my mother took me to see my pediatrician.

"Why do I have to cough so much?" I asked Dr. Zwanstra.

"Oh," he said and then looked like he was struggling to find his next words, "You have a dry cough." I thought that was about as ridiculous an answer as possible. *And you went to med school to learn this?*

Dr. Zwanstra then asked me, "Do you smoke?" I looked at him incredulously.

"Do you even know me?" I thought. I was a straight A student. "No," I answered emphatically. I hated cigarette smoke. I specifically used the bathrooms in the school gym because of kids smoking in the bathrooms.

His next question blew me out of the water: "Do you smoke pot?" This was 1972 and I thought that perhaps Dr. Z was smoking pot.

"I have a dry cough, and of course I don't smoke cigarettes *or pot.*"

"Hmm…," he began slowly. "You may have just a bit of cystic fibrosis." My jaw dropped.

"What do you mean 'a bit?' How do you have 'a *bit*' of cystic fibrosis? You either have it or you don't. It's genetic." I felt like I was giving my pediatrician a medical lesson. Of course I knew quite a bit about CF, as David had died with it two years previous. And Dr. Z had been David's doctor. I could see he was having difficulty telling me the truth. It didn't matter to me what his motives were; when I asked a question I expected a straight answer.

I told my mother on the way home that I needed a new doctor. She finally agreed and later arranged for me to see an allergist at Kaiser, Dr. Damron. Allergists at Kaiser were inclined to be more informed at that point about the care for cystic fibrosis than standard pediatricians. Very little research had been done on the disease at that point but a correlation with allergies had been established. So if one could treat a patient's allergies his lung function could be improved. That was the hope.

I was eventually placed on the same medical regimen my brother David had been on. I could see the road ahead, as it were. I realized that I too would "grow old" early in life, and that I would die young as my brother had. A dry cough leads to a productive cough. A productive cough leads to repeated lung infections. Failure to absorb nutrition meant inability to gain weight. I would stay skinny; my bones would be thin and my muscles pathetic. Eventually I would be too weak to play in sports. I would be in the hospital frequently and have trouble keeping up in school. A CF hospitalization was a two-week course of IV antibiotics as an in-patient. You quickly fall behind in class when you're gone for two weeks. I had seen my brother perish with double-lung pneumonia. I began to think about my future. I could see it would be short. I had to think about how I would live it. That's a lot to process when you are fourteen.

And then I had a life changing experience. I attended a seminar with my mom and brother entitled Basic Youth Conflicts. I thought the name was kind of strange, but the majority of the material that was taught over the week was outstanding. It gave me as a young person a foundation to live my life according to the will of God. That is very important for any young person; for me it was critical. It saved me from a world of trouble.

It is true that children with serious or terminal illnesses mature faster. I think what really happens is that incredible responsibility is thrust upon them. I had to deal with issues of living that most children never think about. Eat right - that means calories, quantities, oils, proteins, and healthy shakes and snacks. Sleep right - sleep enough hours, perhaps in a mist tent. Exercise - do physical therapy on a strict schedule. If I missed one postural drainage treatment (now called Chest Percussion Therapy) it meant I was going to be fighting to breathe. My airways would simply be clogged shut. That encouraged discipline. If I didn't do it I couldn't breathe. I also learned to be disciplined as a Boy Scout and as a musician, but my primary teacher was illness.

As it turned out I remained pretty healthy in high school. I did have to be enrolled in special PE as a senior, however. It had been absolute torture for me when I tried to run the mile. And the mandatory two-mile run every month was a killer. I would be one of the very last students to finish. I felt like soccer was a cruel game because of all the running. I preferred basketball, badminton, or tennis with the shorter jumps and sprints. Plenty of time to catch one's breath.

When I got sick at age 14 I was given oral antibiotics and told I had "walking pneumonia." I understood that meant I could still walk around and go about my daily activities. I had no idea that I would fight lung infections for the next twenty-four years. Sometimes I would be sent back to a hospital for IV antibiotic treatments within weeks of being discharged. I grew accustomed to using all my energy for study or work. I quit playing.

I didn't actually miss any classes in school until my senior year in high school. I was hospitalized in the second semester for two weeks. I was able to catch up in all my classes accept college calculus. I loved math, and was delighted to take a college class while in high school - at 7 am every morning. But after missing those two weeks in February, I totally bombed out in Calculus. I had no idea what 'e' was. The teacher kept referring to it in differential equations and all the new formulas. I still don't know, for that matter. I had to drop the class; it was humiliating. I had perfect A's in all my other classes, and the one withdrawal from the college course. I managed to graduate in 1976 from Leigh High School as valedictorian.

But more significant than the awards I received for grades or activities was the inner peace and assurance I had received from experiencing illness and finding comfort, peace, and purpose from the word of God. "For I know the plans I have for you," declares the Lord, "plans to prosper you and not to harm you, plans to give you hope and a future." [4] I was not placed on earth to get high grades, or get a great job, I was here for a divine purpose. Knowing God has a purpose for me, gave me strength to face insurmountable obstacles with my health. And I was going to need that strength very soon.

---

[4] Jeremiah 29:11

Chapter 5

Brain Surgery

Pretty girls. Lots of pretty young girls. And they all had come to see *me*! No this was not a dream. It was June 1977, I was almost nineteen, and was an inpatient at the Santa Clara Kaiser Hospital. It was the same place where David had died. The story begins after a simple game of racket ball the previous week.

I came home with my best friend Bill Colton from the gym all tired and sweaty. I had finished my first year of college and I was looking forward to a summer with my friends and to landing a couple part time jobs. I plopped down on a black bean-bag chair on the blue shag carpet in what used to be David's bedroom. Bill began telling me a funny story that he had told me at least two times before. He had a penchant for doing this if it was a really good story.

I began to feel a bit dizzy. *"Put your head between your knees,"* I remembered from my scouting first aid training. Bill and I were Eagle Scouts so we knew a few things about first aid. The dizziness didn't go away. Hmmm. I felt myself kind of drifting away, getting more and more dizzy, slowly tipping over off the bean bag chair and onto the floor. My last thought as my younger brother Doug entered the room was, *"This doesn't seem right."*

Doug had been studying first aid as a sophomore in Health class at Leigh. He had just studied grand mal seizures that week. He had had a quiz on it that very day. He looked at his brother lying and shaking on the floor and recognized the symptoms immediately. He also knew you were supposed to put a comb or something rigid in the person's mouth so they don't bite on their tongue. And he knew you had to call for an ambulance right away.

(This was before the phone number 911 had been instituted). Doug knew it was serious.

I guess there was a bunch of activity in my bedroom of which I am oblivious of course; I even missed the drama of the ambulance ride. I had been in an ambulance just one time in my life. Let me digress... On that occasion it had been fun. I wasn't sick. It was an emergency disaster drill that the county healthcare system was running. I was a volunteer who was acting the part of a critically injured burn victim from a bus accident. They had professionals do our makeup and even burn my pants up with a blow torch. (Not while I was in them.) They were testing the emergency disaster preparedness of the nearby hospital. I now look back and realize my whole life has been an emergency disaster drill. The disaster is - I am going to die. The drill is - am I ready?

My first waking recollection after the seizure was of a physician, Dr George Huertas. He was telling me they needed to get something called blood gasses. It would test the amount of oxygen in my blood. I would have smiled at the mention of gas, being a college kid, but the doctor was holding this huge very thick chrome syringe in his hand. It looked like a hypodermic needle, the kind you might see in a horror movie. The needle itself looked to be about six inches long. I could not believe that he was serious. He placed the tip against my wrist after wiping me down with a cotton swap moistened with alcohol and began to penetrate the flesh. The needle was perpendicular to my arm. I had never felt pain like this; it was complete agony. I didn't shout in pain, but the tears were flowing fast down my face. I watched as he pushed the needle deeper and deeper into my flesh. I was sure, and I am not exaggerating here, that he was going to come out the other side of my wrist. Finally he hit something, because he seemed pleased and he drew back a bunch of arterial blood. He finally pulled the instrument from my arm and pressed another cotton ball against my skinny arm. Slowly a large black bruise developed.

If I had known at that time that he was going to do this to me each day I was in the hospital (two weeks) I would have checked myself out immediately and gone home and died. But I didn't know then that a patient has the right to check himself out of a hospital. I figured they were like prison. Once you are in, you have no recourse but to stay put until they let you go. It was during this hospitalization that I began to call hospitals, "white prisons." That is because the walls were white, the linens and gowns were white and the doctors and nurses all wore white. And I was locked inside like prison.

The doctor said there was something wrong within my brain. My brother surely felt this was an affirmation of his former assumptions. Dr. Huertas did not know whether it was an infection, or a tumor, or an abscess, or just exactly what. But something was putting pressure on the brain and causing the seizure. He announced that a new technology had been developed in Britain that would allow them to take a "picture" of the inside of my skull. It was called an MRI, which stood for Magnetic Resonance Imaging. He continued to tell us that prior to the development of this imaging device the only way to tell what was wrong and where the problem was located was to actually remove the top of the skull and take a look around. That sounded pretty barbaric to me so I was very glad for the MRI. I found it quite a relief to just lay on a very skinny platform, be rolled inside a giant canister that filled the whole room, and listen to the racket of the machine as it rotated around making magnetically created "sliced images" of my brain.

The results indicated an abscess in the back left quadrant of my brain. The team of doctors decided the best way to remove it would be to drill a hole in my skull and suction it out with some special device. It was probably just a fancy turkey baster. I remember the doctor telling my dad that the drill he used was just like the one you could buy at the hardware store for thirty bucks. Only this was a medically approved one, so it cost $900.

Dr. Huertas came into my private room to explain the surgery to me. He carefully and fully explained the risks of the operation. This is something surgeons always do so that if something goes wrong they can say in so many words, "Well... I told you so." It isn't that crass of course, but that is essentially the purpose of the talk. It is sort of like the commercials on TV when they are selling some new drug. They talk real fast and recite a litany of horrible things that always end with "a possibility of death." Well Dr. Huertas didn't mince his words. He said, "There is a 25% chance of survival. There is a 0% chance that you will be normal after this surgery. You most likely will be paralyzed on one side of your body. If you are not paralyzed you will probably still have to learn to walk all over again. You may lose your ability to think clearly, to reason, or to talk. He went on with a lot of other awful things. It all sounded pretty bad. Especially the 0% chance thing.

I know this sounds really stupid but my first question to him after his recitation was, "Will you have to cut off my hair?" In retrospect this sounds like a vain and foolish question. And it is. But you have to consider that this was the seventies and I had really cool hair that went down over my ears. I carried a comb with me at all times and kept it combed so it would look just right. Okay, it still was a stupid question. But it does reflect the fact that I wasn't afraid of the dying part of his speech. I had an assurance that I would be okay, whether I lived or died. I knew my life was safe in the hands of Jesus. I had asked Him to be my savior when I was six. I understood that through Jesus my sins had been forgiven, that He loved me, and that I belonged to Him. I had prayed on my knees with my mom on the hardwood floor beside her bed. I had learned to walk with Him and had really developed a close relationship with God when I was in my teens. So I knew beyond a shadow of a doubt that if I didn't survive the cutting, drilling and sucking procedures (25% survival) I was going to be fine. But I was definitely going to lose my hair. Yes, they had to shave my head.

Word got out at First Baptist Church and at Leigh High School, where I had been the student body president. "Dan was likely going to die." People began to pray and many came to visit. Brain surgery was quite a big deal, especially in 1977. I was hooked up to an IV and was getting an IV antibiotic, but the doctors weren't sure which medicine to give me because they couldn't get a culture to see which bacteria was present, causing the abscess. I began to get more and more visitors as they realized it could be my final days. And this is the part where the young pretty girls come in.

As a high school student I naturally made a lot of friends. I played tuba and then trombone in the high school band. I was in the honor society and in student government. Girls would say I looked just like my younger brother. Other people would tell me that Doug was really cute. I did the math and figured I must be good looking too (I certainly couldn't tell; all I saw were the pimples). Anyway a steady stream of female visitors came into my room bearing gifts. It was really quite miraculous as there were never two girls visiting at any time. The nurses chided me because they would see people coming in and out. "They must have passed in the elevators," they said. One gal brought me a cake in the shape of a train; (I worked as a conductor on the train at an amusement park). There were plants, flowers, and of course candy. I was a really skinny kid (6 foot tall and still 125 pounds) so food was always welcome.

The day came when I was to get the surgery. As I was wheeled out of my room and placed on the gurney, I handed my surgeon the book, *Born Again* by Chuck Colson. Dr. Huertas said he was Jewish, but the book was very popular at the time and I hoped he would read it. I don't remember much more about going in for surgery, but I woke up after the operation and felt pretty normal. As I regained consciousness I was given Jello.

To this day I have a special fondness for Jello. Whenever you have surgery you get to eat all the Jello and drink all the grape juice you want. That's about the only perk of having surgery.

Then I was given a funny hat to wear to cover my bald head; it was sort of like a stocking cap. It was crocheted by somebody with a good heart. I guess it was to keep my head warm or maybe to keep me from seeing myself or messing with the bandages. Dr. Huertas came in to my hospital room to do a post operative exam. He asked me how I felt.

"Fine," I said. "Do you want me to get up?"

"Oh, no. Just lie there while I do some simple tests." He looked in my eyes, squeezed my hands and feet. "Can you feel this? Can you feel this?" He went to all my extremities, checking my sense of touch. He poked my toes with a sharp instrument. "Do you feel that," he asked?

"Oh yeah," I replied. "I can feel that. I feel great!" Then he held both his hands up and touched his thumbs to each of his fingers in succession.

"Can you do this," he asked? I then lifted my hands up and repeated the motion back to him.

"I can do that." Then I moved my two middle fingers back and forth sideways while the forefinger and little finger each stayed still.

"Can you do this," I asked him? He was not amused and didn't even try.

When he saw that I was completely normal and had no damage from the surgery he was quite astonished. I replied that surely God had done something extraordinary. He did not look too pleased. I did not mean to diminish the super work he had done during the surgery, but I did and still do believe that God uses the hands of gifted men to do His work. He gives us the intelligence and the skills to accomplish great things. Even the technology that is developed is just a fraction of the wonder of the creator God. "For He created all things, and by His will they were created," Revelation 4:11 says. So surely when man comes up with a new invention or finds a drug that allows a cure, it is knowledge that has existed since the beginning. And God always has existed, even before creation. God gives wisdom and knowledge to mankind. Yes, even to Dr. Huertas as he is drilling a hole in my skull.

It must have been a pretty big deal for Kaiser Santa Clara to do the brain surgery because there was a team of about ten doctors evaluating and discussing my case. They would stop by and see me from time to time to check on me. The problem was they each told me something different when they came to visit. I remembered this really upset my parents. One doctor was very optimistic and would tell me I would be able to go home in a couple days, then another would say it would be at least several weeks before I would be released. It was an emotional roller coaster.

In the end I was discharged exactly two weeks after I had had the seizure. I was learning that doctors are all very human. Medicine is not as exact as patients wish it could be. And doctors are all experts but certainly not always in agreement with one another. In fact, it's not unlike a lot of theologians. It has something to do with being human.

It was turning out to be quite a summer. But the excitement was far from over.

Chapter 6

Being Bald

I don't like to sit still for long. Two weeks laying on the couch after brain surgery was like boredom on steroids. Prior to my brain abscess and subsequent seizure I had landed two new part-time jobs. One was in a berry-pie place as a waiter. I had worked a total of two days on that job, one of which was training. The second job was with my buddy Bill. I worked the midnight shift as a security guard at a data processing firm. They had hired Bill and I to walk around their building, up and down corridors and inside offices, punching time clocks. It was extraordinarily boring, but at least I

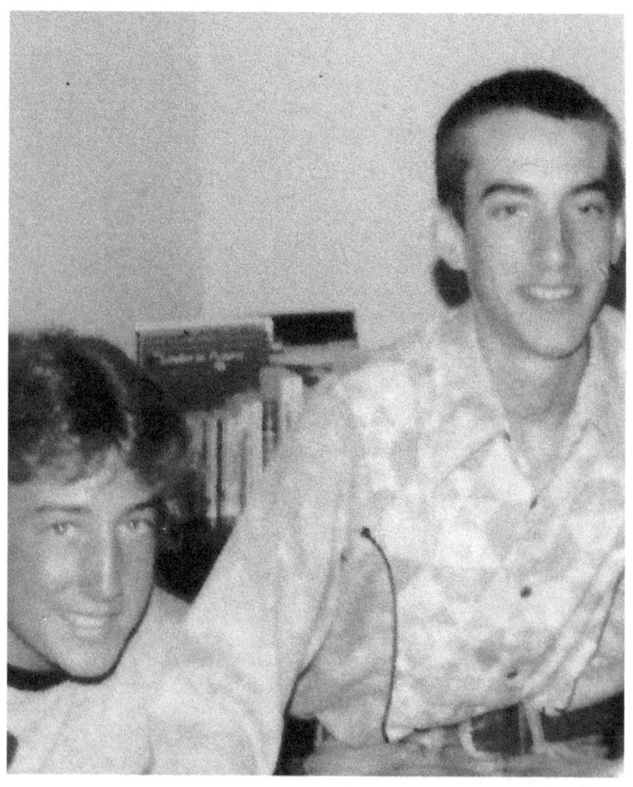

DOUG WITH HAIR AND DAN WITHOUT

earned something. I had worked two graveyard shifts at that job also. The next day was the night of the seizure. I had had to call in "sick." But now a month had passed and those jobs were history. I was alive, however, and ready to get back to work.

So I got off the couch and went looking for employment. I knew I would not fare too well in an interview with a massive bandage on a bald head. My loving mother went out and bought me a wig. Only women bought wigs in those days. She took it to a beautician and had it cut to the style young men wore in the late seventies. The wig covered my ears, touched the collar, was parted in the middle, and when blow-dried it had just the right look.

I landed a job at an upscale restaurant on Hamilton Avenue in San Jose. The dress code for waiters was black pants, white shirt and a black tie. I felt a bit funny wearing the wig, but nobody seemed the wiser for it. Then on the third night a waitress asked me if I had really long hair. I was taken aback.

"No, I don't - actually. Why do you ask?"

"Well I know that long hair is not allowed at this restaurant, so I figured you were covering it up with a wig." I was at once embarrassed that she could tell I was wearing a wig, but then in the awkward position of explaining the truth. I have, however, found that most people can accept the truth. What they cannot accept is a lie once the lie has been discovered. And lies will always be discovered. Still, any young man wants to be accepted, especially by a pretty waitress.

I decided to tell her the truth. "I am actually wearing a wig because I am bald." In 1978 nobody was bald unless they were in their eighties. She gave me a funny look. I continued, "I had brain surgery and they had to shave my whole head. So I got a wig." I thought she might be mortified.

However, instead of acting strange she followed up with, "Why did you have brain surgery?" To have brain surgery in the nineteen seventies was almost unheard of. I told her I'd developed an infection and an abscess and surgeons had to remove it. She seemed to accept it at face value. People are more compassionate than we sometimes think. Even teenagers. It seemed a bit out of place to discuss all this while holding a tray full of food so I moved on.

I clocked out just short of midnight on my fourth night of work. My drive home was only four and a half miles, and although I had to work late each night the job paid well. I was glad I'd figured out and memorized the huge menu. I was driving my dad's new yellow Datsun B-210 toward our home. I was on Los Gatos Almaden Road and preparing to turn left onto Pinehurst - a block and a half from home. As I waited to turn left I could see two pair of headlights a couple blocks away. (It was just a two lane road.) They seemed like a long ways away and I could see I had plenty of time to make my turn. As I finished my turn onto Pinehurst I heard a loud squeal of tires.

In the next millisecond there was a huge impact as a grey Celica GT slammed into the right rear quarter panel of my parent's car. My body twisted violently in the seat. The Celica bounced off my car and slammed straight into a telephone pole. My vehicle spun in a complete circle and landed atop some juniper tams that were planted on a parking strip on Pinehurst. I felt my brain inside my head actually bounce around inside my skull. It was weird. I realized that the Datsun engine was still running so I shut it off. Over and over a question played in my mind, "Why did that guy turn his car towards me? Why did he turn into me? Why didn't he just keep going straight?" My new stereo system (which I had wired to the battery) continued to play a song by Chicago Transit Authority. I turned it off too.

I could smell gas. People from the neighborhood heard the huge impact as the car hit me and they came running out of their homes. I looked out my window to see a woman smoking a cigarette.

"Hey, put that out!" I yelled.

I released my seat belt, feeling a huge pain in my side where the belt assembly had pressed into my side. It felt like someone had landed a direct punch to my right kidney. I opened my door and crawled out onto the ground, not wanting to be caught in the car if it ignited. I didn't know how badly I was hurt. I wasn't bleeding. My main thought was, "What is Dr. Huertas going to do when he hears what happened to his precious brain surgery patient?" He had wanted me to go home and take it easy for a whole year.

Somehow I figured going back to work after two weeks wasn't going to sit too well with him.

Moments later I saw a familiar car. It was my mother's bronze colored Ford Pinto. My brother had been a mile down the street working an evening shift at the drive-up window at Jack-in-the-Box. He saw the commotion down the block so took a small detour to see what was happening. His heart leapt into his throat when he saw the Datsun. He knew it was me. He came to my side, but what could he do?

The police had arrived and an ambulance was called. The driver of the Celica was pacing up and down in the street swearing loudly at me. He told the police it was obvious I had been drinking.

"Look; he's all dressed up. He's been at a wedding reception." I was still in my waiter's uniform of black pants, white shirt and black bow tie. Moments later a second car, with whom the Toyota Celica had been racing, returned to the scene. The driver stopped in the single driving lane. It was a beige Mustang Mach 1. He wanted to see what had happened to the Celica and probably see if his friend was okay.

I yelled from my prone position on the sidewalk to the bystanders, "Hey stop the driver of that car! He was racing against the Celica! Get his license plate number!" I could not get up from the ground and I couldn't see the policeman beyond the bushes.

A lady approached me and said in sympathetic tones, "Now you just take it easy; an ambulance will be here in a bit." Nobody listened. The Mach 1 drove off.

The officer took note of the hundred-fifty-foot skid marks that left the driving lane at an angle and he could see where the impact took place - on the side street. I explained about the race. He said he would not cite me. (Later I received a citation in the mail, but with careful diagrams and measurements I showed in court that I was not at fault.) My brother had just served the two teenagers burgers and fries at the Jack in the Box. He knew both boy's cars from our high school. They were never cited.

It was my third ambulance ride. After a long wait and some x-rays I thankfully learned that I had a bruised kidney. The Datsun did not fare as well as I did; it was totaled. I am afraid that was also the end of my work at the steak house. I was unable to return to work for a while. However, I still like to eat a good filet mignon now and then.

I think about my brother Doug standing in the middle of Pinehurst Street looking at me on the ground and the totaled Datsun B 210. Sometimes we are helpless to come to the aid of a family member who is in dire straights. It might be a car accident or cancer. But in the end there is nothing physical we can do to change the outcome. We offer all the support and love possible. I cannot tell you how many hours my wife has spent in waiting rooms, how many weeks lying beside me in hospital cots, how much time was spent in cars ferrying me to and from appointments and surgeries. My father and mother also suffered as I suffered, as did my brother. Ultimately the best thing we can offer is our physical presence, expressions of love and support, and prayer. Because prayer does make a difference in the outcomes of life. "Therefore confess your sins to each other and pray for each other so that you may be healed. The prayer of a righteous person is powerful and effective." [5] That is what I most often request from friends and what I always offer to others when confronted with illness. Prayer.

We do not have control over the destiny of our loved ones. And even our own destiny comes down to events not of our own making. I had no control over the brain infection and abscess, or of the car accident. Regardless of the circumstances we face, God is near if we seek him. God says, "You will seek me and find me when you seek me with all your heart." [6]

1 John 5:14 tells us, "This is the confidence we have in approaching God: that if we ask anything according to his will, he hears us." So praying does make a difference. And discovering his will is critical too. An honest reflection will often reveal that our time and money is not spent on God's will but on our own. When we pray, "Thy will be done," we have to also be open to finding his will for our lives.

---

[5] Jeremiah 5:16

[6] Jeremiah 29:13

Having brain surgery and being bald was teaching me humility. Surviving the auto wreck? That was about the prayers of loved ones who prayed according to God's will.

7. Pancreatitis

Shortly after the accident I returned to Santa Barbara to start my second year at Westmont College. Westmont is a small Christian Liberal Arts college. At the time there were just eight hundred students. It wasn't long until I recognized everybody on the large campus. I had chosen to live in the dorm where mostly older students lived because I liked the atmosphere better. Nobody told me I was more mature than most students. I learned later in life that facing death makes you grow up quicker. As is often said, trials can either make you bitter, or better. It made me take life seriously.

While in college my roommates gave me chest percussion therapy. It was humbling to have to ask another student to pound on my chest. But if I didn't do it twice a day I simply couldn't breathe anymore. That's a strong motivator.

In the fall of 1977 I had a new roommate. Jeff Mathews was a clean-cut athletic third year student. He was five foot seven, had short black hair, and drove a slate grey (always clean) BMW. He was willing to share his room on campus with me, a lowly sophomore because I was, "so organized." He told me this himself. I was a little perplexed. So I asked him what he meant.

"Well," he began, "I was over at your room last year visiting your roommate. I saw you open your file drawer and I could see inside. I said to myself, "Hey, a guy who keeps his files that neat and alphabetized, and in such logical sequence.... *that* is the kind of guy I want to share a room with."

I was impressed that somebody appreciated cleanliness and orderliness to such a degree. My prior roommate only changed his sheets when they became green down by his feet. Then he would take them off and turn them over to use for another couple weeks. So maybe Jeff also had had a bad experience. Getting a college roommate is a bit of a crap shoot.

After we'd shared a room for a few months I noticed a few unusual behaviors. Mathews subscribed to the Wall Street Journal, which made sense since he was a business major. But he would fold them back up after reading them - just like when they'd been delivered. Then he'd stack them in chronological order on top of his refrigerator. *"Okay, that's a bit odd,"* I thought. *"But no big deal."*

He kept his desk totally devoid of anything at all, accept for the desk lamp and a single finely sharpened pencil. *"Well, at least it looks nice and it's not embarrassing when I have guests over,"* I thought. Each morning he'd rise at five am and go down to the basement where he'd do five hundred jumping jacks. *Wow, now that's discipline.* Then he'd run five miles. I was impressed. I hated running, still do in fact. I sat with him at dinner one evening in the dining commons. He had a huge serving of canned corn, which being cafeteria corn was not particularly desirable or palatable. Then he ate a plate of lettuce. No dressing or add-ons, just head lettuce. He drank several glasses of water and excused himself.

These were the days before people had defined OCD, obsessive compulsive disorder. At least I'd never heard of anything like it. And George Costanza of Seinfeld had yet to become famous. I was, however, living with a George, only without the quirkiness. Mathews was nothing short of amazing. His personal discipline was record setting. But then there were the rare evenings when he would come home with sourdough french bread. One night when I was at my desk typing a paper (yes, on a typewriter), Mathews arrived from Von's grocery store with a large loaf of freshly sliced sourdough french bread.

He sat cross legged on his well made bed, with its brown bedspread neatly tucked in, and carefully opened the loaf of bread and select just one slice. He took small bites from the slice, obviously savoring each delectable swallow. Only he didn't finish with one slice. He eventually consumed the entire loaf in one sitting. I did not say anything; I saw no reason to create conflict. I knew Mathews was a "private person." He'd told me as much one evening when I asked him if he were going out on a date. He was too kind to say, "None of your business."

So after avoiding my inquiry in various ways he finally said, "I am a private person." Okay. I get it. *Just don't ask.*

He did confide in me on one occasion that he would never ever throw up. This came up in discussion when our suite mate Rich got violently ill. Mathews was so distraught at the sounds of retching in our shared bathroom that he had left the dorm for the evening. I asked him if he had ever tossed his cookies, even as a child.

"Absolutely not!" he answered. "That is the most disgusting thing in the world. I would sooner die." I knew he meant it.

I hadn't been back in school (after the brain surgery) more than a couple months when I had sudden severe stomach pains. No, I did not throw up. But I was laying on my blue plaid bedspread on my side holding my gut, groaning loudly when Mathews came in.

"What's the matter, Dan?"

"I don't know. My stomach just hurts something horrible."

"Did you call nurse Divilbiss?" he asked. Lois Divilbiss was a wonderful sweet woman who had seen me regularly. As the school nurse she had even given me intramuscular injections of antibiotics twice a day so I could finish semi-finals or finals without being admitted to the hospital. One butt cheek in the morning and the other in the afternoon. I couldn't afford to miss a week or ten days of classes to get hospital IV's to combat lung infections. So she gave me intramuscular injections twice a day. Cystic fibrosis was taking its toll on me. But nurse Divilbiss kept me going.

"No, Mathews. I haven't called the nurse." He made a quick phone call to her office.

"She says you need to get to Cottage Hospital."[7] That hospital was thirty minutes across town from the college. Westmont is up in the hills among luxury mansions just on the southern edge of Santa Barbara in a community named Montecito. It has an incredible view of the ocean. But right now all I could see was my brown headboard. The abdominal pain was intense. Getting to the hospital meant driving to the northern most part of Santa Barbara.

---

[7] www.cottagehealth.org

Mathews half carried me, and half led me to his shiny BMW. I thought I might pass out. The guys in the dorm were helpful but at a loss of what to do. Mathews drove his BMW down the hill, through the S curves, (and no, I did not throw up) and out to Highway 101. When we reached the hospital he handled the admitting details for me and I was taken from emergency into a private room. What a guy. I'm still thankful for him.

After the requisite questioning, probing and testing, it was decided I must have pancreatitis. I had never heard of it. Over time I figured out that anything that ends with "itis" means I am in deep trouble. It means that something is inflamed and spreading bacteria out of control. In this case it was my pancreas. I did not really know what the pancreas did, or was supposed to do. I learned that the glands in cystic fibrosis patients produce fluids that are very viscous. They have a tendency to clog up, just as mucus did in my lungs. That meant that my pancreas also could clog up from time to time.

The doctor explained that when the pancreatic enzymes are not allowed to flow through the pancreas and work on the food in the intestines, they simply start digesting the pancreas. Hence the pain. Got it.

"What can you do?" I asked him. This is the question every patient wants answered. Doctors are supposed to have fixes for everything; that's why patients treat them as some kind of gods. Well this god had a surprise for me.

"We are going to give you an injection of Demerol, which is a powerful pain killer and then try an enema, and see if that helps."

I will spare you the details of the enema, but suffice it to say that it did not help. It humbled me, but my bowels did not move. And the Demerol had absolutely no effect. My pain remained a steady 10, as medical professionals like to label pain. I just lay there on the pathetic mattress that most hospitals put on their beds. In those moments the bed could have been plywood and it would not have mattered. The whole world became a blur. I did not look at faces, remember names, talk coherently, or even try to have a good attitude. It is amazing what a bit of serious pain can do to ordinary people.

The doctor surprised me further with his next method of treatment.

"We are going to put you on a three day fast. We will be giving you nutrients by IV but you will receive nothing by mouth, not even water." He explained that every time we swallow food or liquid our pancreas responds by emitting some enzymes. That would make the pancreatic pain only increase. Also, by stopping all food, there was the hope that the inflammation and swelling would decrease and allow the destructive enzymes to eventually pass the narrow ducts.

I am not sure I understood all of this, but at the time the absolute last thing on my mind was eating. So I didn't argue. It was a waiting game. I was put on antibiotics and fluids and was of course subjected to the regular blood draws for lab work. When I became thirsty my nurse brought me a ridiculous lemon swab that I was supposed to suck on. It seemed like a sick joke (pun intended.) When that didn't help she would put a couple ice crystals in a tea spoon and allow them to melt on my tongue. And that is how I spent the next three days.

I am happy to say that Jeff did come to visit me, in spite of his abhorrence for hospitals. He was glad to see my health improve and I was glad to feel the pain subside. Within a few days I was allowed to begin drinking clear liquids, and eventually was discharged and allowed to resume my studies. The Bible says, "There is a friend who is closer than a brother." [8] Jeff was definitely that friend. But his trials with me were not over.

A couple months later I was in our bedroom preparing for bed. I pulled my covers back and lifted my feet off the new blue rug that my parents had purchased for our dorm room. I began to lay down and rest my head on my pillow. I started to feel dizzy. Very dizzy. I remembered this feeling from the previous June. It was the day I'd been rushed by ambulance to Kaiser in Santa Clara - with the brain infection. I realized I was going to have another seizure. Those few moments before the seizure is called an aura. It felt like my brain was sending confusing signals. I felt lifted from reality, where thoughts stopped having meaning and language lost its

[8] Proverbs 18:24b

content. I entered a type of floating, helpless, buzzing state. It was terrifying. I lost control of every human function as I once again fell helplessly into a gran mal seizure.

Jeff happened to be with me in our dorm room. He shouted to the dorm mates. Everyone scurried in trying to figure out what to do.

"Put a comb in his mouth or he'll bite his tongue." "Keep him on the bed so he doesn't hurt himself." Somebody called an ambulance from the dorm pay phone. My last memory as the seizure began was that I was dying. Earlier that evening I had been leading a Bible Study in my dorm room with other students.

I had a ridiculous thought, *"Is that why I came into this world, Lord?"* I asked. *"Did you bring me all this way just so I could lead this one Bible Study?"* Then just as I was passing out of consciousness I puked on the new bedroom rug.

I don't really remember puking but I heard about it later in no uncertain terms. One doesn't puke on Jeff Mathews's floor without some consequences. I can still see the spot on the blue green carpet in my mind. It was an area about three feet across, judging by the spot that remained there even after Mathews had given it a thorough scrubbing and then had rinsed it with many cans of lysol. I can picture poor OCD Mathews cleaning my puke out of the rug that lay between our single beds. Poor sap. And the smell of Lysol is forever imbedded in my mind.

I will confess I was just a bit pleased when Nurse Divilbiss told me years later that Jeff had gotten sick with a flu bug in his senior year at Westmont. And yes, he threw up. I had to smile at the thought.

Doctors told me later that after a brain surgery there is a build up of scar tissue at the site where the infection was. This scarring establishes an unusual surface upon which electrons build up. These electrons are supposed to fire around in the brain as we think. But when they build up in one place on the scar, they develop a significant electrical charge. And when that charge reaches a certain tipping point, boom! The electricity fires around the brain stimulating every muscle via the nervous system. The body has a seizure. As a precaution from it happening again I was put on Phenytoin, and when better drugs were developed my prescription was changed to Gabapentin, which kept me seizure free.

But the experience caused me to ask a question, "Can we evaluate our role on earth from a single experience, such as that one Bible Study which I had led?" It was in some ways a ridiculous thought to have at that moment. But many of us judge our lives by the final moments we have in life, or the one mistake we make. It is foolish.

Our lives are more like an entire book, not one solitary chapter and certainly not the final period in a sentence. And we are not the final judge of our lives. A great reminder about final judgement comes from the writer Paul, "Therefore judge nothing before the appointed time; wait until the Lord comes. He will bring to light what is hidden in darkness and will expose the motives of the heart. At that time each will receive their praise from God." [9]

I remember the memorial service for my father, David Lagasse. He lived to be seventy eight. Doug and I performed the memorial service. When people came up to share about our dad we realized that of the twelve people that came forward spontaneously to share a few thoughts, all were men. The message was clear, our dad was a man's man. He lived to enrich the lives of men. His career as a probation officer and administrator of justice was to bring men into their right role on earth. His retirement was spent leading men into ministry roles. He lived to not only mentor his three sons, but to mentor men wherever he met them.

One of the men who shared at the service was a guy our dad had met just months before at our local gym. He was an African American who'd fallen on hard times. He was working at the desk at the gym checking people in. He remembered my dad as someone who took time to talk to him, to listen to him, to give him advice and guidance.

It's not what we do in our final moments that matters; it's what we do with our whole lives. Another thought comes to mind as I think on that final moment when I thought I was dying.

I had posed a question to God, *"Is this why I was created?"* I was talking to Him in my final moment of consciousness. I didn't

---

[9] 1Corinthians 4:5

say, *"Amen"* or *"Dear God,"* or *"Our Father..."* I just spoke to Him in my thoughts. This is how I live. It is typical of the type of dialogue I have with God from moment to moment. God is present; He is not distant. When we seek Him he responds. When we place our faith in Him He puts his Holy Spirit inside us. He promises never to leave or forsake us.

Practice the Presence of God, is a very old book by the Catholic monk Brother Lawrence. Insights from this book helped me understand the teaching of Jesus when he told his followers to pray without ceasing. Brother Lawrence lived as a Carmelite Prior in Paris as a simple cobbler and cook. He was uneducated in the popular sense of the word, but full of wisdom in the Biblical sense. He recognized God's active role in our lives. It is we who must actively engage with the ever-knowing God.

I have sought to always be aware of my Creator and loving Father. Psalm 139:2 and 3 says, "You know when I sit down and when I rise up; You understand my thought from afar. You scrutinize my path and my lying down, And are intimately acquainted with all my ways."

It is of great comfort and assurance to me, even when I think I am dying, to know I have such a caring conscious Father who knows me - even my innermost thoughts.

Chapter 8

Psychiatric Ward

When many people think of mental illness, they might have a rather judgmental attitude. I know I did. It is true that some have destroyed their minds through drug or alcohol abuse or some other self inflicted cause. Many of course have had trauma in life that caused their illnesses, but I, in my immaturity didn't really understand that. I also couldn't grasp how mental illness could be an inherited tendency. An experience I had in the fall of 1979 changed my perspective.

It was in London, England. I was studying English literature and poetry with 18 other Westmont College students under the tutelage of Professor Delaney and his wife. Westmont has a semester abroad program where one can get much of the English degree by studying in England. Dr. Delaney was a good man, intelligent, caring, diligent, and an excellent professor. I had the misfortune of having a lung infection before my departure that fall as I was preparing for the program abroad. I was faced with the choice of heading to Stanford Children's Hospital in Palo Alto, and missing a semester of college, or flying to London, England (while sick) and starting my third year of college. I chose the latter.

I still remember sitting in the airport in San Francisco with my dad and mom and contemplating the decision before me.

I asked my loving parents, "What should I do?" I already had a fever, felt fatigued and congested, and knew I had a lung infection. That is life with cystic fibrosis. "Should I walk through the departure gate and head off to England, or go home and head to the hospital?" I asked my dad. We discussed the pros and cons of each option.

Then he looked at me and wisely said, "Son, it is up to you. We will support you in whatever decision you make." Wow. That was a tough one. I wanted so much for someone to tell me what to do. But in his wisdom he knew I should, as a young adult, make the decision for myself. It was part of growing up and being a man. I chose to fly to England. I figured it was a modern country and they'd have hospitals too. I was sort of right.

The flight over was terrible. I was coughing and gasping for breath. I finally asked for oxygen from the flight attendant and she brought me a bottle and cannula. I knew it would mitigate the effects of the altitude and my lack of oxygen due to the crud in my lungs. When I landed in London I exited the terminal and took a taxi straight to Brompton Hospital[10]. As I entered the massive hallway I was impressed with the hardwood floors, the 18 foot ceilings, the two-foot thick walls, and the feeling of antiquity that pervaded the place. I soon became accustomed to the unending tea that was served - seven times a day, no kidding. And every time with milk. Brompton Hospital was the top notch lung and heart hospital in the country. I was told it was the queen's hospital. I guess if she got sick she would be treated there. Nurses came there to train from all over the world. I met young women from every continent with all kinds of strange English accents.

I was to find myself admitted five times during the course of my three month stay in England. It made keeping up with my studies rather difficult. Each time I stayed just seven days until my temperature returned to normal and my lungs sounded better. Then the doctors would decide I was healthy and they'd discharge me. I would then board a train and travel the two hours south to the place where the other Westmont students were staying/studying. As a result of my frequent admissions I missed out on much of the other travel the students did and some of the course work as well. Instead of 16 units of classes I reduced my class load to just 12.

It was during my fourth admission that I was given a new treatment. My British doctor knew my lungs were inflamed from all the coughing and infection. He decided to try a dose of pred-

---

[10] https://www.rbht.nhs.uk

nisone. He gave me 20 milligrams a day. I swallowed the tiny white pill – completely unaware that it would have a disastrous impact on the next six months of my life and bring me to the verge of death. He did tell me that in the future I should never stop taking it "cold turkey" or it could be fatal. He said I should taper down one millimeter at a time each week, over the course of twenty weeks.

The night after swallowing the pill I had the most disturbing night's sleep. I dreamt of all kinds of crazy things. I had been reading a trilogy by C.S. Lewis called, "Out of the Silent Planet." It is a kind of mystical fantasy filled with all kinds of bizarre creatures and landscapes. I too, had bizarre dreams. I thought my dreams had all sorts of deep meanings and wonderful secrets. I began, upon waking, to write my dreams down as fast as possible, filling pages and pages of notes. When I read the stuff many months later I was completely perplexed. It was all a pile of nonsense. Nevertheless, at the time I truly felt that it was wonderful and full of deep and mysterious meaning. I had reached a deeper level of knowledge and understanding. I felt ecstatic, happy, even exuberant.

My doctor was pleased with my lung's progress and discharged me. My plan was to return to Herne Bay Court, in the south of England, where my fellow students and teachers were residing. I gathered my things and left the mammoth hospital and boarded the train. I felt wonderful and was really enjoying the scenery out the windows. I had ridden this line many times before but it all seemed fresh. In my semi euphoric state I missed the train's stop at the Herne Bay station entirely. Soon I was seeing signs out the train window with all sorts of unfamiliar names. I finally got up from my seat and went and found the conductor. He explained that I had missed my stop. At the next train stop he allowed me to exit the train, cross the tracks, and board on the return train without paying another fare. That was pretty decent of him. I traveled back past several towns and found the right platform for Herne Bay and got off.

Back in class, my fellow students and my professor found me to have changed. But I felt fine. I remember showing up for class one morning with all kinds of clothes on that didn't match and looked odd. I had a hat on, a red scarf and a brightly colored vest over my long sleeve shirt. Then I had put all kinds of buttons (which I had collected from the various places we had visited) all over my clothes. Nobody said anything to me at breakfast. Later I took a 100 foot rope and tied one end of it around a souvenir from Ann Hathaway's cottage (Shakespeare's birthplace) and placed it outside my professor's doorway, and then I ran the rope all the way to the student's dormitory.

When Dr. Delaney called me aside and asked me the meaning of it all I asked him, "What is truth?" About that time he decided he'd better bring me back to the hospital. I packed a bag and we headed for the train station.

All along the two hour journey I remember wanting to touch his arm, as a child might do his parent. I had in my mind that he was going to help me, so long as I remained close to him. I was feeling disoriented and he was my connection to getting help. I am afraid this really freaked him out. He most certainly got some strange looks from the other passengers on the train. (Thirty years later he was still nervous when he saw me at a reunion.)

Brompton hospital admitted me again and put me in a private room instead of the behemoth four-patient rooms of my prior admissions. I think they were uncertain of how to treat me. They gave me a special nurse who sat outside my door at all times. I knew she was sitting out there in a chair but didn't understand why. She also stood outside the door to the bathroom in the hallway whenever I had to use the "*loo*." While I was inside the *loo* on one occasion I deliberately sprinkled water on all the walls of the bathroom after I washed my hands. I was doing it for some special purpose. I have no idea now why I did it. I don't think the staff appreciated it one bit.

The following day they decided I had to be sedated. I am sure I'd done or said some other really strange things. They didn't explain this to me, however. I recall a nurse coming into my room with a plastic kidney tray with a big syringe in it. I saw the needle, took the syringe right out of the tray and broke it. She left the room in a rush. When she returned she had a male assistant. He was there to hold my arms down as I lay on the bed. The nurse then again tried to administer the medication. I kicked my foot up and sent the tray and needle flying across the room. I clearly remember thinking - being surely convinced – that whatever they were about to do to me was bad, really bad. The next time they came into my room there were four of them. They took my legs and arms and pinned me to the bed, then they flipped me over and jabbed the needle right through my clothing into my buttocks. An instant later I was in a deep sleep. I vaguely remember being loaded into another ambulance - or perhaps it was being unloaded. It was all a blur.

When I came to my senses I found myself in the psychiatric ward of the London Hospital. It was a different hospital in a different part of London. I had again been placed in a private ward. But this one had windows that were double pane and did not open. The door to my room was also locked from the outside so I could not leave at will. This was a totally new and unpleasant experience for me. All my belongs, even my clothing, had been taken away from me. I was left with nothing but a pair of gym shorts, a tee shirt and flip flops. The surprising thing is that the euphoria and bizarre imaginations I had been experiencing were completely gone. I was thinking and feeling normal. The sedation I had been given to transport me between hospitals had reversed the chemical effect of the prednisone. I was thinking and acting like my normal self.

But now I was in a psychiatric ward and I knew nobody. And nobody came to visit. The Brompton Hospital doctor who'd transferred me never came to see me. I can assume he ordered the transfer, but I have no idea what was communicated. And as for my fellow students who were studying with Westmont, they and their two professors had left England entirely, and were continuing their studies in Israel. I was alone. It really shook me up. I was all alone, in a foreign country, locked up in a psychiatric ward. And as far as I knew nobody even knew where I was or who I was. I realized that all I had was Jesus. He is my rock and my fortress.

The nurse came around to check up on me. I explained that I needed to see the respiratory therapist for treatment for my clogged lungs. This was new for them. They did not have CF patients in their ward normally nor did they have experience bringing respiratory therapists into the psychiatric ward. So they did not come. My lungs began to fill up with mucus. My high calorie diet that maintained my skinny frame was also gone. I asked for some food to supplement my diet and was given a single piece of white bread. I then asked for the enzymes that were prescribed to aid my pancreas in digesting food. The nurse was unfamiliar with the drug, but she brought me four capsules. I explained that four capsules are taken with a full meal, not a snack.

She treated me like I was crazy and said, "Take all four; that is what is prescribed." I tried to tell her that four pills are taken with a full meal and that with a snack I should take just one pill. She insisted I take all four. We went back and forth; she clearly was not listening to me or understanding what I was explaining. Finally in frustration I told her to take the bread and the pills and leave. I can only imagine what she wrote in my chart.

Later that afternoon I was called to participate in group therapy. I went obediently. There were sixteen people sitting in chairs in a circle. Half of them looked like they were sleeping or severely doped up. Most of them were smoking. The room became cloudy with all the smoke. The topic was, "How to deal with depression." I was a Psych major at Westmont, (as well as English) and so I began giving some input. There was one individual who was at the center of the discussion so I began to ask him a series of questions. I asked him to imagine himself in bed that morning. Then I asked him if he thought he would have the energy to just sit up on the side of the bed.

"Don't think of all the tasks that are before you, just think of sitting up." He said he thought he could do that. Then I asked him if he could imagine going to the bathroom and after he said he could I asked about brushing his teeth. He said he could imagine doing that. I took him step by step through his morning routine until he was involved in his daily tasks.

The social worker or counselor was very pleased. She said, with the most patronizing and insipid tone of voice you can imagine, "Thank you very much for sharing that, Daniel. Those are very good ideas." I felt demeaned and it upset me. She was treating me like a child. Between her attitude and the smoke filled room I decided I had had enough. I excused myself and left the group and went back to my solitary confinement. Again I am sure she had some observations to mark in her report about me. I felt like I had stepped right into the movie, *One Flew Over the Cuckoo's Nest*.

The next day a respiratory therapist arrived and began an aerosol treatment. During the inhalation the glass device that held the medication (today plastic disposal ones are used) was dropped and shattered on the floor. The therapist discontinued the treatment and left the room. It was not her job to clean floors. Later I asked about the glass that remained on the floor day after day. I was told that many of the hospital staff were on a one week strike, so they would not be coming in. So I had to carefully step into my flip flops when getting out of bed, to avoid getting my feet cut.

I began losing weight. The diet was clearly not designed for someone who needed 3000 calories a day. I still weighed just 125 pounds. But after those crazy days at Brompton Hospital and then four days in the London Hospital psychiatric ward I was down to 106 pounds. The physicians became concerned that I would die (though they did not discuss this with me or offer me more food), but somebody called my parents in Los Gatos, California. My mom and dad decided to come immediately. It was shortly before Christmas and the airlines were all booked. In spite of the travel crowds they managed to get a standby flight to London.

I shall never forget the moment my parents walked into my secured hospital room in the psych unit. They saw their skinny son in the isolation ward, standing among the broken glass, wearing nothing but gym shorts and a dirty tee shirt. They hugged me tightly and we cried. I sobbed like I never had before. I felt suddenly safe and comforted. Then we sat on the edge of my hospital bed and I coherently related to them what I had endured. My parents could see that I was mentally healthy and should not be in a psych ward; I belonged in a place where I could get some care for my infected lungs.

My dad went to the main office of the department. He asked to see the psychiatrist in charge.

"I am sorry; he is not here today. He will be in tomorrow." Frustrated, but respectful of their policies, he came back into my room and explained that he and mom would be back the next day to work out my discharge with the department head. The following morning they returned and were told that the psychiatrist was playing golf that morning.

"The patient cannot be discharged without a psychiatrist's evaluation and approval," they said dismissively. "He will be in tomorrow," they were told. My dad and mom were indignant, but felt powerless to do anything. Again they left me alone in my room to spend another night in hell.

The next day they were again put off by the lady in charge.

At that point my dad said quite clearly, "I am taking my son *now*. If the psychiatrist cannot come in now then I am taking my son out whether you like it or not."

At that point the receptionist made some phone calls and then replied, "Someone will be here shortly." A few minutes later someone appeared in her office. I was retrieved from isolation and the four of us stood as my father demanded action. The lady, (I do not know her official position) began asking some questions about my medical history. She explained that the hospital had to keep me in the ward because they did not have a diagnosis for me. They could not find anything wrong with me.

My father and I explained what had transpired with the prednisone, the sedation, the transfer to the London Hospital and my sudden decline in health. The entire time the lady never looked at me nor listened to my input. She spoke about me in the third person, as if I was not present, as if I had no value or dignity. She treated me with a bias that we too often give those who have psychiatric issues. I was less than a full person. I was crazy. I did not deserve to be listened to because I must be mentally living in another world.

At length she said, "Oh, he must have had steroid psychosis. His euphoria and confusion was a result of the medicine. That is a side effect that sometimes happens." And then she simply said, "He is free to go." Finally I was discharged.

My father and mother then joined me in a taxi and we went back to Brompton Hospital for another week of proper treatment for cystic fibrosis. I began to taper off the prednisone that had caused the psychosis. We flew back home together just after

Christmas and I checked into Stanford Children's Hospital to get a final tune up, as we CF'ers liked to call our regular inpatient stays.

Psychological scars are some of the most difficult to live with. Especially those that are rooted in traumatic life experiences, abuse and so forth. From my time experiencing a psychosis I can tell you that someone who is psychotic really believes with all their heart that *their* understanding of reality is the right one. They are not intentionally playing games, nor can they be cognitively convinced of their false ways. No amount of logic can convince them of their delusions. What can you do to help such a person?

First of all there is usually no reason to be fearful. All of us need love and acceptance. Look for practical ways can you aid them. They may be standing at an intersection holding up a cardboard sign asking for financial help. They often are blessed by meaningful eye contact and an honest greeting, and a kind word, as well as money or food you might give them. Listen to them, even if it doesn't make a whole lot of sense. Look them in the eye. Showing dignity and humanity can mean more to them than one can imagine.

Jesus dealt with people whose mental health problems needed supernatural healing, and he gave it. He treated all people with dignity, love and understanding. He cared for their physical needs and accepted them, in spite of the pressures and bigotry of the religious leaders of the day. Praying for those who are mentally ill is as important as praying for any other illness. And showing kindness and compassion is the most basic expression of our common humanity.

Chapter 9

Purpose in Life?

It was the spring of 1979 and I was completing my psychology studies at Westmont College in Santa Barbara, California. My degree required doing an internship. I chose to spend three months as an intern at the Santa Barbara Mental Health Day Treatment Center. That is a pretty long name for what sometimes seemed like a baby-sitting and activity center for people who had been in mental hospitals. Patients at the center participated in group therapy sessions, and they saw the psychiatrist and psychologist. They could also participate in occupational therapy.

They spent their nights at half-way houses that had marginal supervision, and during the day they would walk or take the bus to the treatment center. They were also free to wander around Santa Barbara, sit on the beach, shop in town, or whatever. Most of them eventually would wander into the center to take part in crafts like leather working or join us for rides to city parks. Occasionally some would try to play ball games. I say, *tried* because most of them were on so many meds that they couldn't catch a frisbee or a ball if their life depended on it. Some had schizophrenia, were simply bi-polar, or had mild psychotic disorders. I was not there to treat their psychosis, rather I was there to interact with them, to observe them, to understand a bit of the mental health system, and to engage with the professionals who were employed there. I spent many days driving the patients around in the passenger van, taking them to various parks where they could have a picnic or take a walk. I supervised many of these activities. But I was not responsible for face to face therapy.

I did try playing frisbee with one fellow who had consistently refused to interact with anybody. He never spoke to anybody, never touched anybody, and never looked at anybody. He just wandered around in a semi-catatonic state, no doubt drugged up on lithium or something. I got a brilliant idea that if an object was thrown at him he might react to it - at least in self defense.

So I hollered, "Mike, catch this. And I tossed a frisbee at him." Now you have to realize that as a college student I prided myself on my accuracy with a frisbee. It was one of the major free time activities of men in my dorm. We used to play in the parking lot right among the cars and never hit any of them (well most of the time.) So I threw the frisbee right at Mike's chest. He shuffled to the side and it went right past him. This told me he could react if he wanted to. Bit by bit I gently threw it until he did catch it. Then I began to teach him how to throw it. He didn't have to touch me, or talk to me, or even look at me. He just interacted with the frisbee and I was remotely present at the other end of the yard. Eventually we were playing catch. I felt this was a big accomplishment. So much for my abilities at therapy.

One time I did try something that I thought was novel. There was one guy who always said he was Jesus. Perhaps he had some sort of religious background and he was confused. Or maybe he was like those described in the Bible who had demons and claimed to be Jesus. I won't try and assess that, but he was diagnosed as having a psychosis. His real name was David. Nevertheless most of the time if you asked him his name he would answer, "Jesus."

On a particular sunny day another patient came in to the center and I greeted him with a simple, "Hi Jim, good morning."

"I am not Jim," he retorted. "I am Jesus."

I said, "Oh," and left it at that. It was futile to argue with patients. I had learned that long ago. But then I got what I thought was a brilliant idea. I called David into the room and had him sit at a small table. I brought Jim over and seated him across the table from David.

"Who are you Jim," I asked?

Jim replied boldly, "I am Jesus." David sat there just three feet away totally motionless, his face devoid of expression.

Then I turned to David, "Who are you, David?"

He replied in his deep voice with a straight face, "I am Jesus." There was silence. I looked at each one and saw no reaction from either of them.

Finally I interjected, "Don't you guys see any possible conflict here?" Still they sat in silence. I explained further, "David you say you are Jesus. But Jim here says he is Jesus. How can that be possible? You can't both be Jesus, right?" I was hoping to somehow cognitively shake them out of their psychosis.

David looked at Jim and said, "Well ... he is lying." And that was the end of my novel idea.

There was one other day that is as clear in my memory as if it were yesterday. It was one of those experiences that remains with one for a lifetime because it was clear that it was the culmination of something for which God had prepared me. I was sitting in a metal folding chair at the very end of an incomplete circle. We were indoors at the center. On the opposite side seated side-by-side were the social worker, the psychologist, and the psychiatrist. Seated next to them all around the circle were all of the patients - perhaps ten - and the final person in the semi-circle was me, the intern. I tried to sit with the patients, rather than the therapists in an attempt to bond with them. Behind me were large glass doors that opened onto a cement patio.

The psychologist began the group therapy sessions by asking if there was anything anyone wanted to talk about on that particular morning. There was considerable silence. Therapists are used to creating this space, because silence is uncomfortable and it often will encourage reluctant people to start speaking just to fill the void. Then they share part of their lives. Most of the patients were not too communicative and certainly not eager to begin a group discussion that focused on them. But one fellow named Ramon was pretty outgoing. He began by saying that he had been struggling with rejection by some of the men he'd been seeing. He explained that he was a homosexual prostitute - something I had never heard of in 1979, and to be honest I wasn't even sure what it was. In 2020 you might think that is unbelievable that I could be so naive. But our society used to be quite different. Anyway, he went on to say that he was really depressed. Then he said he didn't have any purpose in life and was thinking of, "ending it all."

This seemed like a good topic of discussion to the psychologist, so he asked the group, "Who would like to talk about 'purpose in life?" This was greeted by silence. I looked around the room at the patients and most of them were sitting there looking at their knees. So the social worker decided to get things going by speaking up.

She said, "I know that I get purpose in my life by raising my children and caring for my family. Of course working as a social worker also gives me purpose. These things are important to me." I thought for a moment. None of the patients were currently married or had kids. None of them had a job.

Then the psychologist spoke up. "My profession and education has given me purpose. Still I look to the future to give me purpose, and my daily responsibilities give me a sense of purpose. I am still assessing what my purpose in life is, however." There was some more silence.

I thought, "If I had to come to this old building each day to hang out with mental patients would I struggle with purpose?"

Then the psychiatrist began to speak. He was tall and confident. I sensed that the patients were listening. At least they were looking at him.

"Of course I get a strong sense of purpose by the work I do. I like helping people. My free time is also important to me. I enjoy playing golf and spending time with my family. These things give me a purpose in life and a desire to live." I thought to myself, *"Golf? Come on; you've got to be kidding."*

The sharing had begun on the far side of the room with the social worker and had proceeded clockwise. Next to her was the psychologist and then the psychiatrist. It was logical that the patient sitting next to the psychiatrist would share next. It was a guy and he did his best to say something meaningful. The talk when on from there and nobody had much to say. Some of them just mumbled (which happened pretty frequently when trying to converse), some said nothing at all and the others said they had no purpose or couldn't think of any. I was the final one to share.

The whole time the professionals and patients had been sharing I had a bit of a struggle inside. I knew what my purpose was and was quite willing to share it, but I also knew the institution where I worked was a secular one. *"Should I speak out about my faith?"* I asked myself. I knew the psychiatrists perceived Christianity as a crutch at best and a source of mental illness at worst. I knew many of the mental patients often worked religion into their psychosis and so the head psychiatrist viewed the Bible (and faith) with great skepticism. He would not let patients bring their Bible into his office when he worked with them. One lady with schizophrenia always carried a giant Bible with her everywhere. And of course I remembered the two Jesus patients.

As I sat at the end of that row of ten patients I knew that in a moment or two my turn would come to share about life's purpose.

Every student at my Christian liberal arts college was required to take philosophy. And one of the big questions that philosophers have dealt with is the meaning of human existence. Through the ages it's been answered in many different ways. "I think therefore I am," (Descartes) "Life has no meaning" (existentialism) and dozens of others. The answer that made the most sense to me is clarified in the Westminster Catechism, "The chief end of man is to glorify God and to enjoy Him forever." This actually is another way of expressing a portion of scripture, Romans 11:36. It says, "For from Him and through Him and to Him are all things. To Him be the glory forever! Amen." The apostle Paul repeats it again in 1 Corinthians 10:31, "So whether therefore you eat, or drink, or whatsoever you do, do all to the glory of God." This explanation for purpose in life satisfies me at the deepest level. A biblical explanation for my existence surpasses that given by Plato, Aristotle, Kierkegaard, Descartes, Hegel, Hume, Berkeley, Aristotle, Thomas Aquinas and a host of others - although each did their best to sort out the meaning and purpose of man. It had been good to study these great men and their noble efforts – because that gave me a deeper understanding of the worldview of many Americans.

So when my turn came in that circle of mental health patients I figured the best answer I could give was an honest one.

"My purpose in life is to glorify God," I said. Then continued, "I didn't come into this world to satisfy my own desires and plans; I was created to fulfill God's plans for my life. Each day that I am on earth I want to acknowledge and serve the One who gave me breath. And because of this I live a full and satisfying life and am fully content." I looked at the faces in the circle. They were listening.

The psychiatrist looked at Ramon and said, "Ramon, I think you should talk more with Dan after our time together." I was surprised to hear him give semi-affirmative support to my Christian worldview. Then he ended the session. Afterwards many of us went out into the patio to talk more.

I knew God had a special purpose for me that moment on that special day, to glorify Him through serving one whom he had also created, Ramon. That is purpose. To love God and to love others. I only had a brief opportunity to talk more with Ramon that day, but I knew that my daily acts of kindness and my few spoken words of faith did have an impact on their lives.

Chapter 10

Falling in Love

Although I dated girls in college, I never thought I'd get married. I never got serious with any of the women I got to know. *Who would want to marry somebody that was going to die in a very short time?* I figured. That'd be a lousy deal.

It wasn't until I finished my undergraduate work at Westmont and returned home that I found the love of my life. After graduating from college I had felt a strong desire to serve others, specifically in a different culture. I had developed a fascination and love for peoples of different ethnicities. But first I needed to find a job and earn something. I returned to my parent's home in Los Gatos, California. I found work teaching junior high at Valley Christian School. Occasionally I would need to have a substitute come teach my classes while I went in to the hospital for a tune up. The school administration was very understanding. Then after a week or two I'd resume teaching. Often I would come home at the end of the day and literally collapse on the couch only to be awakened by my mom for dinner and therapy. Since I carpooled with three other teachers to work I often slept in the car on the thirty-minute ride home.

I was in my second year teaching when I met a petite brunette at a college Bible Study in somebody's home. Her name was DeAnna Van Tuyl. As we chatted I discovered that her cousin Karen was one of my students, my best student in fact. Standing just five feet tall DeAnna was beautiful and cute at the same time. She had the most wonderful big brown eyes. Wow. She was sensitive, caring, patient and had a soft and gentle disposition. We went for ice cream with a group of other students after the study. And over the next few months I invited her on a few casual dates.

But a couple of hospitalizations and the demands of teaching had me distracted from pursuing our relationship. Then something happened.

It was a Sunday morning in May of 1982, and we were chatting in the fellowship hall at church, surrounded by four-hundred other students. She told me rather casually that she was leaving for Peru in a month. I was shocked.

"How long will you be gone," I asked?

"A year," she said. I was astounded.

"A year? Why so long?" I was thinking how very far Peru was from Silicon Valley.

"I am going to live with a missionary family that works high in the Andes. I will study Spanish and Biology as well as work in the Peruvian church." She continued to explain how she'd come to this decision. "My family has known this missionary, Bob Whatley for many years. He is part of Baptist Mid Missions. He, his wife and his seven kids have been church planting in Peru for decades. I'll be living in Cusco."

I was immediately fascinated. Not so much with Peru as with this slight young girl who had such a big heart, a plan for her future, and a determination to serve people of a different land. My interest was piqued.

Mustering up some courage I asked DeAnna, "Would you like to go to lunch?" She said yes. I took her to the Good Earth restaurant in Los Gatos. (I probably had a coupon).

We dated every day for the next thirty days. We went sightseeing in San Francisco. Then roller skating with my junior high students along the boardwalk in Santa Cruz. She made Mexican food for my Spanish class students in my parent's home. We had dinners with her parents at their big table. She helped me grade papers from my junior high kids. Her younger sisters Judy and Janine were a bit leery and amazed that she was dating a teacher! They were students at Valley Christian high school and they considered teachers to be a different species. The days seemed to go by so very quickly. Soon DeAnna would be leaving for Peru.

My eyes were moist when I stood with the Van Tuyl family and said goodbye at the San Jose International Airport. As we parted I gave her a silver rose that I'd cut from our garden that morning. It was from a bush my dad had transplanted into our garden. The rosebush was a hundred years old, named "Mr. Lincoln," by whomever names rosebushes.

Our relationship marked the beginning of a battle, fought not between us, but a fight against illness. Would we be victorious? Would God do a miracle? Or was I soon to join my older brother David in heaven?

She was a courageous woman to fall in love with a dying man.

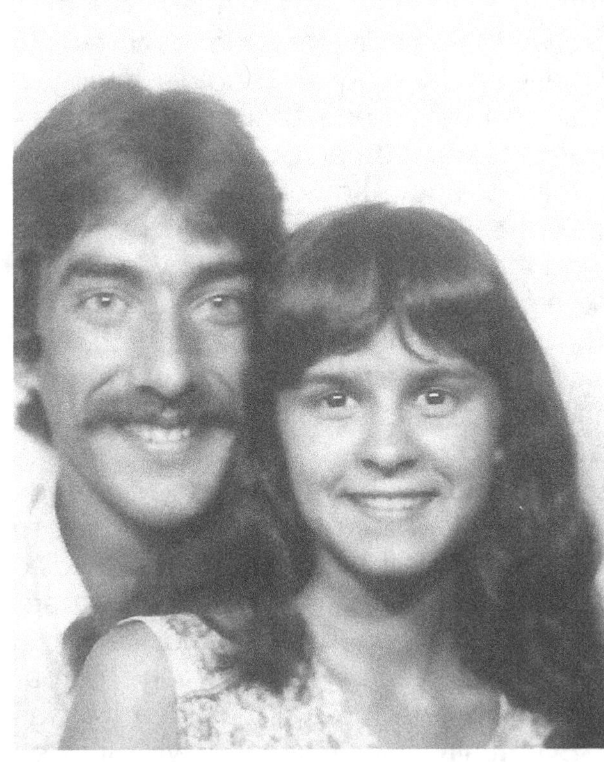

KIOSK PHOTO FROM THE MALL

Finding DeAnna, was another key spiritual experience in my life. After college I had prayed and asked God specifically that he lead me to a wife that was not just godly, but was a woman committed to go serve at the ends of the earth if necessary, as I pursued a life of cross cultural service. I had met many wonderful women, both in school and at church, but there were only a few who were willing to answer God's call to go to the unreached and difficult places. DeAnna Van Tuyl was special.

But isn't it a bit unrealistic to think of going to remote places when you know you have a terminal illness? Cystic fibrosis is an illness that afflicts mostly caucasians. Most hospitals in the world don't have CF patients. And what about getting married? I had never heard of anybody with CF getting married. All the kids at Stanford, with whom I'd shared communal hospital rooms while growing up, had all passed away.

What kind of future would I have?

DeAnna's departure for Peru marked the beginning of a lot of letter writing. We were unable to make telephone calls, as the cost was prohibitive and she didn't have a phone in her apartment in Cusco. I realized this was a great opportunity to ask questions and get to know one another better. In the two hundred letters (and dozens of audio tapes) that we exchanged over twenty months of separation, we really got to know one another deeply.

We were each committed to trusting one another and remaining faithful to our commitment to each other, even if our ability to communicate might fail. I think this is a key element to any successful relationship. We talked at length what it would be like to be separated for so long and the importance of honesty in our relationship. This established a groundwork of trust. We agreed that neither of us would date anyone else during our separation, until we'd written about our desire (and received a response) from the other person. Because mail service was so slow, getting that answer would take at least a month!

During DeAnna's time in the mountain city of Cusco and then later in the tiny remote village of Paucartambo, I continued to prepare to someday go overseas myself. I had been motivated to share God's love with people who had never heard or experienced the love of Christ. I was encouraged by Arnold Palmer, a pastor at my church, to spend a year living with one of our church's missionaries. That would give me a better idea if I was cut out for work overseas. Eventually I was invited to live with Ben Siaki in the Philippines. He worked with Philippine Crusades, which was called OC Ministries in the US.

DeAnna had been in Peru for about four months when I flew to Manila. It would be another 16 months before I returned home to San Jose.

My mentor in the Philippines, Ben Siaki, was fond of quoting a poetic verse toward the end of his motivational sermons, "'Tis only one life, will soon be past. Only what's done for Christ, will truly last." It makes one think about all the frivolous things we do while we are young and healthy, (or while we are old and frail.) Will they last, will they matter? What are we doing that will last for eternity?

I started feeling old while I was still young. But it does not matter if we are seventy, eighty or ninety. While we live, we can live for Christ. The apostle Paul said, "For to me to live is Christ, to die is gain."[11] There is nothing in that verse about feeling sorry for oneself because we are weak, or have failing health, or reduced capacity. When I look into the Scriptures I don't read about retiring at a certain age and then kicking back until Jesus comes. I see some old men and women who are greatly used by God; in fact they are pivotal in history. They did not give up; they did not quit when they were tired or weary. In fact their strength was renewed and they "Rose up on wings like eagles."[12] It is for God's purposes that we press on; our mission may change but the one we serve will not.

Repeatedly in life we are faced with a choice. Faith or fear. It is truly a choice, and it is dictated by the path we choose in our relationship with Christ. It is certain that we will all get old and usually get sick. And then we will die. The immediate question is, "How will we live with the life we have been given?

---

[11] Philippians 1:21

[12] Isaiah 40:31

Chapter 11

Ceiling Rats

September 13, 1982 was a momentous day. It was the day I said goodbye to my parents for good, as in, forever. At least I thought so. I was on my way to the Philippine Islands. I stood in the San Francisco airport at the departure gate (that was before security prevented families from entering the departure areas) and gave each of my parents a huge hug. I looked at their faces, my dad and mom smiling to hide their emotions. I had been sick all through my teens and young adulthood. They knew and I knew, that when I got sick in Asia the health care would be a far cry from Stanford Hospital. To fly to the Philippines was to say goodbye to top notch healthcare. It was to head into the unknown. I honestly assumed I would die on the other side of the planet. Really. But I would rather die serving others than live comfortably for myself.

I had a very vague idea of the city of Manila. It was a word, a concept. I tried to picture a large bay, probably some palm trees and traffic. It was orange on my map. I was pretty far off. When the airport doors slid open and I faced downtown Manila my first impression was a hot blast of heavy humid air. I thought it was an anomaly, perhaps something that was blowing from an air-condition evaporator overhead. But it was the normal outside air. It was stifling. And it was dirty polluted air from all the traffic. My second immediate perception was the noise. There was a non-stop cacophony of sound. It was mostly horns honking. I really couldn't see the point of everyone honking their horns simultaneously but I was to grow accustomed to it during the next sixteen months residing in this foreign land.

My third immediate impression was a crowd of men pushing at me and my luggage cart and shouting, "Taxi, taxi, taxi! Carry your luggage, sir?" "You need a hotel, sir?" "You want a tour, sir?" And on it went. It was overwhelming as cards and signs and brochures were waved in my face. I couldn't take one step forward as the crush of men pressed in on me and my luggage cart. *Welcome to Manila.*

Behind the crowd of five foot dark haired Filipino men stood a six foot white guy. He stood out like a sore thumb. He had a big grin on his face and a head of wavy blond hair.

With a smooth American sounding voice he shouted, "Dan?" I could not have felt more relieved. Unless you have flown across an ocean and landed in a foreign land without the slightest idea of who is going to pick you up, you cannot imagine my joy and relief.

Paul Newman (not *the* Paul Newman) greeted me and said, "Welcome to the Pilippines. (Yes, he pronounced it with a "p".) Do you have pipty pesos for the parking?" he asked in his best impersonation of a Philippine accent. He was making a joke and I had no idea what he was laughing at. I would soon learn. Filipinos speak English, which is one of their national languages. They incorporated the language during the occupation of the Philippine islands by Americans following the second world war. But they retained their unique accent and inability to properly pronounce the consonant "f." It always sounded like a "p." Paul thought this was hilarious.

He drove me through the crowded streets with acumen. He was right at home. I had never seen such random and crowded traffic. The lines that delineate lanes were ignored, as were red lights and any car or bus that wasn't immediately ahead of you. Cars wanting to turn left at any intersection would drive around the cars waiting to turn until the whole intersection was blocked with a mob of cars trying to make the turn. After about an hour of stop-and-go and weave-and-dodge we arrived at his house. His wife Nancy greeted me warmly and we entered their air-conditioned home. It felt like heaven compared to the hot humid air outside. She gave me a glass of water with ice cubes. What hospitality!

When your breathing is compromised, trying to get oxygen from hot humid air becomes quite an exercise. I could feel the congestion in my lungs after traveling for twenty hours without therapy. Nancy led me to a guest room. It was spacious and comfortable. But as a guest in their home I was embarrassed to hack and cough in my traditional manner. I wanted to be polite and gracious but I was actually feeling quite awful. I knew that without twice daily lung clearance it was going to be difficult to stay alive. I closed the door to my room, laid across the bed and tried to do chest percussion therapy on myself. It is hard to pound on one's back and be very effective, especially when laying on my stomach with my butt in the air. My coughing was pretty loud and echoed off the concrete walls. Nancy kept asking through the door if I was OK. I tried to explain my situation. I am afraid she assumed I was a very sick traveler.

In fact I was quite congested, having endured all that travel without any lung clearance at all. Plus there was the fact that Manila had some of the dirtiest air in the world. Cars didn't have catalytic converters; ancient busses were everywhere and spewed clouds of diesel exhaust as they stopped and started

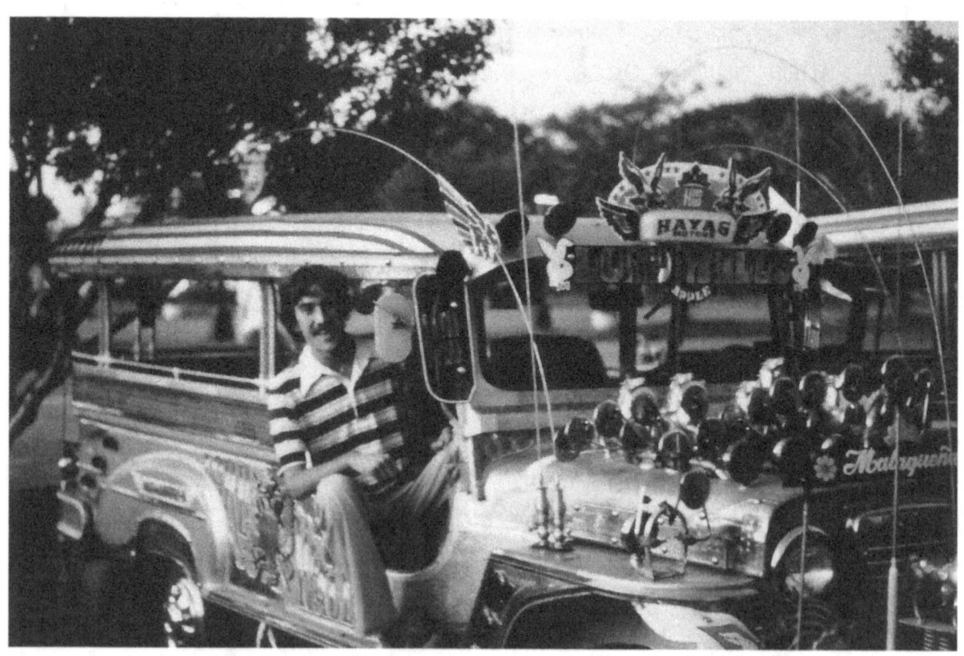

JEEPNIES IN MANILA WILL PICK YOU UP AND DROP YOU ANYWHERE ALONG THEIR ROUTE

every few feet. Jeepnies did the same. Jeepnies are an extended and highly modified version of the American army jeep. They are typically twenty feet or more long and can accommodate seventeen passengers. In addition there was a cement plant just outside the city limits that dumped tons of toxins in the air daily. I really wondered where and how I was going to live amongst all this pollution. After some discussion it was decided my permanent housing should be up above the city center in an area called Antipolo. It was adjacent to a private school, Faith Academy.

I knew I would be working with Philippine Crusades and that I would be interning for about a year with Ben. I knew who Ben was as I'd heard him preach at my church. But I didn't really know him personally. It was a decision I'd made by faith. When Ben spoke at my church during a missions conference, I had made a personal commitment to serve God anywhere he called me to go. But I knew precious little about the Philippine ministry or Ben. I knew he was a really big guy, even by American standards, and he was absolutely huge by Filipino standards. He was born in New Zealand and was from the Maori tribe. He had won the national championship as a boxer in his homeland and was well known for his big hands and his deep voice. He also had a huge smile and an ability to speak with authority and conviction. I also learned that he loved to eat. He would talk with incredible excitement and regale us with tales about people who had served him enormous steaks. (Beef was very expensive in the Philippines, since it was flown in.)

Ben's primary ministry was evangelism and church planting in the outlying villages and remote areas of the 7000 Philippine islands. He and Nestor, a Filipino missionary, would regularly take two week journeys with an old rusty red Ford F-100 truck to specific areas where local pastors wanted to expand their ministry. Soon I began to join them on these trips.

The bed of the truck was loaded with a generator, movie projector, giant screen, sound equipment, food, and our personal belongings. We would set up in a remote Filipino village, accessible only by miles of single lane dirt roads. There was an enormous contrast between the overcrowded capitol of Manila and the wide open provincial towns and villages. The movie screen might be positioned right in the middle of the dirt road perpendicular to the roadway. But nobody had cars in some of these villages and there was no traffic so it didn't hinder anyone. When night fell the local resident pastor would introduce us in the local dialect, then introduce Ben and me, and then translate what we said into their language. I shared the story of my life and how I found faith and strength in Christ and Ben preached about how a person could receive God's gift of salvation. He had a powerful voice and persuasive speech. We showed evangelist movies to the audience, who were seated on either side of the screen in the dirt road. The films explained basic truths from the Bible. All about us was pitch black night, with nothing but a candle or two alight in some of the nipa huts[13]. Everyone in the entire village came to watch the

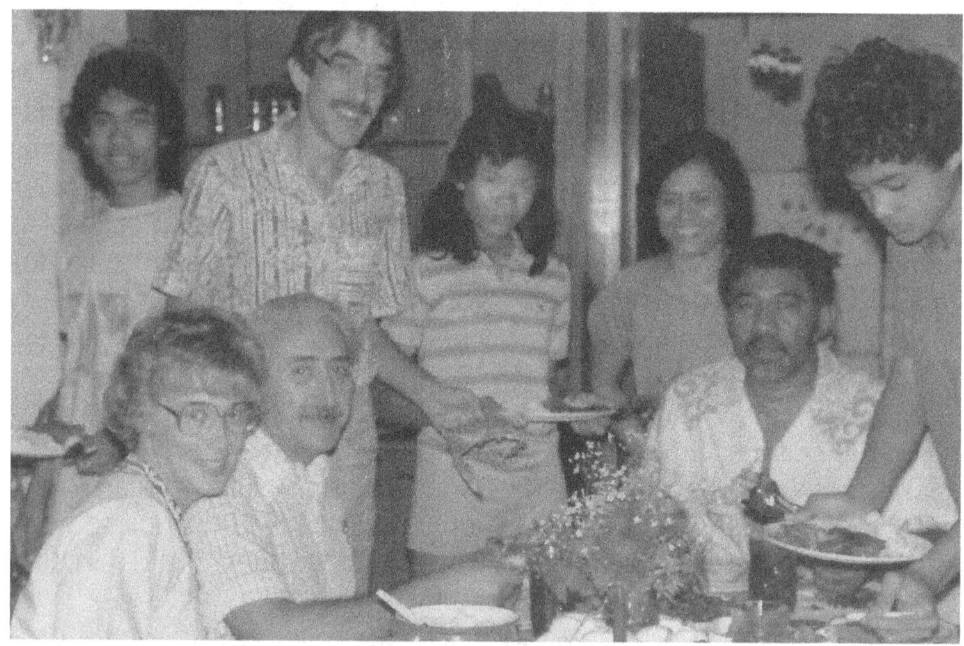

MY PARENTS CAME TO VISIT AND WE SHARED THANKSGIVING WITH THE SIAKI FAMILY (PAUL, ANGELA, PERLA, BEN AND DAVID). MY DAD BROUGHT A TURKEY ON THE AIRPLANE.

---

[13] homes made from bamboo and woven palm branches

movie and hear the foreign speakers; we were the only show in town, so to speak.

The local pastor would pass out an invitation to gather on a regular basis and discuss the Bible in a small study. From these small studies churches would eventually be born in the weeks to come. Ben, Nestor and I would hit the road early the next morning and drive to the next village. In some of the larger towns where there were multiple small churches we invited all the pastors from the various denominations to come together for a luncheon. We purchased the meat (canned corned beef) and they brought the rice. We would "feast" together and Ben would speak about church unity and the possibilities if we worked together as the body of Christ. For many of the men present it was the first time they had met the pastors from the other denominations, even though their churches were in the same town. They had always kept themselves at a distance and were somewhat distrustful of one another.

But before we even took our first trip, while I was still in Manila, I began to get a fever. It was decided that I should go to the Polymedic General Hospital (now called the VRP Medical Center)[14]. The name sounded pretty funky to me, and it was on Edsa Boulevard in Mandaluyong, which was right down the street from our missions office. The Polymedic General Hospital was a nine story building made of concrete. It was very basic inside and understaffed; I soon learned that each nurse had thirteen rooms to oversee.

As mentioned before, I have always been skinny and underweight. When I endured the heat of Manila I also began to get dehydrated. One would think that with all the humidity that dehydration would be unlikely but it is actually quite common unless one is consuming lots of water. It becomes even more difficult to start an IV when a person is dehydrated because the veins collapse. The needle may be in the vein but the nurse or doctor cannot tell because no blood is flowing back up the line. So they keep pushing or twisting or backing out and going back in, sometimes at one angle and then at another, hoping to get some blood flow.

---

[14] www.vrp.com.ph

This is unpleasant for the patient. (Understatement intended.) I apologize to my CF readers who are right now feeling that familiar agony.

My Filipino doctor was beside himself after trying repeatedly to get an IV going. He was having no success. I was beside myself too. The bandages from all the previous attempts were collecting all over both arms. I began to count the number of sticks I had received. After sixteen sticks I had had enough.

"Here give the thing to me. I will try," I said. In the US you will always get a fresh needle for each stick, but in the Philippines they were short on supplies, so the same needle was often re-used. This invites infection of course, and the used needles are not as sharp.

The needle and plastic line leading to it was filled first with saline, so that the blood would immediately disperse into the fluid and "show" in the line. The doctor watched for this flash of red color to know he's in. The IV tubing was full of saline too, and was connected to a bottle (which was glass) and attached to a metal IV pole. The pole was welded to a base with four arms on wheels. The doctor was sweating profusely, not only because of the heat and humidity but because of the stress. I think most physicians hate sticking patients more than the patients hate being stuck. It is harder to inflict pain for a medical professional than it is to endure it; as least that is my experience as the patient. So this Filipino doctor was sweating like crazy, having stuck me so many times. I could see he was having a rough go of it. So I was being genuine when I said to let me give it a try. He was right at my side and he simply handed me the needle. I didn't really think he would let me try or that I would be successful, but I figured, *"What's one more failed attempt? It should be kind of fun - in a morbid sort of way."*

Well guess what? With my right hand I pushed the needle into my own left forearm, right at the sight of a bulging vein (facing the opposite direction of course) and I got a blood return. I was really jazzed. So was the doctor. He then took a step backwards. That step was fatal for my IV. I shall never forget that step for as long as I live. The tube that extended from the needle to the IV pole was wrapped around the doctor's back as it headed up to the hanging bottle of saline. The needle ripped right out of my arm with his backward motion. The pain was not as bad as the disappointment. I think I would have liked to stick the doctor with the needle at that point but I probably said something unpleasant instead.

At that point they sent another doctor in to try. The whole procedure had taken well over an hour. After six more sticks I had a working IV. Without an IV I could not receive the necessary antibiotics to fight the lung infection. Without killing or at least degrading the bacteria in my lungs, the infection would continue to spread and my lungs would fill with more mucus. Essentially I would drown. So it was critical to get the IV started.

Three days later I was feeling much better and was beginning to get a bit bored. But at night time I was always worried that my saline bottle would run dry. The nurses kept the saline flowing very slowly and connected to my arm in between antibiotic infusions. It is something nurses call KVO. That stands for Keep Vein Open. In other words, let a drop or two of saline flow in every second so the blood doesn't back up in the line and form a clot in the vein. A clot in the vein ruins the IV and you have to call the doctor again and begin getting stuck all over again. I was not too keen on that idea.

Since there was only one nurse to manage thirteen rooms I didn't see her that often. I was always afraid my bottle would run dry while I was asleep. This occurred a couple of times, and it was pretty unpleasant. Each time I had to have a new IV started. And this is where Filipino hospitality and friendship saved me.

I had met some great guys during my ministry trips with the church youth in Manila. I had taught at their retreat in a place called Baguio up in the mountains. It is somewhat akin to heaven for Filipinos because it is cool and the humidity is very low and it has fresh strawberries. There are also pine trees and the whole place seems like a vacation retreat. The high school youth endured a six-hour hot smelly bus ride up to Baguio because they looked forward to a week with their friends.

I had made some great friends at the retreat. Two of these guys, Kenneth Ola and Ronaldo Figueroa, moved into my hospital room in Manila to look after me. They had discovered that I didn't have anyone to stay with me in the hospital and this mortified them. Patients are never hospitalized without a companion or family member at their side. In Filipino culture it is unthinkable for a person to travel alone, eat alone, sleep alone, or I guess... be alone. It is a very relational culture. To be isolated in a hospital bedroom without a companion and someone to look after you is incredibly sad. So they took it upon themselves to be my *casama*, friend. They brought me peanut butter (it's an American thing), sat at my side, told me stories, made me eat *balut* (which is 96-hour-old unborn duck egg) and other delights. Most important they watched my IV glass bottle hanging from the IV pole to see when the saline was getting low. When it got real low they fetched the nurse. That enabled me to sleep peacefully.

During the day I kept my windows open because there was no air conditioning (air-con) in the hospital. There was, however, an incredible racket outside as jeepneys vied for space on the street below. I could hear roosters crowing at all hours, as each family kept their own chickens for eggs and food. Cats fought and people hollered as they tried to sell various wares. "Zapatos, zapatos," somebody hollered every morning as he rolled a wooden cart down the street, hoping someone would buy a pair of shoes.

One night it stormed violently. I could hear the wind howling and see huge flashes of lightning and hear loud cracks of thunder. The single pane windows rattled. Manila is no stranger to typhoons and massive storms. The neighboring district (Quezon City) flooded often when the typhoons hit; and all the residents fled to the second story of their homes as the first floors were completely inundated by the flood waters.

Mandaluyong, where my hospital was located, sits on higher ground so it did not flood. But the wind blew ferociously. Out my window I could see the palm trees swaying violently back and forth. While the storm was beating about, I could also hear some incredible racket in the ceiling above me. There were some sort of animals having a fight right above my bed. The ceiling tiles (it was a dropped ceiling) were sagging dramatically above my pillow where I lay in the semi-darkness. I could see the brown water marks in the tiles from previous water leaks and wondered if the tiles would break. The whole tile above my face shook violently and it looked like it was going to drop down on top of me. I couldn't move out of my bed because my IV line was attached to the saline bottle and that was anchored to the top of my IV pole. The pole was permanently stuck into the corner of my steel bed frame. So I just lay there looking up from my pillow in the darkness wondering what was causing all the screeching and hissing. The tiles were sagging lower and lower. They bounced up and down. I could not fall asleep as I imagined that whatever was fighting up there was going to come crashing down on me.

The next morning I asked my friendly physical therapists what they imagined the source of all the chaos to be.

"Oh," they smiled and said, "Those are the rats. There is a restaurant right below and the rats are always digging through the garbage. Sometimes they come up inside the walls and ceilings." I could just imagine the ceiling breaking and a couple enormous rats falling in my face on my pillow.

That was Polymedic General Hospital.

After two weeks of IV therapy I should have been well enough to be discharged. But I was still spiking temperatures which meant the infection was still active. After some discussion they called my physician in Palo Alto at Stanford Hospital. My Filipino doctor, Dr. Sarmiento, (the most wonderful doctor I've ever known) was surprised when Stanford told him I was receiving too small a dosage of antibiotics. Filipino patients are smaller than Americans and receive lower doses of medicine. Also cystic fibrosis patients require the maximum dose of antibiotics possible. Doctor Sarmiento was incredulous when he was told that I should be given so much medicine, nearly twice the amount he'd been giving me for two weeks. He increased the dose and I recovered after another couple weeks.

I had three such hospitalizations at Polymedic during my time in the Philippines. But immediately after that first admission the leaders at OC wanted to send me home. I could think of nothing that would be worse. I was devastated at the thought of having to leave after such a short time. I persevered (and gave every reason I could think of) and was allowed to remain. I could not imagine that God could guide me all the way around the world for just a couple weeks and then be sent home. I really wanted to serve Him abroad. Following that admission, I was then healthy for the next seven months. When I traveled with Ben he did my physical therapy, whacking me with his giant hands for thirty minutes twice a day. When I was at home in Antipolo I appealed to my house-mates Mike Haus, Steve Reid and Roy Sheffield, and they took turns giving me chest percussion.

I think the abiding lessons I gained from my admissions to Polymedic actually came from the selfless service of the hospital personnel, as well as from Ken and Ronaldo. I was absolutely amazed at the zeal with which the respiratory therapists did my chest percussion therapy. They learned the techniques for doing CPT's from me, then applied them 200%. There were always two of them, pounding away like crazy, sweating in the intolerable heat.

These guys were amazing. When they found out I didn't have any slip-on shoes in my hospital room one of them had me trace my bare foot on a piece of paper. I really didn't understand why. A few days later they presented me with a pair of custom made slip-ons. A gift of ingenuity and love.

The apostle Peter tells us, "Each of you should use whatever gift you have received to serve others, as faithful stewards of God's grace in its various forms."[15] These guys really demonstrated that to me. And with passion. This was not the first, nor the last time, that hospital staff treated me with above-and-beyond care. Such acts of kindness do not go unnoticed and they shall be rewarded in due time.

---

[15] I Peter 4:10

Chapter 12

Fever Out in the Boonies

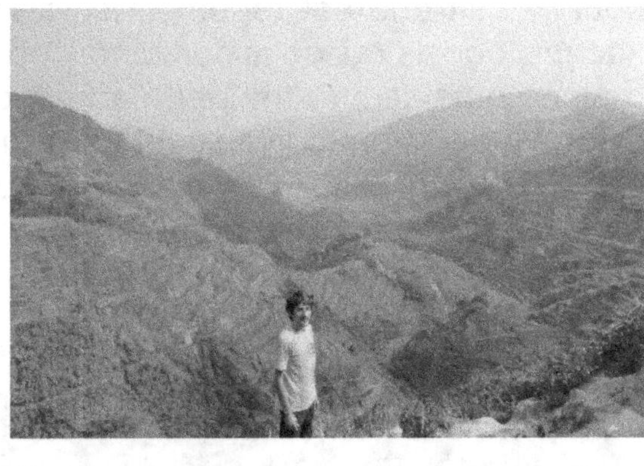

High in the mountains of the Philippine Islands are the most amazing terraced rice fields in the world. They are over two thousand years old and Filipinos often called them, "The eighth wonder of the world.". It was a tribal people, the Ifugao, who constructed them and who resided in simple huts built above the ground. The terraced fields are fed by natural rain forests and the rock and mud walls were made entirely by hand. It is estimated that these walls would, if put end to end, circle the globe. However, when I went there in 1983 I was told they were six thousand miles long. So I guess nobody has really walked them off.

In June that year a buddy and I decided to leave our home in crowded noisy Manila and take a vacation among the Ifugao tribes. My friend Tim Bascom was in Manila for three months doing a sociological research project for his studies at Wheaton College. His research had him living with a Filipino family in one of the largest squatter areas of the city. At the time it was estimated there were a million squatters in Manila. Most of them came from the provinces (anywhere that is not Manila) in search of education, work, and a better life in the big city. When they arrived - to find the better life - they discovered they had to live in abject poverty in a huge slum. They took menial jobs wherever they could find them but they were happy their children could go to school and have a better future.

Tim was fortunate to have found a Christian family who hosted him in their shack in the slum. They even built a western toilet for him outside their simple two story house. Then they walled off a room inside their one room home that was three feet by six feet so he could have his own space. The walls of the house were made of one quarter inch fiberboard. This family was wealthy, and by that I mean they had a piece of clean linoleum on which they could all sit and eat together. It's also where they all slept. Their kitchen consisted of a horizontal board with a hole in it, which drained outside into the dirt. I admired (this family) and Tim greatly for his decision to live such a sacrificial life - so he could understand a people, a lifestyle, and a sub-culture. He grew to love them deeply, and to appreciate many spiritual qualities lacking among the affluent.

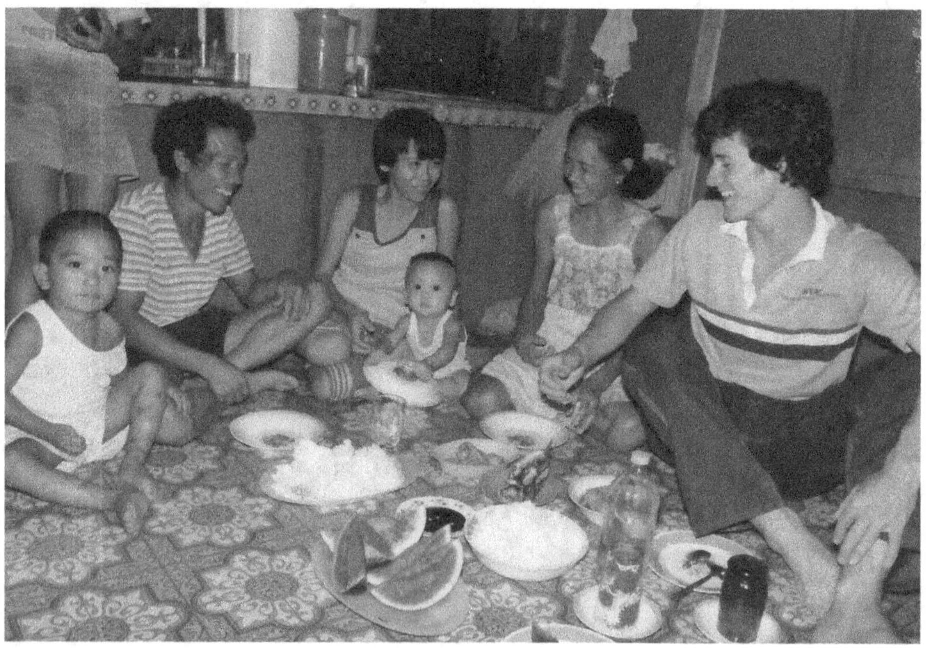

I spent the night with Tim once in the squatter hut and was amazed at how clean everyone and everything was. Outside their home it was all dirt and mud and filth. But inside they managed to keep everything clean, even without running water (they carried it in).

It was time for our little trip. Tim and I took a public bus out of Manila and headed north to the Ifugao province. It was a nine hour bus ride. No air-con of course, with school bus type seats. The first time I boarded one of those long distance buses I couldn't understand why all the passengers were sitting on just one side of the bus. I gladly sat down on one of the wide open bench seats on the empty side. Then, once the bus was underway (and full of passengers) I figured it out. I was sitting in the direct sun for the entire journey!

Even after living in the RPI for nine months the countryside never ceased to impress me. My travels with Ben had taken us to many provinces, particularly in the northern islands of Luzon. There were endless fields of rice, towering volcanos in the distance, and attractive towns that we passed through.

Most foreigners who meet Filipinos are impressed with their warmth, kindness, generosity, and huge smiles. Smiling is actually their non-verbal body language for greeting, so it seems everyone smiles at you. They are especially appreciative of Americans, even forty years after Douglas MacArther returned with the US army and liberated them from the Japanese. As we stopped to eat a bite at a roadside restaurant we were often greeted with, "Hi Joe," as if we were all GI's just passing through.

Leaving the main bus route we boarded a jeepney that would take us up into the Ifugao rural areas. Jeepnies are manufactured in the Philippines. Each one is individually painted inside and out in bright colors with images of saints and loved ones, stripes, and of course their route/destination. They have no windows or doors. Their drivers honk the horns constantly to let people know they are coming. It is an ingenious form of transportation; all one has to do is raise a hand and they stop and pick you up. When you wanted to stop you just flick a finger against the steel ceiling and the driver pulls to the side of the road and lets you out. I rode many of them standing on the rear bumper or on the back step, because it was already too packed inside. A short ride cost (in 1983) about the equivalent of fifteen US cents. The wonderful thing about jeepneys was they seemed to be everywhere; you seldom had to wait for one and they would pick you up anywhere on their route.

We had a destination in mind for our first night, a certain boarding house that a friend had recommended. After sleeping there we would drive higher into the mountains on another jeepney. We ate a light breakfast the morning of our departure from the guest house: some mango jam on toast with a cup of tea. In these remote areas traffic was sparse, or non-existent might be a better way of putting it. We waited a good thirty minutes for the first jeepney to pass; we didn't want to miss it.

The jeepney that finally drove by was full of passengers when it came alongside the guest house. Rather than slow down when we waved it began to just continue on. I am sure the driver assumed that the two Americans would want to sit inside on a bench seat, and not hang on to the rear or stand on the bumper as many locals did. But I stepped out onto the roadway and waved him down. He pulled over.

"I'm full," he said.

"No problem," I replied. We can ride on top. I had seen others do this and I figured, *"Why should we be any different?"* We put our light backpacks on, put a foot on the open doorway, then on the corner of the hood and pulled ourselves up onto the luggage rack. A tire was tied to the rack so we sat on the tire.

It was just a one way rutted dirt road but it accommodated two way traffic. If an oncoming jeepney was seen up ahead, our driver either pulled way to the side and stopped, or if necessary backed up to find a wide spot in the road. Many times I was looking straight down from my perch atop the vehicle - into a gorge - with no edge of the roadway in sight.

"These guys are good drivers," I assured Tim. I'd no sooner said it when a tire blew. The driver jerked to a stop.

Everyone piled out of the jeepney and began to search for spots in the shade to sit and wait. Tim and I helped the driver pull the spare off the roof and lower it to the ground. It was not a new tire by any means, but it was a tire. After he had put it on the car we took our places again, this time sitting on the flat tire. Many times we had to duck as low branches whipped us in the face. The good thing was the travel was pretty slow as the dirt road was pretty nasty. This gave us plenty of time to navigate our heads around the low hanging limbs.

Then another tire blew.

The roadway was very rough and the load was full. People who travel in the mountains are always carrying something. They don't travel for pleasure. I had seen a full grown pig in a motorcycle side car. A friend of mine got slapped in the face by two live chickens in the grip of a woman entering a jeepney. Huge bundles of belongings were often strapped to busses or jeepneys as people moved or bought stuff to resell in the provincial areas. This jeepney was no different. It too was loaded to the gills. But we had no more spare tires. I was in for a lesson in Filipino ingenuity.

Again everyone disembarked. The driver started to build a

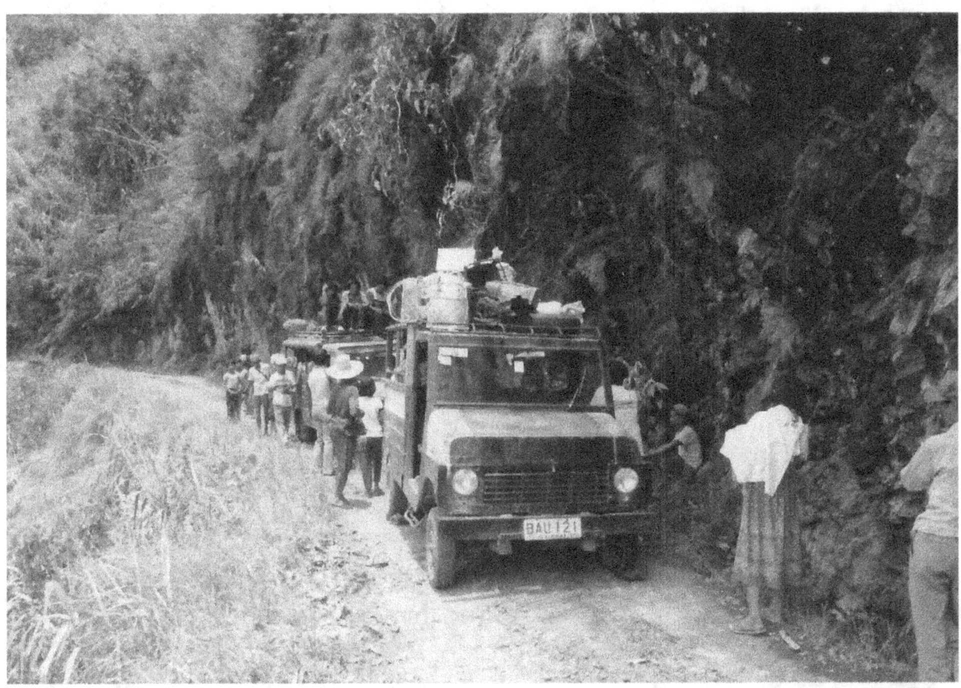

small fire in the middle of the one way road. A short while later another jeepney came up the road from behind us. Of course he had to stop, as there was no way to get around. Everyone from that jeepney disembarked too. Nobody said anything. People got their lunches out and began eating and talking. Nobody was upset or complaining. This was everyday life, pure and simple. Especially simple.

As a foreigner in a foreign place one of the first things I had learned was to keep my mouth shut and just observe. Somebody famous once said, "Even fools are thought to be wise if they keep their mouths shut." That was King Solomon and it's recorded in Proverbs. So we just watched and learned. The driver proceeded to use his small wood fire to vulcanize the tire. I had never seen anything like it and I was impressed. Nobody seemed to blink an eye and as soon as he was finished and had hand pumped the tire back up everyone re-boarded the jeepney and we continued on our journey.

After a couple hours of getting a really sore bum I saw our stopping point. We slapped the roof of the jeepney and he stopped. We climbed down at a trail head. The dirt path led practically straight up a steep cliff. It was the spot where people who lived in the distant village could walk/climb over the mountain to get to their homes. There were no roads to their village, just this trail. Women with seventy pound bags hefted their load up the narrow trail. Tim and I were huffing and puffing our way up, stopping frequently, with our thirty pound bags. Many sections were washed out so badly that we had to hang onto tree roots and pull

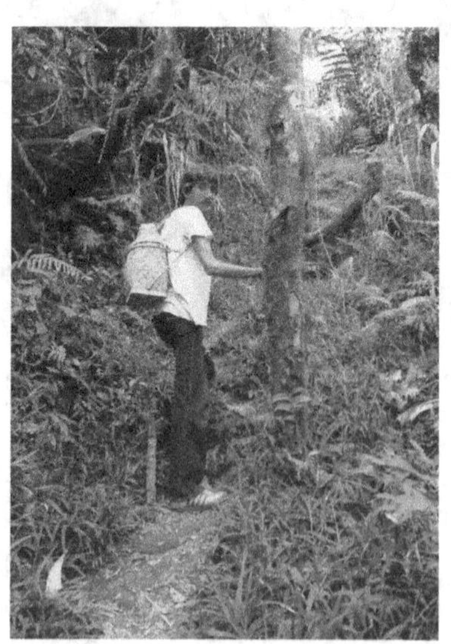

ourselves up the incline. It was a couple hours of sweating profusely in the ninety five percent humidity. Mosquitos were delighted with the slow moving meals we presented. Every muscle was burning when we finally reached the top of the ridge.

Then the trail leveled out and appeared to wrap around the mountain slope. After descending about a quarter mile we saw women with sticks poking holes in the hillside. They were planting a purple yam known as an *ubi*. *Ubi* is a popular food in the Philippines. It's sort of like a round purple yam. I had even eaten *ubi* ice cream at Magnolias (a great ice cream parlor) near my home in Antipolo, Rizal, outside of Manila. This was my first time to see it planted.

The Ifugao tribal people are not normally happy about foreigners visiting their homes or villages. The don't see themselves as curiosities or their homes as a tourist destination. They are people living out their lives. However, Tim and I were not tourists. We were followers of Jesus who desired to teach others who follow Jesus how to know him more, how to serve him more and how to grow their church. This group of Ifugao were delighted to meet us and hear about our lives. Almost the entire village had chosen to follow Jesus years ago and had built a simple church with a corrugated steel roof. It was the nicest building in the community. They were delighted to meet fellow Christians.

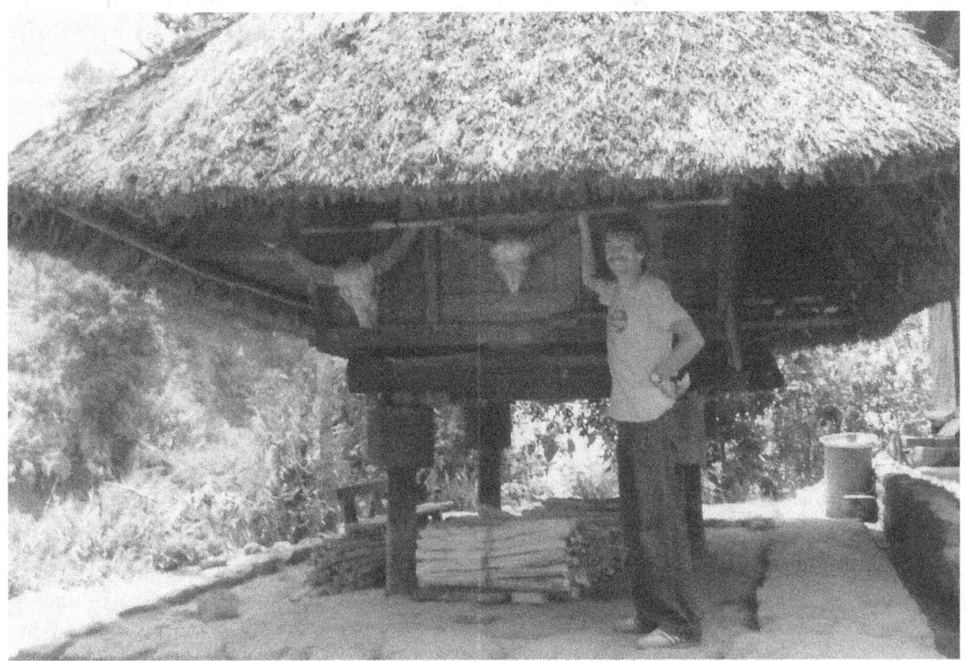

The *nipa* homes were elevated from the barren earth on four sturdy posts. A simple ladder led up to the one room interior. Beneath the fenced-in home roamed chickens and sometimes pigs.

We were warmly welcomed. We chatted as best we could; I spoke a little Tagolog as did they. A few of the older men also spoke some English. I wasn't feeling all that well, however, and I asked if I could retire early.

First, however, our host insisted she serve us dinner. It was a bowl of delicious *ubi* soup, with a one inch cube of pork fat in the bottom. The chunk of fat still had hair on it. Of course I ate it. Although these Ifugao grew rice, they ate mostly *ubi*. Their rice fetched a better price at the market and so they lived off of *ubi*. Sometimes they boiled it in a soup. They also fried it and ate it like potato chips. They even roasted it. On special occasions they would splurge and cook some of their own rice. With their earnings from the rice they grew in the terraces they could buy oil and other items from town. It just so happened that the chief had slaughtered a pig the week we arrived, and of course he shared it with everyone in the entire village. So we were blessed with that piece of fat in our soup. I was glad I had kept silent about the hairy piece of fat and had eaten the soup with a smile of appreciation. One never knows what sacrifice has been made for you as a guest, particularly in a foreign culture.

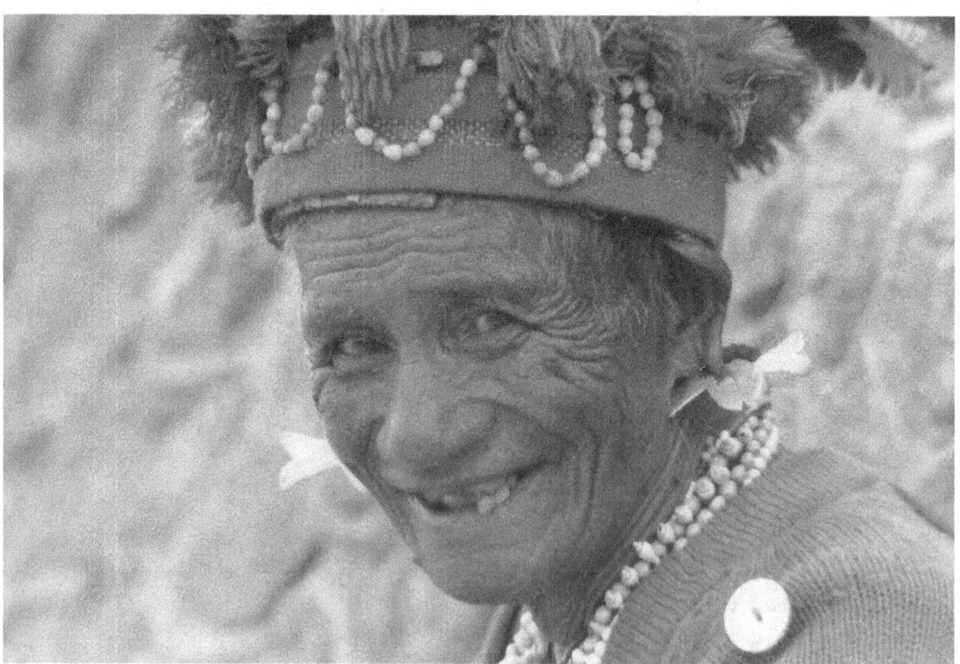

As I lay down on the split bamboo floor to sleep and pulled my sleeping bag over me I was feeling poorly. I didn't know if it was the exertion or the altitude or something worse. And I did not know what tomorrow would bring.

The next day was Sunday. I was feeling much better. We joined the family for their church service at the top of the hill. It was very moving to see them worship God in their own way - to see them communicate with their Creator in a context that had meaning to them. It was different for me, but I did not come so they could make *me* comfortable; I had come to enjoy what was real for them. The singing in their mother tongue was particularly impressive.

My heart was full as we climbed back down terraced walls and along the tops of stone walls to reach their home for lunch. Little paths run along the tops of the terraces permitting foot traffic. Different terraced ponds had rice in various stages of growth.

After lunch Tim and I felt up to do some exploring and hiking. We set out in a northern direction, toward what looked like some impressive waterfalls in the distance. We hiked single file for a couple hours, climbing down terraced walls and following worn narrow pathways to stay headed toward the waterfall. The final descent to the bottom of the falls was particularly tricky. There were no more terraces in this canyon. There was a lot of loose rock. Tim was wearing flip flops, the most common footwear in provincial Philippines. I had a pair of old tennis shoes on. We clung to branches and bushes on the hillside as we descended the shale like surface.

The view of the falls from the bottom was breathtaking. As we approached the pounding torrent we knew we had to celebrate our hike by standing directly beneath the falls. It would be a refreshing break from the sweat and humidity. It was the culmination of our strenuous feat. The water coursed over our tee shirts and shorts, soaking us from head to toe. We did not notice the dark clouds gathering on the horizon.

Having finished with our shower we stepped carefully over rounded stones in the river bed to head back out of the canyon. We thought our bodies would dry off quickly. But it began to sprinkle. Since we were already drenched it didn't seem important. Then the temperature began to drop pretty dramatically.

"Hey Tim; let's take some shelter and wait out this storm," I suggested. Climbing up the left embankment we spotted a cave. A European tourist appeared around the bend smoking a cigarette.

"Excuse me," I began, "Do you have any matches?" He had just two remaining in a wrinkled matchbook.

As an eagle scout I knew how to build a fire, even in wet conditions. But everywhere we turned things were thoroughly drenched, not just damp. The man handed me the matches and we crouched together in the narrow cave. It was standing room only for the three of us. We bumped heads. I assembled some tinder from grass growing in a crevice, but it was green. I began to shiver, my wet clothes pulling the heat from my slender frame. I lit the first match. A blast of wind swept up the cave entrance and put it out before I could even reach down to touch the tinder.

We looked at the final match as our only hope for some heat. We had to get a fire going. I thought briefly of Jack London's short story, *To Build a Fire*. A story that did not end well.

"We might have to spend the night in this cave," Tim said. Bunching the remaining tinder together I was skeptical. It looked too wet.

"Let's huddle close together to stop the gusts of wind, then cup our hands around the match when it's lit." I struck the paper match against the matchbook. Nothing. Again. Nothing. The matchbook had gotten wet when it was handed to me. I remembered that a good way to dry a damp match was to run it through your hair. But then, that only worked if your hair was dry. Our heads were all soaking wet.

One more strike and the match lit. Our hopes raised a notch. I put the match to the tinder. It would not light. I held it steady, hoping against all odds that it would light. "Please..."

The match went out.

The European stood up and said, "Well, I'm heading out." And he left. I looked at Tim.

"What do you think we should do?" The rain was coming down hard now. The sky had become black. I remembered the treacherous rock that we had clambered over to get down into the canyon. It would be a pure disaster if we twisted an ankle trying to come up that steep incline.

"If we try to stay here, Tim, we will get hypothermia. At least I know I will." I was shivering uncontrollably.

"Then let's go," he said. We climbed out of the cave and began to hike out in the torrential rain single file. I was most concerned when we got to the shale rock because Tim was just wearing flip flops. We took it slow, one step at a time, hanging on to anything, even each other.

Water was dripping off our faces and running down our backs. Our ankles and feet were soaked. The only consolation was the weather was not as cold as a California rain. But with the wind and my already frail state I was feeling the cold sapping me of energy. I wondered if we'd become statistics. I recalled it had been a two hour hike to get to the falls. With the rain and our slow progress I figured it would be at least three hours before we reached the village. It had been around one p.m. when we left; then we'd spent about an hour playing in the falls.

"It must be four," I said to Mike. The sun was no longer visible through the dark clouds. We were moving as fast as we safely could.

The last mile we hiked was in complete darkness. Of course we had no flashlight. Each step was in search of the next, as we followed the edges of the terraces. Some terraces dropped ten or twenty feet off to our left. Many times we used our hands to find the ends of one terrace and then to find the next one. There was no trail; we just followed what seemed to be the general direction from which we came.

In the pitch dark we finally found the *nipa* hut and our host family. They were very concerned. I was shaking, from the cold I assumed. The hut was wonderfully warm, as was the soup we were served.

Before bed Tim helped me with my respiratory therapy in the one room dwelling. It was never easy to ask a friend to help me in this humbling routine. But if I did not do this twice daily I could not breathe. The Ifugao family no doubt thought the Americans had some very strange habits.

I had learned long ago that it was best to be up front with my friends and co-workers about my illness. I did not hesitate to ask them to help me clear my lungs by doing physical therapy. I can only remember one friend, a roommate in college, who declined to help. I asked for helpers to pound on my torso when I lived in England, when I lived in the college dorm, and when I lived on the road with a team in the Philippines.

People were willing to help, even though it required their time and enduring the retching sounds of me coughing and spitting. Tim knew how to do therapy because I had stayed with him in the squatter home in Manila. And of course he had pounded on my back and chest when we stayed in the guest house. The fact that we were now in a one room *nipa* hut, that measured maybe fifteen feet by fifteen feet, and there was our host and his wife present… well that made it somewhat awkward. But what choice did I have? Be uncomfortable or not breathe?

I awoke in the night with chills. I knew I was in trouble; I had a fever. My host family understood that I was sick. Tim gave me Tylenol. My temperature dropped some. At least I stopped shaking. Early that morning, with Tim carrying much of my gear, we began the long walk out. It was hard to say goodbye to our wonderful hosts. We felt a kinship with them that was deeply spiritual.

Again I wondered if I could make the journey. I was exhausted. It seemed to go on forever, but at least we recognized the landmarks. Finally we slid down the steep embankment to find the main road. I was never so happy as when a jeepney rounded the corner and splattered mud on us. This time we got to sit inside.

It seems to me that people are often ashamed of the wrong things in life. Should I be ashamed that I needed to cough and spit in order to stay alive? Should I be ashamed that I had a terminal illness? Was it shameful to ask my friends to help me keep breathing by giving me physical therapy? How ridiculous. The things I should be ashamed of are the things I do that are wrong, that hurt people, or that break laws whether human or divine.

After the jeepney ride we faced a long bus ride. The fever made it misery. I lay on the bench seat at the back of the bouncing bus for the late night drive back to Manila. The name of the bus line was, "The Rabbit." That particular bus line was famous for exceeding speed limits and caution. We had often passed burned out carcasses of the red Rabbit buses while we traveled up and down Philippine roadways. When oncoming drivers saw a Rabbit bus coming they pulled to the side of the roadway to give them room. We made good time.

When we pulled in to the loud dirty chaotic transit station in Cubao in the middle of the night it was like coming home. And when I was admitted to the Polymedic General Hospital I was very relieved. Feverish certainly, but delighted to get an IV started and serious antibiotics into my body. And no rats came to visit this time.

A few weeks later I was healthy and fit. *"Thank you again Doctor Sarmiento."* It was so good to be able to take a deep breath, to get a lung full of oxygen. I still did chest percussion therapy to keep the airways clear, but the pseudomonas bacteria was beaten down a bit. I remained healthy for the next seven months of my

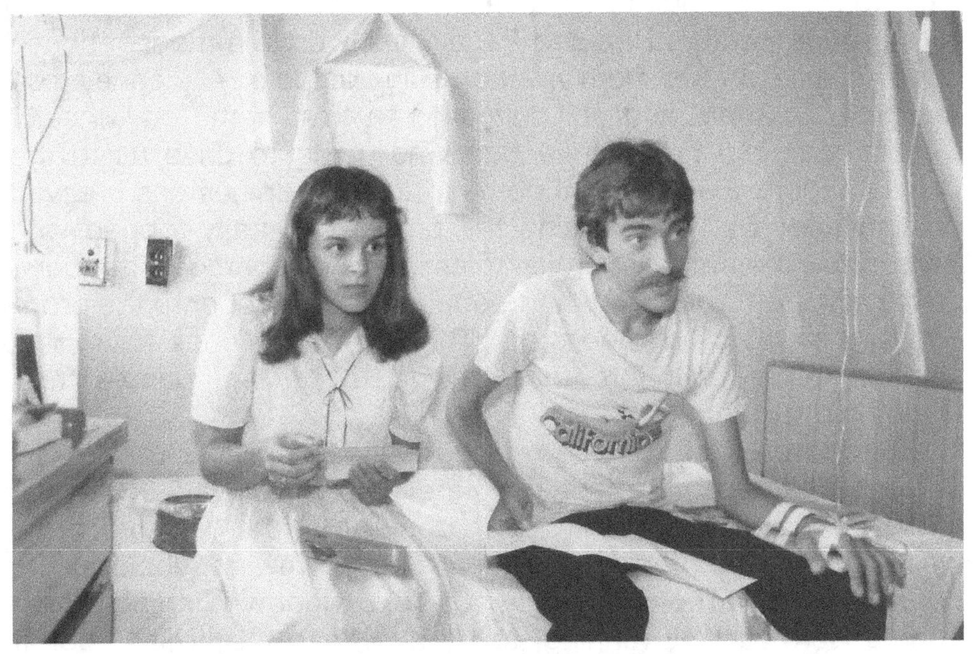

DEANNA WAS SURPRISED TO SEE MY HOSPITAL ROOM ALL DECO-RATED WHEN I BROUGHT HER FROM THE AIRPORT

time in the Philippines, including a three month stint in the southern island of Mindanao.

I was delighted when DeAnna decided to come to the Philippines after she returned home to California from Peru. The day she flew into Manila I was in the hospital for a tune up. I was thankful they released me so I could pick her up from the airport. Then we returned to my hospital room. To my surprise, my friends Ken and Ronaldo had decorated my room with toilet paper streamers and signs as a welcome to her. She was able to join a team of 45 students who came that summer to work in 16 Filipino churches as volunteers in Davao City, in Mindanao. It was a fabulous time.

On my way to Davao, however, I got injured. There is a special scar on my right arm that reminds me of my own foolishness. We were going to fly from Manila to Davao City - about 600 air miles, or 1500 road miles. To drive would have been a mammoth and lengthy undertaking. There were no freeways, many islands to pass through, and dangerous areas with rebels. It was faster and safer to fly. Plus I didn't own a car.

My dear mentors Ben and Perla Siaki lived in a modest house about a mile or two from my home in Antipolo. A jeepney ride took me, DeAnna, and our suitcases to their home on an early August morning. From there Ben was going to drive us to the Manila airport. Every typical home in the Philippines has a seven or eight foot wall surrounding the property, usually topped with barbered wire or at least broken glass. This discourages intruders. Gates, through which cars and people travel to get onto the property, are made of painted steel. The decorative ones have long vertical spikes built into their design to prevent people from climbing over them.

We approached the gate with our suitcases. Ben's house was set back perhaps fifty feet from the gate. I hollered to let him know we'd arrived. There was no doorbell at the gate or on the wall. I hollered louder and waited. Then I threw a pebble at the house. Still no response. I could see their window-hung air conditioners were already running, to try and keep the house cool. It was no wonder they couldn't hear us. I looked at my watch and realized we would be late for our flight if Ben didn't come out.

Perhaps he was still asleep and had forgotten. In desperation, and perhaps with a bit of impatience and foolishness, I decided to climb over the gate.

To go over the wall would have been insane, but the six foot high concrete posts that held the gate were about ten inches square. I figured I'd climb over at that spot. I anchored my feet in the metal hinges and pulled myself up until I was standing on the top of the concrete post. So far so good. The easiest way down from the top would be to jump. I readied myself and to keep my balance I spread my arms a bit. Big mistake. As I descended the six feet of space to the ground I was aware that my arm had come to a sudden stop behind me. Yes, my right forearm was impaled on one of the metal spikes.

I don't remember it hurting. I just remember hearing a "thunk" as the steel went into the flesh. My right forearm was impaled at the height of my head at a ninety degree angle to my body. My feet were solidly on the ground, however. Using my left arm I grabbed my right forearm and lifted it up off the spike. I was expecting a huge flow of blood to come from the wound. I knew one should never pull a nail from a puncture (let the ER do it) but I couldn't remove an entire fence and bring it to a hospital. I immediately put pressure on the wound.

Since I was now inside the gate I went up and knocked and shouted loudly on Ben's front door. Several times. Perla answered pleasantly; she was making a nice family breakfast. I explained my problem quickly and she ran off to get her first aid kit. I went to the bathroom to wash the wound. Amazingly it didn't bleed at all. I could see a deep penetration and a half-inch wide slit. We dried and dressed the wound and then made our way to the airport.

I still have the scar forty years later. It reminds me to think before doing stupid things. Better yet, just don't do stupid things.

While in Davao it was DeAnna who came twice daily to the home where I was a houseguest to do my physical therapy. It was a humbling experience. Here was the woman of my dreams watching me sweat, cough, and spit for thirty minutes every morning and evening. It was a time when she saw how I behaved when most vulnerable, and I saw her at her strongest - selflessly serving and accepting. We could not have learned these lessons any other way.

As DeAnna was leaving the Philippines we both knew we wanted to be married, but we wanted to wait until we were together in the US to become engaged. I came home four months later and asked her to marry me. It happened to be right before my brother Doug's marriage to Dawn Ely on February 10, 1984. Our wedding took place four months later on June 23, 1984. She is still the woman of my dreams.

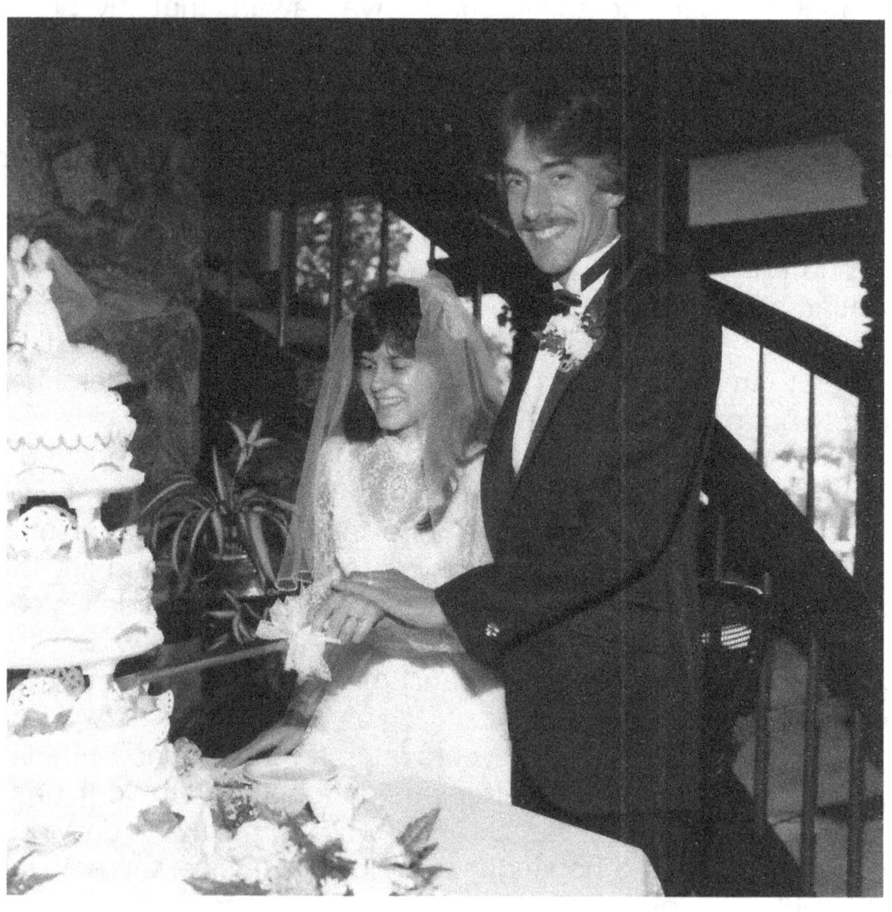

Chapter 13

"Got Any SAM's ?"

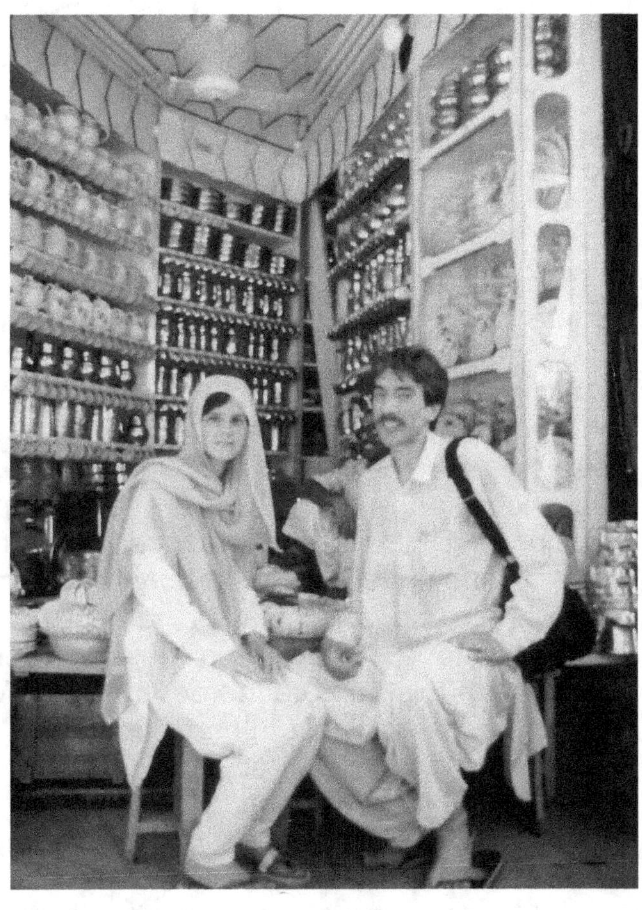

Wearing traditional Afghan clothing (*shalwar kameesh*), the pajama-like baggy pants and long-sleeved long-bodied shirt that men in rural Pakistan wear, I stooped to enter the six by eight foot tent. We were out in the dessert a long way from civilization. The floor was just dirt covered with an old carpet and there were clay walls about three feet high, leaving the front open to enter and exit. A large canvas tarp was erected overhead, giving the Muslim men seated inside a bit of relief from the blazing sun. Around the room as I entered were ten Mujahadeen. These men were fighting the guerrilla war against the Soviets who had invaded Afghanistan. The heat in July in northern Pakistan on the Afghan border was unbearable, especially for a California boy. Forty degrees celsius I was told. All I knew was that no amount of orange soda would quench my thirst or cool me down. There was no way I was going to drink the local water, and bottled water wasn't available. I accepted a glass of hot sweet tea as I took my seat near the open doorway. Introductions were made.

My young wife and I had traveled to this region to explore opportunities of helping the three million Afghan refugees that had fled the Russian invasion of their country. It was July, 1986 and we were in Peshawar [peh Shower], Pakistan. Peshawar is part of the Northwest Frontier Province. Between Peshawar and Afghanistan is a vast area that was under no government's control. Local tribal militias, such as the Taliban, reigned in that territory. The government vacuum along the border had allowed refugees to flee the war in Afghanistan and enter Pakistan somewhat freely.

I looked around the small tent/room where I was seated. Innumerable AK47's were propped against the mud walls. This was not uncommon. After all, Peshawar had its own gun manufacturing facilities. It was all illegal, of course. But nobody was there to uphold the law or they were too afraid to attempt it. I assumed these men were Afghans. I thought my host had brought me to meet them so we could assess the humanitarian needs of their community. Did their families need assistance? Was their children's health in jeopardy? Did they have family members that had been lost in the scramble for safety? Did they have adequate shelter and food? Discovering these answers was our purpose in traveling to this remote border region. We exchanged simple pleasantries, as my host translated for me.

I was then caught totally off guard by one of the men as he looked intently into my face.

"We need SAM's (surface to air missiles). We need them now; the Russians are slaughtering our people. When can you bring them?" I was dumfounded. I was ignorant of the fact that the CIA had been supplying the Afghan Mujahadeen SAM's to fight the Russians. I wasn't even sure what these men meant at first. I certainly didn't have any weapons. Then they asked if I was with the CIA.

It is assumed that every American who is in Muslim or Communist controlled regions, particularly in difficult war-torn places, is with the CIA. This seemed ridiculous to me, but it is a genuine sincere belief these people swear by. Who else would risk their life to travel to such a place? I would have found it laughable except for the desperation and hard core looks in the eyes of the men seated around me in the cramped tent on the tattered carpet. Then there were the guns in the room. This was not a social visit for these men; it was a military strategy meeting. I was surely out of my element. It seemed like some sort of crazy dream.

I assured these men that I had come to Pakistan to help refugees, not to supply an army with weapons. They did not believe me. I was not accustomed to the ways of the wild west of Afghani culture. Lies are told as a way to negotiate, and deception is considered an honorable trait. So they assumed I was playing their game.

"Thou shall not lie," was not in their theology. They asked again. And again. I finally realized they had no interest in helping us with our humanitarian need assessment. They were fighting a war and all they could think about was weapon procurement.

This was a long way from my Christian heritage where lying is wrong and deception a trick of Satan. But these men were radical Muslims. In the Koran it says that God is the greatest deceiver of them all.[16] That was certainly a switch for my mind. What about, *"God is love?"* In Islam, a lie is not wrong as long as one's purpose is achieved. To be caught in a lie is to lose honor, and that brings shame on one's family. The preservation of ones honor and name leads not just to lying and deception, but to the humiliation and oppression of people, especially women. When foreigners saw Afghan women their first impression was the black tent. In Peshawar the rare woman in public was covered head to toe, with

---

[16] Surah 3:54, Surah 7:99, Surah 27:50 The word for deception is "makr" according to answering-islam.org. It means "to practice deceit or guile or circumvention, practice evasion or elusion, to plot, to exercise art or craft or cunning, act with policy, practice stratagem."

nothing but a woven screen of fabric through which to watch her way (called *a burka*). Men did all the shopping for their families, so women would not be in the rough and tumble of the local markets. Women were kept in seclusion; the word for it is *purdah*. Quite simply, women were not to be seen. It would be dishonorable for a woman to go into a market, because men would be staring at her. And that would also bring shame on the family.

Later when we were seated in the Green Hotel (green is the color of Islam), where my wife (also wearing a *shalwar kameesh)* and I were staying, there was a floor to ceiling scrim across the back half of the hotel's street-side restaurant. Whenever a woman was in the party of guests coming into the restaurant, the host would seat that group at a table behind the screen. So this is where we were seated. This was actually a blessing, although at first I did not appreciate the discrimination. Then I realized that had we been seated out front, along the dusty street, every passing male would have been staring at my wife, even though she was also dressed like many local women (though her whole face was not covered.) There were simply no women at all to be seen in public. One did see figures draped entirely in the black *burkas* (in the 115 degree heat) as they walked in tiny groups down the dusty streets, but one actually saw no women. In Pakistani culture to be so completely covered is considered protection. Every male protected his wife and daughters (above around age twelve) by requiring them to wear the *burka.*

Some women valued this protection, even when it meant they could not be educated above grade six (because they would be with boys.) Consequently they remained behind high stone walls that surrounded their home, with only family and female guests allowed inside. They removed their coverings when with family or a group of women. Boys were raised learning to protect women and keep them sheltered within the high walls of a compound. This would preserve the family honor.

I was just learning these things as we toured various facilities that had been established for refugees. There was a camp for widows and orphans that my wife DeAnna visited. Then we went to an eye clinic where doctors dealt with the plethora of eye injuries and infections. We learned that people were even contracting cholera from the ever-present dust that was constantly blown about. We stopped at an NGO (Non Governmental Organization) that was building hexagonal shelters out of concrete for the refugees to live in (Shelter Now)[17]. The concrete slabs had to be cured in huge vats of water because it was so hot and dry they would crack if left to cure in the open. Another NGO (Serve)[18] had designed solar ovens to use the blazing sunshine to cook and bake. Finally we went to a micro enterprise that taught women to weave carpets, which are highly valued the world over.

What had brought us to the Northwest Frontier Province of Pakistan, particularly when my health was tenuous at best? It began with the front cover of the June 1985 National Geographic magazine. Known simply as the "Afghan girl"[19] the photo was of an Afghan girl with penetrating grey green eyes and an expression that seemed cut off from existence, like she was living a nightmare and afraid to show the horrors inside. At least that is what her face said to me. The article said much more, as it detailed the plight of the Afghans fleeing their country and pouring into the Northwest Frontier Province. DeAnna and I also happened to have friends who were living in Peshawar. Pakistan was reeling with this influx of humanity, and it seemed incapable of handling the addition of three million desperate people.

We had felt God calling us to work with oppressed and displaced people for several years. The plight of Afghan refugees was in the headline news and it had touched our hearts. So we gathered our savings and flew to the furthest reaches of Pakistan to find out if we could become involved.

However, the heat had been overwhelming for me in particular. It was regularly 115 degrees and we were busy from morning until night visiting people and researching opportunities to serve. I did not realize I had become dehydrated. Plus the ever present dust was compromising my cystic fibrosis lungs. I realized I was getting sick after just one week in that climate. I wondered, *"What*

---

[17] https://www.shelter-now.org/welcome/

[18] https://www.om.org/en/country-profile/pakistan

[19] https://en.wikipedia.org/wiki/Afghan_Girl

use would I be if I moved with my wife from San Jose, California all the way to Peshawar, Pakistan and then died shortly after arriving? Would God guide me to do such a crazy thing?"

With our research complete, we checked out of the Green hotel and headed back to the Peshawar airport for the flight to Karachi. After we boarded we noted that everyone on the plane was changing out of their village garb and into their western clothing. A man would go to the tiny restroom wearing his *shalwar kameesh* and later appear wearing jeans and a shirt. We talked of doing the same, then decided not to change. Our next stop wasn't California, it was Hong Kong. My brother Doug and his wife Dawn were living there learning Cantonese. Our flight plan would take us from Peshawar to Karachi, then we'd fly to Singapore, change planes and on to Hong Kong. We discovered too late that we should have changed our clothes like the locals. In the far north of Pakistan people wore the traditional clothing, but in the big cities, like Karachi, people dressed in western attire. When we disembarked in Karachi we stood out like a couple of country bumpkins.

Karachi has a customs inspection even for people arriving from within their own country up north. Afghanistan is, after all, the poppy and heroin capital of the east. I hadn't thought of that. I tend to see myself as I see myself, not as others see me. I'm not a drug dealer, nor with the CIA, so I figured the customs officials would see me for who I am. I was interested in humanitarian needs, so why was the official digging into my stuff like I was some kind of criminal? After thirty minutes of tearing through all our luggage I realized that two Americans dressed like locals probably aroused greater suspicion than usual.

We made it through customs after every one of my many 35 mm film canisters had been opened, emptied, and searched. Then we took the one-hour trip into Karachi in a motorcycle driven pedicab. It is basically a flimsy metal trailer shell containing one narrow bench seat - attached to the rear of a motorcycle. One is seated directly behind the back of the motorcycle driver.

There was an eight-hour lay-over before our flight to Singapore and we decided rather than pay for a hotel room we would just sit in an air-conditioned lobby of a nice hotel in downtown

Karachi. It would be far better than sitting uncomfortably in a dirty hot airport, and not as expensive as paying for a whole night in a hotel.

After eight hours of sitting around we returned to the airport in another pedicab to board the next flight. We were both exhausted as we boarded the plane. We lifted our bags into the overhead bins and I began to cough. I sat down, leaning forward to open my airways and trying to relax. Coughing was of course not unusual for me but this was a really hard cough. I was gasping for air in between hacking.

I reached for the little barf bag in the seat pocket so I'd have somewhere to spit. As I spit I was shocked to see that I was coughing up blood. DeAnna was just getting her seat and noticed it at about the same time as the flight steward passed our seats. Other passengers had also noticed (I was making quite a bit of racket) and I imagined they were worried for their own health.

The Pakistani steward asked us with evident concern, "Are you alright?" Both of us thought the same thing, *"We do not want to be kicked off this plane."* In addition I remember thinking, *"I don't want to die in Karachi."* We had seen the streets, the buildings, the chaos and the poverty. I could only imagine the quality of their hospitals. Of course they would have no concept of cystic fibrosis or how to treat it. It was a disease of Europeans and Americans. At the time there were no known cases from other ethnicities, certainly not Pakistanis.

DeAnna turned to the flight steward and said in steady and even tones, "Oh, he always coughs like this." It was completely true. Only I never coughed up blood; it was always sticky green mucus. I was gasping in gulps of air between coughs. I couldn't speak. The steward looked into my wife's eyes and saw she was calm and without concern. He let it go and continued down the aisle. I breathed a huge sigh of relief.

The cabin door was closed and after taxiing down the runway the plane left the ground. Moments later, when the plane had leveled off I pushed the button overhead. The same flight attendant appeared in a flash.

"May I get some oxygen," I asked? He brought me a small bottle with a nasal cannula. I knew oxygen would relax my lungs as they would not have to work so hard to get air. My coughing had slowed but I was still bringing up blood. An airplane cabin, due to altitude, pressurization, and the confines of so many bodies has less than 75% of the normal oxygen in room air. For somebody with compromised lungs the extra pure oxygen I was given was salvation. The bleeding stopped.

In Singapore we had only ten minutes to change planes and catch our flight to Hong Kong. As we ran to find our new departure gate I began to cough blood again, but not as severely. Again, when the Singapore airline plane reached cruising altitude I requested oxygen and things mellowed out. My thoughts returned to think over the purpose of our journey, *"Why did God make it clear that we should respond to the great need of suffering Afghans, but then not give me the health to carry out this calling?"* Scripture says, "In their hearts humans plan their course, but the Lord establishes their steps."[20] God was certainly directing our steps, but they seemed to be directing us away from such a great need. Why? It was a question that would be in our hearts for many months.

Sometimes, in spite of our good intentions, and sincere prayers, we do not hear from God. We do not get clear direction or answers to our requests. Sometimes we have to wait upon Him, have our strength renewed, and learn patience and perseverance.[21]

The captain announced that we would have turbulence while landing in Hong Kong's downtown airport. There were typhoon warnings. Indeed our plane was the last to land before they closed the airport. As the plane dropped and danced toward the runway we looked straight out the plane windows into the windows of apartments. The runway had been built before the thirty and forty story buildings had been erected. Hong Kong was the most densely populated city in the world. A United Airline pilot

---

[20] Proverbs 16:9

[21] Isaiah 40:31

later told me that landing at that old airport[22] was one of the most difficult in the world he had to do.

As we exited the terminal building the full extent of the typhoon rain hit us like tiny pebbles flying sideways. Our thin cotton *shalwar kameesh* outfits were drenched in a flash. We looked ridiculous in Hong Kong wearing the clothing of Pakistan's Northwest Frontier Province. But more significantly it was hugely impractical for a typhoon! My brother hustled us and our luggage into a van he'd borrowed and asked how we were doing. I mentioned to him I was sick.

He said, "Well I was going to stop for my doctor's appointment while we were in this part of the city, before heading out to our home in Kowloon. Perhaps my doctor can look at you too."

Doug took us to the Peace Clinic, where we both were examined. His doctor decided I should be checked into the Prince of Wales Hospital. He made a quick phone call and we were on our way. They had never treated, nor even seen a person with cystic fibrosis, though they had read about it in their textbooks. A little army of doctors passed through my room to have a look at the real deal. I found it amusing.

Not so amusing were the nurses. They did not speak English, and I do not speak Cantonese. One incident was remarkable. I was prescribed intravenous Tobramycin. It can cause deafness if a dose is too high for the patient. Blood samples are drawn before and after the one hour infusion. The blood levels are taken to be certain maximum efficacy is reached, without going beyond a safe threshold. When I was a patient at Stanford Children's Hospital in California this threshold had been surpassed on an earlier occasion and I woke up with ringing in my ears (tinnitus). I still have this today as well as partial deafness in my left ear. The damage is permanent. So I knew about the risks.

My Asian nurse hooked me up with the computer pump to receive the Tobramycin dose by IV. She did not speak English. As she left the room I noted the pump was set to run for thirty min-

---

[22] A new airport was built on a man-made island and completed in 1998. It is home to 100 airlines and employs 65,000 people. https://en.wikipedia.org/wiki/Hong_Kong_International_Airport

utes. I knew (from many previous experiences) that the medicine should infuse over one hour. If the medicine went in too quickly levels would go too high in my blood and it would cause more permanent hearing loss. I also knew how to program and run the pumps, since I had been a patient so many times before. (They used the same infusion pumps as Stanford.) So after the nurse left the room I reprogramed the pump to infuse for one hour.

The nurse came back to check on me after just a few minutes and found the pump was running at half the rate. She was confused and upset. I explained how I had changed the settings. I explained why, but she did not understand. She chastised me in very broken English and reset the pump to infuse over thirty minutes. As soon as she left the room I reset it again for an hour. After the thirty minutes was up, she came back in, expecting the medicine to be gone. It was only half infused. I explained again that I had reprogramed it. She was furious. I asked to see the doctor and she marched out of the room. She understood what I had done, but could only admonish me in Cantonese. I too was frustrated, but knew that it was my body and I had to do what was right.

A few moments later she returned. Her entire countenance had changed. She had spoken with the doctor and found that I was right. She apologized for her mistake. That was remarkable. I have had thousands of encounters with nurses and there have been plenty of mistakes, some that could have been extremely serious. I commend this Chinese nurse for her humility and act of contrition. It is easy to forgive when forgiveness is requested. It is hard when mistakes are denied or excuses made. Even when negligent errors are made Jesus tells me to forgive. "For if you forgive other people when they sin against you, your heavenly Father will also forgive you. But if you do not forgive others their sins, your Father will not forgive your sins."[23] This nurse was very apologetic and said I'd been correct. The medicine should be infused over a sixty minute period. It was easy to forgive. She also forgave me for my interference!

---

[23] Matthew 6 :14,15

Each morning I was served a Chinese staple called *congee*. It is a type of rice porridge that is cooked a long time so that the rice pretty much disintegrates. Tiny bits of rice-size pork are added. It is a dish traditionally served to the sick, much like chicken noodle soup is served in America. Unfortunately, for a cystic fibrosis calorie-starved person, it does not contain very much nutrition. So my brother, his wife Dawn, and my wife brought me some great delicacies - from local fast food restaurants!

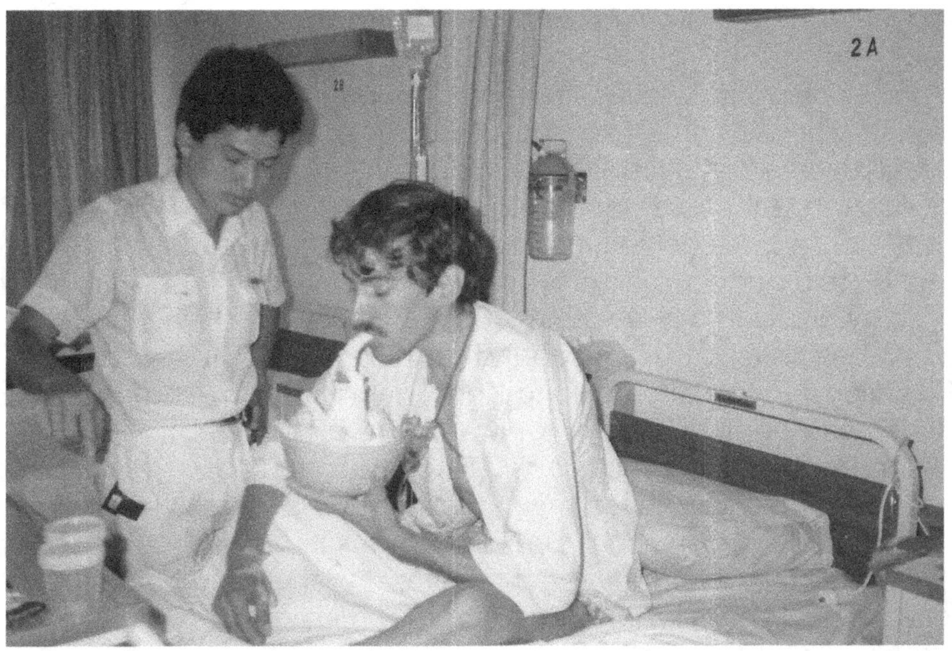

A couple times a day the respiratory therapist would appear with a large ceramic bowl which was put on my bedside tray. In the bowl was an enormous ceramic pipe device. I was instructed to inhale from the pipe. It contained some medications no doubt, and the very hot water in the bowl created a steam that helped the medicine get absorbed as I inhaled. I didn't know if it worked to loosen secretions in my lungs, but it was most interesting. I had no idea what the medication was, but it was my first experience with a water pipe. "When in Rome..." Having a willingness to learn new treatments in various countries has helped me innumerable times.

After a dozen days I was released in much better health and enjoyed a final few days with DeAnna, Dawn and Doug, in Kowloon and also in the bustling city of Hong Kong. Receiving a proper course of strong antibiotics as well as hydration and respiratory therapy had brought me back from the edge of terminal pneumonia. This cycle of health and illness was my three to four month routine from the time I was seventeen until I was thirty-eight. I would eventually see hospitals in nine different countries, and be admitted around eighty-five times for chronic lung infections.

But could God have a purpose for me in all of this? Did He have a plan for somebody that was chronically ill? Would it be a better course of action to just live close to excellent health care facilities in San Jose and avoid great risks? Should I make survival my goal, or should I instead chose to live a life of purpose, of service and perhaps sacrifice?

Why on earth did we make such a stressful and risky trip anyway? It is true that I chose (and choose) *life* not just existence. This trip to Pakistan and Hong Kong was both risky and rigorous. But I was not afraid of dying. I was more afraid of not living well. Theodore Roosevelt once said, "Only those are fit to live - who do not fear to die." And even my older brother David artistically drew and framed a quote from Benjamin Franklin which hung beside my mother's bed for the rest of her life: "I wish not so much to live long, as to live well." This philosophy of life resonated well with me.

But then I realized something equally significant.

We had been planning a life that would take us to oppressed Muslims in really tough countries, countries where Christians were not generally welcomed. However, we are first and foremost followers of Jesus, and Jesus was guiding our steps. First he led us to Pakistan. But his next steps for DeAnna and I would be elsewhere. He was not finished with us yet. In a matter of months we would become aware of another oppressed people group, the Kurds. And they were not only living in the Middle East (where there was no CF care) but they also resided as guest workers and refugees in Germany. And Germans have excellent medical facilities and are well acquainted with CF. Living there would allow me to get my regular "tune ups" in excellent hospitals.

And so our next step was to join an organization called OM (Operation Mobilization) and move to a ghetto in West Berlin, where tens of thousands of Kurds were living.

Chapter 14

Kinderklinik Kranken-
haus Zehlendorf

I purposely titled this chapter with words which will be absolutely foreign to most of the readers of this chapter. You are thinking, *"What on earth does that mean?"* That is exactly how I felt when I first entered a German hospital. I was led down large white super-clean hallways and saw neat little signs that meant who-knows-what. I realized I was completely at the mercy of a system for which I had absolutely no preparation. None of these words were in our Introduction to German class. That class had simple little phrases like, *"Ich trinke Bier."* And this hospital didn't even serve beer. I was more likely to see something like *"Rontgenabteilung."* That means X-ray department. Germans always string their words together so that all the nouns are combined to make one giant noun. And nouns are always capitalized. This looks very impressive but is also intimidating to foreign patients. Some words could have thirty of forty letters. But the point of this book is not to teach you German.

The title of this chapter translated means, "Children's Hospital in Zehlendorf." Zehlendorf is the name of the suburb within West Berlin where I most often went for medical care. *Kinderklinic* means Children's Clinic. *Krankenhaus* means hospital. The best care for anyone with CF was in the children's hospital, as the disease affects children. Recently there have been adult clinics established, but in the 1980's (although I was over thirty) I was always put in a private room on the children's ward.

Zehlendorf is a nice little wealthy neighborhood on the outskirts of West Berlin. It sits comfortably on the edge of a beautiful lake by the name of Wannsee. Surrounding Zehlendorf on three sides is a beautiful forest. The homes adjacent to the hospital are enormous and grand, each with a nice little front lawn that stretches down to the water's edge. A quiet yacht harbor is filled with elegant sailing craft. The hospital itself is a block away from the infamous lakeside home where senior officials of the Nazi regime met together on January 20, 1942 and came up with the "Final Solution to the Jewish Question." It seems that everywhere one went in Berlin there were reminders of its grim past. The city has some pretty sordid history.

But I wish to back-track a bit here. My first experience in a German hospital was far less auspicious, but still a shock to my expectations. It was June of 1988 and we had just arrived in Germany. DeAnna and I were living temporarily in a borrowed camping trailer in a West German town called Herborn. We were meeting secretly to study Kermanji, the language of the Kurds. Why secretly? Because the language was illegal. Yes, really. Our goal for living there was to learn this forbidden language spoken by a million Kurds in Germany and over ten million Kurds in eastern Turkey. It was so forbidden in Turkey at the time that politicians and journalists in Turkey had been imprisoned just for using the word "Kurd." However, an American couple had learned the language in Germany from Kurdish guest workers, and agreed to teach a few of us new-comers some of the basics - in secret. So they established a very private one month class. However during our first week together I developed a lung infection.

This was a bad time to have pneumonia. For one thing we were new to Germany and were eager to get to know our new home. For another, this was the first time in history that somebody was teaching Kermanji to English speakers. We would never again have this opportunity. But I needed medical care, so after just one week of class DeAnna and I climbed aboard a train and went to a big city hospital in Giessen, where I was admitted. It was during my first day as an inpatient that I had a big surprise.

"Don't cough!" the therapist exclaimed during the morning respiratory therapy. I looked at her and laughed. Her English was quite good, but her instructions were ludicrous.

"I have been coughing continually for the past fifteen years," I replied. *"Surely this lady is from another planet."* I thought.

"It is bad for your lungs," she said.

I argued, "How on earth am I supposed to clear my lungs of mucus if I can't cough it up?" I had always done chest percussion therapy, which involved laying in various positions while beating on various parts of the chest and back with cupped hands. And then violently coughing to bring up mucus. This is the treatment – the *only* treatment – that Stanford had taught my family. It was definitely not the treatment that was used in Germany. It was a reminder to me that the American way is not the only way, and I soon realized that it wasn't always the best way.

Over the next two weeks the therapist taught me something that in English translates "autogenic drainage." This therapy discourages coughing, which irritates and inflames the lungs, the therapist explained. Instead the individual focuses on the muscles of the chest cavity. One takes a very deep breath. Then after holding one's breath for a few seconds to let the air penetrate beyond the congestion, one slowly exhales while squeezing the chest muscles, the mucus is slowly forced up into the bronchi. Once it is there it can be expelled by a "huff." No coughing, no hacking away, and no dyspnea (shortness of breath). It sounded too wonderful to be true.

I was learning to actively listen. Hmmm. *There are actually other ways of doing things.* Before I could truly learn, I had to let go of my bias that I already knew the answer. It required humility. I had to release my American way (even though it involved hanging on to something as critical as my next breath) and trust a complete stranger. And surprise, surprise, it worked. In fact, for the next ten years I cleared my lungs using autogenic drainage, except when I was an inpatient back at Stanford Hospital. There it was forbidden - as a foolish foreign idea.[24]

---

[24] It is, however, allowed today at Stanford, although most therapists are not willing to take the time to learn or teach it to patients.

When I was finally discharged from the hospital, DeAnna met me and we took the two hour train ride back up to Herborn. I was in time for the final week of class. Then it was time for the two of us to leave our temporary trailer-home and to make our way by train to West Berlin. I remember arriving in the *Bahnhoff* (train station) in West Berlin with our four overseas suitcases. I was too weak to drag them through the station. DeAnna hustled them on to the escalator one by one and I rode to the top and stood watch over them. Again a lesson in humility.

This trait, humility, is an often overlooked aspect of learning to live with a serious illness, such as cystic fibrosis. In the book of Philippians we are exhorted to, "Do nothing out of selfish ambition or vain conceit, but in humility consider others better than yourselves." I was guilty of having "vain conceit," which I understand to mean that because of technology, education, and our superior American ways, we know better than others. I was guilty of thinking I was better than others, whether they were German health care providers or impoverished and rural Kurds.

Yet because of my chronic illness, my frequent bouts of pneumonia, and general weakness, I was unable to present myself as robust and self-confident. I can well remember huffing and puffing my way up eight flights of stairs to knock on somebody's door, which we frequently did as we visited Kurds in the ghetto where we lived in West Berlin. I would often stand on the landing with my hands on my knees, trying to catch my breath before knocking and somebody opened their door. And when I did talk to people, I was often out of breath. I would cough; I was weak. I was forced to be humble.

I shall never forget when a Kurd, whom I had gotten to know quite well, told me (in German), "You know, Dan, I would never have had the courage to talk with you if you hadn't been sick." He saw me as someone whom he could approach. I didn't intimidate him. I wasn't the big mighty American with all the answers. I was sick. I was weak. I didn't want to be humbled but cystic fibrosis made me so. It reminded me of the verse, "For when I am weak then I am strong."[25] People aren't looking to the high and mighty

---

[25] 1 Corinthians 12:10b

for life's answers; they are looking to the lowly that persevere through the most difficult times.

It is a well known fact that people are most open to change when they are new to a community. Immigrants or refugees are most open to respond to the love and kindness of strangers during their first two years in a new country. It is when they are groping for life's basics, for friends and connections - that they will respond to simple acts of kindness. This is why we wanted to work with refugees in West Berlin. It was also where we could learn their forbidden language. In Berlin we were able to take courses at the *Freie Universität Berlin* (Free University in Berlin - as opposed to the other Berlin University in communist East Berlin.) to learn Kurdish. And finally it was a place where I could receive knowledgeable care for cystic fibrosis.

Which brings me back to where I started: Krankenhaus Zehlendorf. I had a very embarrassing experience while a patient in this hospital. DeAnna often stayed with me – even overnight-while I was an inpatient. During the early years of our life in Berlin we did not have children.

Later it was impossible for her to stay with me because our daughters (adopted) had to be cared for. Still she would bring them to visit. The hospital was a good hour's travel from our apartment in Kreuzberg, West Berlin. DeAnna would bundle our little girls against the freezing cold, walk to the *U-bahn* station (avoiding the abundant "dog dirt") and ride the train as far as possible. Then they would walk to a bus stop, sit on an icy bench and wait again. Next they'd catch a bus and ride past the end of lake Wansee and the marina to the pleasant town of Zehlendorf. After walking a few blocks up and down residential hills they'd reach the four story modern hospital and come up to my room.

However, after about ten minutes our energetic girls would be climbing the walls. All they were really interested in was watching the TV, so we would go for a walk. I would drag my IV pole along the asphalt paths and the girls would jump, skip and run to and fro. They were amazingly active for wearing snow boots, heavy coats, scarves, mittens and winter hats. It seems like it was always bitterly cold, or maybe those are the memories that are the most vivid. I know there were days when it was warm in Berlin because we did take hikes in the forests from time to time. But mostly I remember how grey the skies were and how cold the wind blew.

Prior to adopting children DeAnna would move into my hospital room. She would be given a cot which was next to my hospital bed in the small private room. She was a real trooper and endured the two-week stays with me. It was an act of love and sacrifice for which I am forever grateful. It is part of what has made our marriage strong, her willingness to walk this journey of health and sickness by my side.

One night I lay in my hospital bed for a long time, unable to fall asleep. I had gotten past the fever and serious infection but had to remain an inpatient to receive IV medication. I was bored. I slid six inches down off my hospital bed to be beside her on her flimsy cot. Just as I was giving her a hug a young hospital nurse came in to check on me. Maybe she wanted to take my temperature or blood pressure. Nurses seem to be required to do this throughout the night. One time a nurse woke me to ask if I was sleeping okay. During this particular night, however, I was just laying there wide awake. Meds sometimes cause insomnia. The poor nurse was quite embarrassed. She turned abruptly and disappeared faster than she'd popped in. Feeling quite embarrassed myself I clambered back up onto my mattress as fast as possible, but of course no more nurses came back into the room that night.

I was further humiliated the next day when the supervisor came in and told me in no uncertain words – she even spoke in English – that nobody else was allowed in my hospital bed except me. And I was to stay there! *Got it.* That never happened again.

The incident does underlie the need for closeness during times of trial. We need one another to be near us when we suffer. The greatest challenge for us as overseas Christian workers was leaving our homes and the ones we loved. Likewise the hardest part of being in the hospital for two weeks was missing my wife and children. A warm hug between a man and wife or parent and child does a world of good.

And *that* remains my most vivid memory of Krankenhaus Zehlendorf.

Chapter 15

The Power to Say No

There are times in life that one has to say *no*. I have never been good at it. I am one of those compliant people who always wants to please the person asking. This is a good quality if for example you are supposed to take a long list of medications, or do an uncomfortable and timely therapy twice a day for twenty years. But it isn't always the best thing. This is a short account of one of those times when I actually said, "No."

DeAnna and I were in Berlin in the mid 1980's. We were living in our apartment on Reichenberger Strasse (Street). The building was in total disrepair. The top floor had been bombed out by the Russians at the end of World War II when the war in Europe was in its last days, and nobody had invested the time or money to replace the top part of the building. They just built a roof over the forth floor. As you looked down the street you saw all the buildings at the same five-story height, except ours. There must have been a point in history when Berliners decided it was acceptable to walk up five stories, but no more. Our building was over a hundred years old. All of prewar West Berlin consisted of five story buildings. Except ours; it was four. We lived on the third story.

That doesn't sound very high, unless you are carrying up four bags of groceries that contain seven liters of juice and milk, etc. Plus our ceilings were thirteen feet high, so that adds a bunch of stairs to each flight. Years later, DeAnna had to also help our small children up the stairs plus carry our groceries… but that comes later.

On this winter day I had a tremendous pain in my side. I don't normally have sharp pains; it's not part of having cystic fibrosis, unless your lungs are so infected that you are having a pneu-

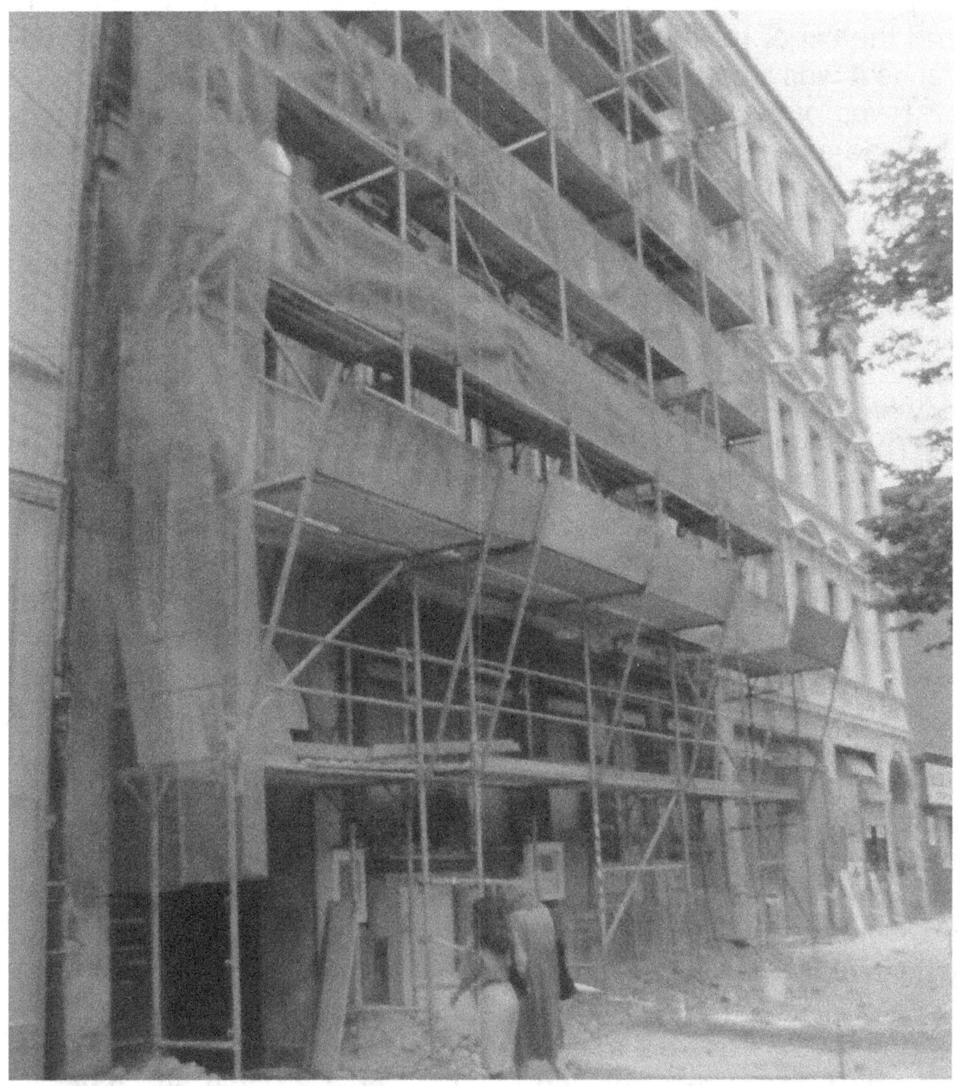

OUR APARTMENT WAS IN THIS BUILDING IN WEST BERLIN

mothorax, which is essentially a collapsed lung. But I had never had one of those, so the pain was causing me concern.

I decided I should get to a hospital, and the closest one was a place called the *Urban Krankenhaus*. All it means in English is, Downtown Hospital. I learned (too late) that it was essentially the inner-city hospital where all indigent and uninsured persons were sent. That obviously had some affect on the quality of the care and the expertise of the personnel. Nevertheless, I went there because it was closest and I was in pain.

I was put in a large room (ten beds) and underwent the standard admission tests. At this point in my language learning the doctor's exam was still a bit of a mystery to me. I was looked over by a physician but I didn't really understand what he was saying, until he used his imperfect English. Doctors always want a person to lie down on their back so they can listen to the abdomen. I understand the point of this, as they want to listen to bowel sounds. They are perhaps the only people who seem to be pleased by bowel sounds.

The problem with me was that because of my damaged lungs (that were full of mucus) I simply could not breathe if I lay on my back. Ever. I always slept on my side, because I could get some air that way. I could not recline straight back and just lay there, unless I completely stopped breathing. This was difficult to communicate to the doctor, so, wanting to be compliant I just laid back – and stopped breathing until the doctor had listened intently with his cold stethoscope pressed against my belly. Then I sat up and began to breathe again.

As the exam progressed I got the gist of what the doctor said and then he left. When the nurse came to see me, however, and began to carry out what the doctor had instructed, I was at her mercy. She did not speak much English, or at least she didn't want to try. One was never sure which it was. She put me in a wheel chair (I always wondered, *why can't I walk? I certainly walked myself into the hospital; I didn't come in on a gurney!*), but I compliantly covered myself with as many blankets as I could grab and began the long trip down a series of cold and mysterious hallways. It didn't help that I was dressed in my underwear and a thin cotton gown - which of course was open at the back and had just a single string to tie it together…

After several turns down many long corridors I was told to sit and wait. The view from the window was of the bleak city. Grey skies, grey buildings, cluttered courtyards behind the long straight walls of apartment blocks, and then behind the courtyards more identical grey apartments. Berlin is laid out in a classic German grid design which minimized streets and maximized buildings. There were entire masses of pure five-story blocks of buildings, accessible only by passing through a series of tunnels into court-yards. The cars would be left out on the main street somewhere, assuming one had a car and that one had found a parking place. The rest was done on foot.

I was wheeled into a room with an X-ray machine. Germans are famous for their construction of state-of-the-art medical de-vices; including the MRI that you will find at most hospitals in America, and of course the CAT scan, and X-ray machines. In the German language an X-ray is called a *"Rontgen"*. (Mr. Rontgen was the fellow who invented the X-ray machine.) Every German carries a *Rontgen* card in their wallet, to keep track of how many X-rays they have had. If you get too many *Rontgens* you can get cancer. Nobody carries a card like this in America, which is too bad, because I got way too many X-rays. And I got cancer. But that is a different story.

After the X-ray I was wheeled back to my room to wait for the next doctor's order to be completed. It started with a urine sam-ple. That is the easy one. Then they wanted labs. I wish those were the cute puppies, because labs in a hospital means they will try and get blood from my skinny arms until they succeed. Of course I tried my best to tell them that my veins were very poor and they couldn't get blood from my antecubital veins. These are the veins on the top side of one's elbows, which are normally quite large and easily accessible. But mine were long ago abused and used by various lab techs, so they can never be even seen no matter how tight you put the tourniquet on, slap my arm, heat it, swing it, etc. After five or so attempts one of the lab techs hit a vein in my forearm and drew out the required amount of blood.

This is of course a very unpleasant experience, and I am sure the reader would rather not even re-live this page of the story. But it is all part of the Urban Krankenhaus experience.

After returning to my room, sporting six bandages on my arms, I climbed into bed and pulled the clean sheets over my scantily clad body. I figure that there are three reasons a patient is given such a thin hopeless garment. One, it keeps a person in bed, because they will freeze if they actually get up and walk around. Theoretically doctors tell patients to get up and walk around. But if a patient actually does this, the nurses all stare at him like he is trying to run away, or he is invading *their* space. So most patients just lay in bed. The second reason is the medical personnel always know where to find you, so that their time is not wasted looking for you in the hallways. And finally it makes the patient *feel* that he is sick and he therefore submits to their authority. This is very important. If doctors are gods, then nurses are right up there next to the gods, and therefore deserve the utmost of respect and perhaps even admiration. At least one should listen to them and obey their commands. I had become very good at this after some forty-five hospital admissions. Please excuse the sarcasm here, but I was not having a good day and definitely had a bad attitude.

The nurse then brought me a small strainer, exactly like the one you use in your kitchen to strain loose tea or other small food items. It measured about two inches in diameter. The nurse told me to pee through the strainer while using the toilet. I found this confusing at worse and interesting at best. Certainly it was something I had never done before and I couldn't quite understand the purpose. Finally it was made clear that the doctor thought the pain in my side was a result of kidney stones. Their intention was that I would pass the stone at some point. They wanted to catch the stones. Hmm.

At first I thought it rather strange that they would want the stones. I wondered what they would do with them. Maybe evaluate them? Count them? Validate their theory that I had kidney stones? Save them for research? As a patient one never knows these kind of things; it's all new and strange. And as a patient in a foreign hospital it is even worse. You can't ask. You can only comply. So I complied. Every time I used the bathroom I held out my little strainer. I noted that other men were carrying little strainers too, so I didn't feel very out of place. Apparently everyone in my ward was thought to have kidney stones. Guys like competitions; maybe we could see who could get a stone in their strainer first.

Another unpleasant aspect of hospital stays is the "standing order." These are orders that the doctor writes that are routinely and automatically carried out without the doctor having to submit them repeatedly. It is very hard as a patient to argue with a standing order. They simply have to be done. So if a doctor wants to know how some aspect of your body is doing, he or she will order a blood test for twice a day, for example.

Then the phlebotomist will come in with their little cart full of nasty needles and say in a pleasant voice, "It's time to take some blood." Many phlebotomists (even in San Jose) speak very little English. It turns out that it is one of the professions for which it is easy to get certified, so it is a good entry level job in the field of medicine.

Unfortunately, however, phlebotomists have to come to work very early – like four a.m. Or perhaps they are at the hospital all night and they think that it's unfair that other people should be asleep while they have to work. So invariably I would be woken at five a.m. for a blood draw. I find it rude to be woken at five a.m. when I've had precious little sleep in the first place, but to wake me up and inflict pain is simply beyond belief. But since I am compliant, I sit up and start rubbing my arms in the hope that today my veins might comply on the first stick.

The phlebotomist in Berlin was not successful on the first stick, nor the second, nor the third, nor the fourth. So I offered my foot to him, which is a huge sacrifice, because there is very little tissue under the veins of your foot. So the pain is insane when that needle is pressed into the flesh on the top of the foot. Most hospitals will require a special order to take blood from a foot, because one also runs the risk of a blood clot shooting up the leg and messing one's brain up. But this vampire at the Urban Krankenhaus couldn't get blood from my foot either. Apparently he was pretty upset (at me?) and left in a huff.

"*Good*," I thought to myself as I lay back down and covered my body in an attempt to get warm again. I had pulled on a pair of grey sweatpants to help my thin frame retain its meager heat. It was probably against the rules, however. (German hospitals are very legalistic.) It was now five thirty a.m. and I was happy to get some more sleep while it was still dark.

Suddenly I was awakened by a big woman in a white coat. I will call her, Hilda-the-Hun. She was a doctor and she seemed pretty upset. I surmised this, because without a word to me she pulled back my bed sheet, grabbed the waistband of my sweatpants and my underwear, right at my hip nearest her and yanked down. To say I was shocked would be a gross understatement. I knew Germans had a different idea of personal privacy, but this was *my* person and *my* privacy she was dealing with! She hadn't yet spoken a word to me.

She then did something that blew my mind (and my pain tolerance). She took a large syringe and (without using even an alcohol swab) pressed the tip of the needle into my hip area, straight down into the femoral artery. Arteries run away from the heart and are large and hard to miss. They are also very precious for a litany of heart surgeries and if damaged they could cause a person to lose an appendage. I had a bit of knowledge about such things so I was aghast. She got the blood she wanted and left.

I placed heavy pressure on the afflicted area after she had gotten her requisite blood. It takes a long time for an injury to that artery to heal, because of the pressure coming from the pumping heart. So I held direct pressure on it for a long time and remained prone on my back.

As I recoiled in shock I began to think to myself, *"What on earth am I doing here?"* I came to this hospital to address the pain in my abdomen. That pain didn't seem so bad anymore. I looked around at my surroundings and thought about the kind of treatment I had received. I had been in a lot of hospitals (in several countries) and never had I been treated with such indignity.

I wondered, *"How much more will I take? At what point will I actually say, 'No. Enough. I won't take anymore of this!"* It is one thing to be compliant. It is another to ignorantly submit.

After several days I still hadn't passed any stones into my little basket, and it seemed rather pointless to sit in a hospital bed for days and days on end simply so I could pee now and then and maybe produce a little stone. Some of my roommates had been there for a couple weeks already. I certainly didn't want to go on with this day after day until I perhaps produced some tidbit of calcium. What if I didn't have a kidney stone anyway?

"I should never have told the doctor that my mother had had kidney stones," I thought to myself. Sometimes the doctor is so eager to obtain a diagnosis they will grab at anything.

So I made a decision that I have never made in fifty years of being in hospitals. I got dressed, grabbed my belongings, and walked to the nurse's station.

"I am checking myself out," I choked the words out. By their immediate (and vehement) reaction I surmised that my statement was not often heard in their realm. I was violating the atmosphere of total submission to the almighty doctor-god. The desk nurse hurried off and moments later the doctor appeared. I was soon surrounded by medical professionals. I knew it was a power play; the more white coats that surround a person, the more the patient is pressed into submission. But the only thing that was clear in my mind was the memory of Hilda pulling my sweatpants down and stabbing me in the groin with a needle. I was ready to fight all of them if necessary.

Argument after argument was made why this was a bad idea. I was told I could not return to the hospital if my kidneys flared up. I was told I would have to pay if I got sick again. I was told that if something happened I would be legally responsible for the outcome; that the doctors could not help me. Blah blah blah. It had no meaning to me. My mind was made up.

I looked the doctor in her face, which was just several inches from mine, and said, *"Ich gehe nach Hause!"* (I am going home!)

"Well you will have to sign these papers," she replied in German. "Fine," I said, "I'll sign anything you want. I completely release you of any liability." I don't think I actually said that, since I don't know the German word for "liability" but I got my message across.

I signed a bunch of yellow papers in triplicate and I walked out a free man. I felt like the Berlin wall had just come down and I was Ronald Reagan. (But that is my next story.)

Chapter 16

The Wall Came Down

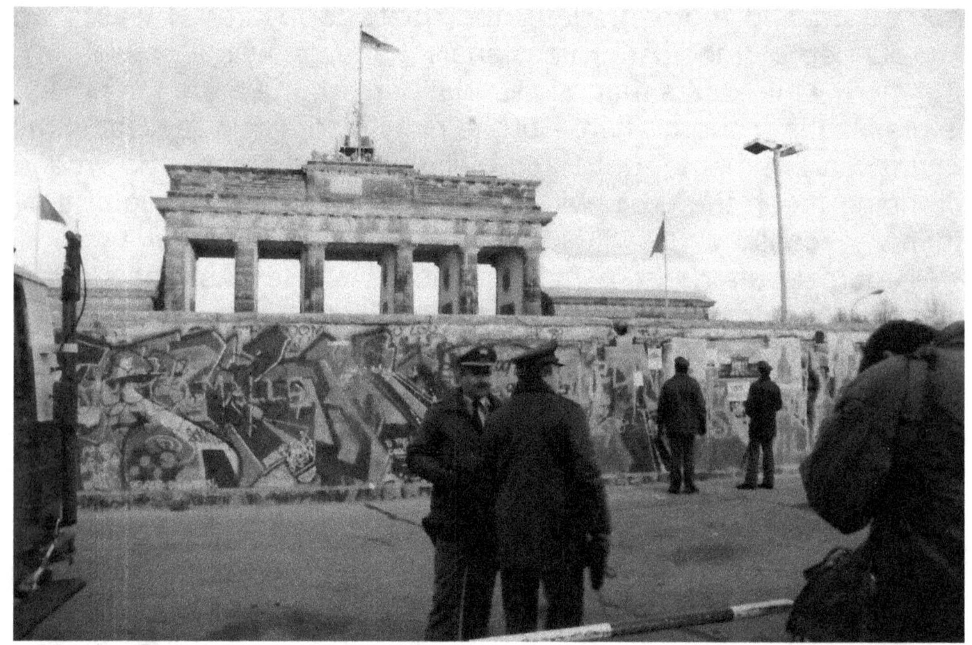

By now I hope the reader realizes that one can have a fulfilling and interesting life even if one has a terminal or debilitating illness. The days of November 1989 certainly lend credence to that fact.

I was serving tea to some young Turkish and Kurdish men in the lower level of a local church on a Thursday night. This was something that the men of our team did to give these guys a clean and safe place to hang out. We played chess, backgammon, or checkers, drank lots of sugary tea and just talked.

The phone rang and I answered it. It was DeAnna calling from our apartment in Kreuzberg.

She said the most unbelievable thing, "Dan, the East Germans are going to open the wall."

Unless you are a student of history, or born before 1980, you won't realize the significance of that sentence. The wall had been erected overnight on August 13, 1961. That was before my wife was born. Communists had built it to stop the exodus of their citizens. Since the time the city had been partitioned (into British, French, American and Soviet sectors), 3.6 million people had fled the Soviet sector to get into the western sectors. There was also an outer wall in West Berlin that surrounded the French, American and British sectors of the city. Then there was another wall (actually a pair of them) that ran the entire length of the country from north to south. This was the very visual and real iron curtain. It was really a concrete curtain, but the seal between east and west was certainly ironclad.

This wall, which was twelve feet high, was a few blocks from our dingy apartment. Our neighborhood was run-down because there was no business near the wall; all the roads had been blocked off by the impenetrable barrier. We sometimes took walks on a path along the wall. It was interesting to read the political slogans that were freshly painted and the graffiti. Sometimes we'd climb the viewing towers the West Germans had built so we could peer over into no-man's land. There we could see the barbed wire, the stretches of sand (that were mined), the towers with machine guns and guards at the ready. In the distance we could see the drab buildings of East Berlin and make out all the identical cars (same color too) that the very fortunate drove. For everyone living in the island of West Berlin, the wall had become part of existence. We felt it would be standing forever.

So DeAnna's proclamation to me on the phone sounded like she was teasing. She had to say it several times and give me the whole back story before I believed her. She had heard the news from a neighbor who had watched the East German's television news. (TV broadcasting does not respect walls.) They were replaying the pronouncement that had been made by their government. It was decided that East Germans who had valid passports would be immediately allowed to travel to the west. This was earth shattering news. That night, November 9th, 1989, would become a demarkation point in world history.

Because it was freezing cold outside, I donned my heaviest coat plus my long overcoat and drove our VW bug to the border crossing at Checkpoint Charlie. This was the closest crossing point near our apartment. After I parked I walked up to the fat white line that was painted on the asphalt street right at the border. Facing me were East German guards standing shoulder to shoulder holding their weapons.

"Was ist los?" I asked one of them. (What's going on?) He had no idea. Of course they had just shown up for a normal night at work and hadn't seen the news on the TV. They were clearly very nervous. There was a huge crowd gathering behind them (behind a cyclone fence) and it was growing by the minute. A film crew (I think they were Japanese) came over to interview me, as if I would know some secrets about what was happening. (Maybe it was my dark overcoat and hat.) I didn't have much to say.

A hundred feet away, looking into East Berlin, beyond the two crossing gates that separated the two countries, was a fenced-in area where foot travelers were normally processed. I could see masses of people pressed up against the fence. They were waiting eagerly to go into the mysterious city of West Berlin - the symbol of capitalism (with all the good and the bad).

Nine p.m. arrived. The gate was opened! As people started coming into Kreuzberg at Checkpoint Charlie crowds of West Germans were there to welcome them. Champagne flowed. Flowers were given. Complete strangers were hugging one another. A few cars came across. West Berliners banged on the flimsy hoods and trunks of the Trabants and Wartburgs as the tiny cars putt-putted across the border. By midnight a special edition of the local newspaper had been printed and was handed out for free. *"Die Mauer ist Weg!"* six inch letters proclaimed. (The Wall is Gone!)

The wall was actually still there, but there had been an opening. (Hyperbole always sells better.) People were seeing relatives whom they had not seen in years, even decades. Families and friends were reunited. It was difficult to convey the emotion of it all. Germans, who are rational and fairly non-emotional by nature, were crying, laughing, shouting, and being - well - exuberant. It was three days and nights of party and pandemonium.

The next night DeAnna and I joined thousands of others and climbed onto the wall itself right next to the Brandenburg *Tor* (Gate). We were a mass of humanity pressed in against one another. Dozens of TV crews were already there on elevated platforms and they had huge lights so they could film the excitement. I greeted Dan Rather. The wall was only eight feet high in front of the historic gate. Plus it was really wide at that point, maybe six feet wide. Somebody put a wooden ladder up against it and we climbed up. We had our little hammer with which we happily made our contribution at demolishing the divisive wall. The fall of the wall is a cherished memory for three generations of people who lived in its shadow.

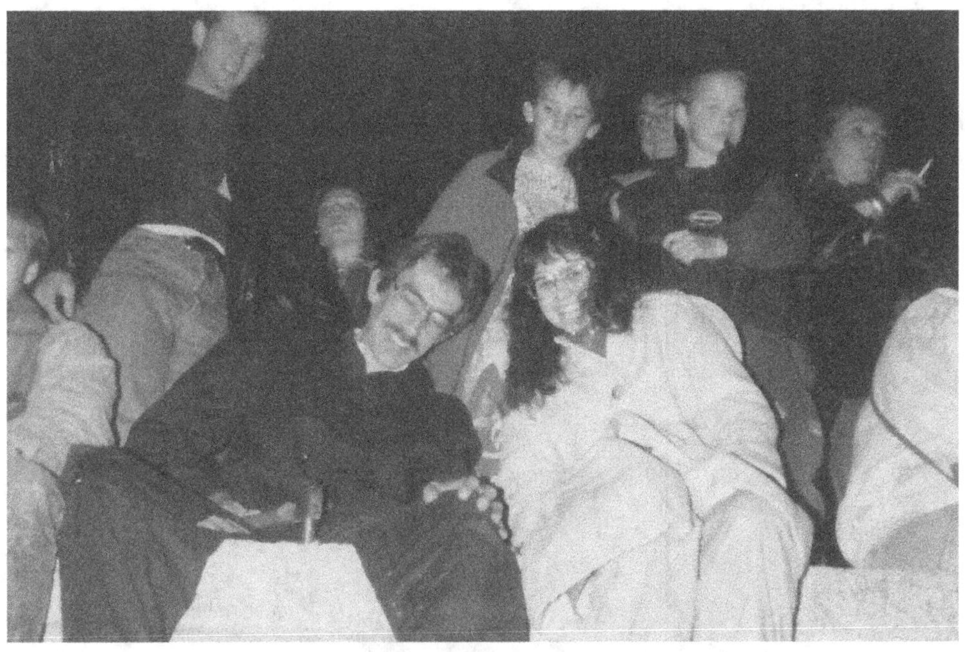

**DAN AND DEANNA WITH A HAMMER ATOP THE BERLIN WALL
NOVEMBER 1989**

The wall stood for division, for separation, and for alienation - dividing humanity. There is another wall, called sin, which separates us and alienates us from our holy God. But Jesus, in his mercy, broke down that wall of sin by his sacrifice on the cross. That cross and the belief in what it represents, means we can be reunified with our creator. The Bible puts it like this: "Once you were alienated from God and were enemies in your minds because of your evil behavior. But now he has reconciled you by Christ's physical body through death to present you holy in his sight, without blemish and free from accusation— if you continue in your faith, established and firm, and do not move from the hope held out in the gospel. This is the gospel that you heard and that has been proclaimed to every creature under heaven, and of which I, Paul, have become a servant."[26]

Such an opening in this spiritual wall of separation made all the difference to my wife and I. It changed our understanding of our world, or humankind, of illness and evil, and of eternity. Accepting the truth of God at his word changed our hearts and minds. The barrier of sin and death that Jesus broke down allows us to live victorious lives in spite of the horrors in this world and the brokenness in our societies. We have a hope for the future and a promise for eternity. There is nothing like a solid hope to give one strength when facing constant illnesses and a terminal diagnosis. The fall of the Berlin wall is for me a metaphor of the enormous wall that the cross of Christ has removed, for those who believe.

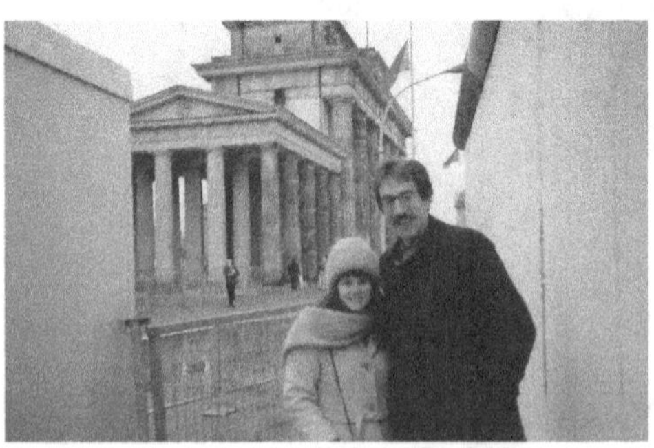

Standing inside East Berlin at the Brandenburg Gate – 1989

---

[26] Colossians 1:19-23

Chapter 17

Apache helicopter

August 2, 1990 is a date I won't soon forget. We were living in Pforzheim in West Germany for a month. DeAnna and I were part of a short term team of volunteers from various countries. Each morning a couple of the team members would go to the local bakery and buy some *Brötchen* (small single servings of bread). This would be our breakfast, with jam and perhaps tea. That particular morning we were listening to the BBC and we learned that Saddam Hussein had invaded Kuwait, claiming the oil rich and prosperous region as part of his country.

The world was outraged and eventually mounted a multinational force which ousted him from that country, leaving a wake of destruction and chaos. In America it was called The First Gulf War. That war was going to change our lives too.

After the war there was an uprising in the Kurdish north and the Shiite south. American generals at the peace agreement gave the defeated Iraqis permission to fly armed helicopters throughout their land. This turned out to be a horrific mistake. Kurds and Shiites were revolting against Baghdad's Sunni ruling minority (in the center of the country). They took cities and towns and were advancing towards Baghdad. However, Saddam's pilots set about suppressing the uprisings with their armed helicopter gunships. They were able to easily slaughter civilians and bomb towns. Kurds began to flee their towns and cities. They feared they would also be gassed by their dictator, as he had done many times before.

The most infamous gas attack occurred in Halabja on March 16, 1988. Mustard gas and other chemical agents massacred at least 5,000 civilians. They died an agonizing death. The chemical poisoning of the region has had disastrous health affects even thirty years later.

The world now witnessed a huge exodus of humanity, over a million and a half Kurds by some estimates. They quickly grabbed what they could carry, fled from their homes, and while the snow was still falling they headed for the Turkish and Iranian borders. US Secretary James Baker was flying high above the mass of humanity and immediately called the White House.

"Mr. President," Baker said to George H.W. Bush (41), "We have a humanitarian crisis of epic proportions. We must respond."

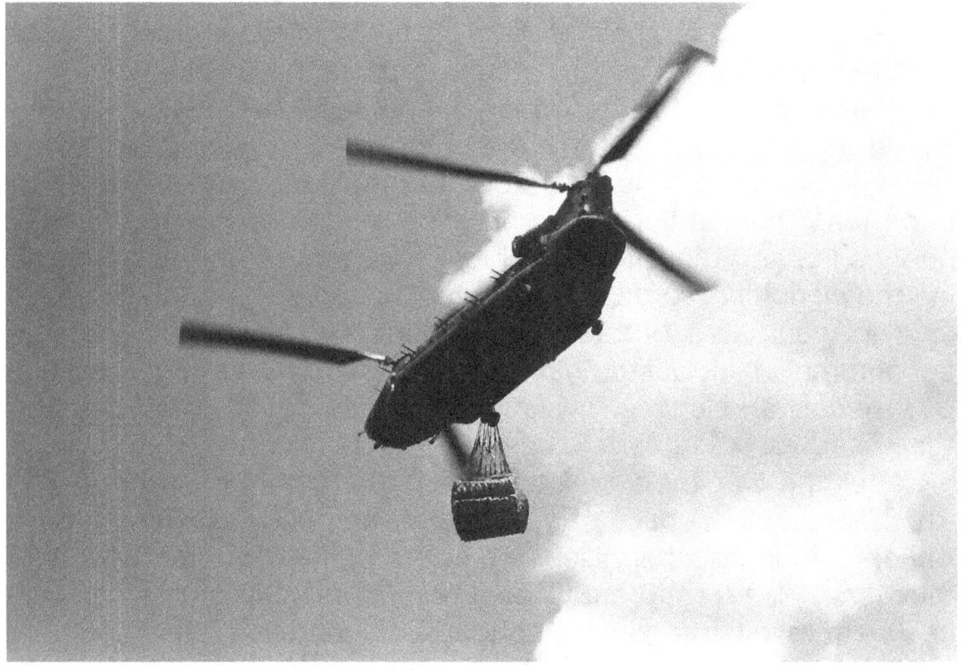

Thus began one of history's most extensive relief efforts led by the US military. Live television showed pallets of water and food being dropped from the back of Chinook helicopters. Mobs of men on the ground were seen clamoring over each other, fighting for loaves of bread to feed their families. Turkish trucks loaded with bread drove up through the mud in the rain and sleet to approach the mobs of hungry Kurds. Men wielding sticks fought off the refugees who attempted to climb into the truck beds to get food. It was chaos.

In the midst of this chaos in Iraq we received a telephone call in Berlin from Julian Lidstone, the leader of the Turkish work with OM (Operation Mobilization). OM was our employer. Julian asked DeAnna and I if we would be willing to fly to Istanbul, connect with a colleague who spoke Turkish, and then travel the breadth of Turkey (a thousand miles) by bus to the far east. Julian explained that a convoy of relief supplies was headed from northern Europe down to the Iraqi border. They needed to be guided to the places where the refugees were in the greatest need. In our hearts we knew that God had prepared us just for this moment in history. We spoke some Kurdish and could connect on a deeper level with the refugees. My health, while tenuous, was good enough to make the journey.[27]

As I mentioned earlier, the Kurdish language spoken by Kurds in eastern Turkey was illegal; it was in fact even illegal to say the word, "Kurd." But in Berlin we had been able to sit in the apartments of Kurds and dialogue in simple ways and create a lexicon of their language. We had a Toshiba lap top (weighing twelve pounds!) that contained all our vocabulary study materials in three languages. We packed as little as possible and flew to Istanbul.

A thirty hour trip on Turkish buses took us from Istanbul, via the capital of Ankara, and eventually way out east to the ancient Kurdish city of Diyarbakir. In Diyarbakir we learned of the route of the convoy. From there we made our way to the city of Van and met up with the relief trucks that had driven from northern Europe. Our next journey was a four-hour drive on mountain dirt roads towards the city of Hakarri. All along the roadway were military checkpoints. The Turkish army was constantly aware of Kurdish separatists who smuggled guns and food to the peshmerga, the Kurdish freedom fighters. When we reached Hakarri it really felt like the edge of the earth. It seemed to us like the wild west. We saw more donkeys than cars. Most men carried a weapon of some kind.

---

[27] To read a complete account of this amazing experience, read the book "Between Iraq and a Hard Place" by Kirk Legacy (pseudonym for this author, Dan Lagasse.) It also tells the incredible story of how the Lagasse's were able to adopt two Kurdish/Arab sisters who were starving.

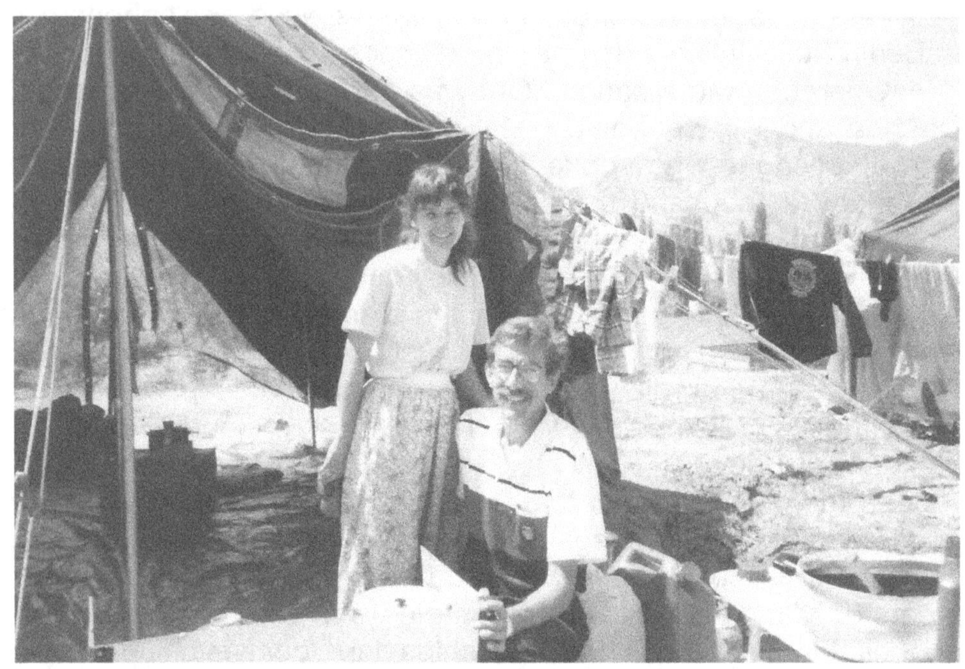

We were told that a large team of men and women volunteers would arrive after the convoy. We knew they'd arrive in a few days to assist in the relief effort. They came from all over Europe and Turkey. Among then were even Christian Turks who, unlike the bulk of their countrymen, had a sincere love for the displaced peoples of Iraq - even if all Kurds were considered terrorists by the Turkish media and government.

Thus began a remarkable period of our lives, where we crossed into Iraq innumerable times, even living there, to help the downtrodden and oppressed Kurds. We spent the next year leading various teams in and out to take part in the work of a new NGO (Non Governmental Organization.)

As winter turned to spring, and spring to a very hot summer most of the refugees left the mountainous border region between Turkey and Iraq to move back to their destroyed homes. With the assurance of a "no fly zone" along the 37th parallel, they began to rebuild their homes and cities inside northern Iraq. I was told by several Kurds that it was the fourth time they had rebuilt their homes after Iraqi air campaigns against them. In June we traveled back to Berlin.

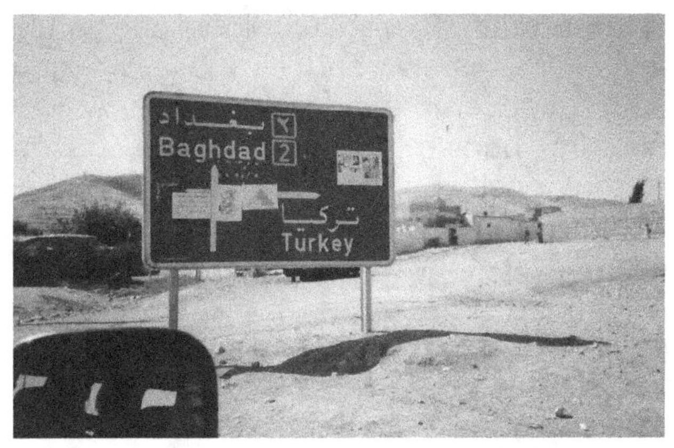

Then in July of the same year some Swiss friends of ours asked me to guide a team into the region and connect them with people so they could begin to work where the needs were greatest. I agreed to go. We flew to Istanbul, and then to Diyarbakir. It was a lot nicer than riding in a bus! Then we took local taxis to the Turkish/Iraqi border town of Silopi, a four hour journey. After exiting Turkey at the border, we immediately crossed a large bridge over the Habur river into Iraq, where Kurds greeted us warmly. *"Ser ça va!,"* [sair cha VAUH] they exclaimed, giving us a blessing that translates literally, "On your head and eyes." You'd have to understand the culture to get the drift of it. Bottom line: it was a happy way of saying, "Welcome; how's it going?"

As July rolled around the temperature soared. We experienced one hundred twenty degree heat during the day. The house the Swiss team had rented had no air conditioning, just a swamp cooler. We tried to stay inside during the day, doing most of our shopping and visiting in the early morning or late at night. We wrapped wet towels over our faces and arms. We lay flat on the concrete floors like the locals. That way we could catch some breeze and avoid the heat that had collected in the rest of the concrete house.

"I hate to say this, but I am feeling bad," I said to Hans, my Swiss friend. "And it's not just the heat."

"What's wrong?"

"My stomach really hurts. And I mean *really* hurts." I recognized the pain. The location was right where my pancreas was. I remembered well the time in the late seventies when I'd had pancreatitis. I feared that if it really was pancreatitis I'd be really stranded. I had only seen one hospital during my travels in Iraq. It was just after the First Gulf War had ended and being a central government hospital it had no staff. There was blood on the tile floor, supplies were nearly non-existent, and all those working were volunteers. All of the Iraqi government officials (Sunni Arabs) and their employees (doctors, nurses, teachers, police, prison guards, etc.) had vacated their positions in town, left their homes, and then fled south into Arab controlled regions. The sectarian hatred ran so deep that any Arab that was in the Kurdish north feared for his life.

This was made abundantly clear to me when I drove by the police office in Zakho, a Kurdish border town in the north of Iraq. It was thoroughly gutted by fire. It looked like it was the first building to be attacked after the no fly zone had been established. The message from local residents to the Iraqi government was clear, *"You have no authority over us anymore. Your lives are in danger."* We drove by an enormous stone prison on the road to the city of Dahok. It was empty; everyone had been released. Most of the prisoners had been political dissidents or men who refused to join Saddam's army. I'm sure there were a few criminals too.

I had tried to find a government official at one point to obtain legal documents (birth certificates) and was told, "I am sorry, since the end of the war there have been no officials in the Kurdish region. None of our babies who were born in the last two months have been registered; there have been no birth certificates granted." It was going to take the Kurds of Iraq some time to rebuild their society.

Fortunately for the NGO's at work in the region, the US government had instructed the US military to offer any logistical assistance necessary so that the NGO's could be effective. That meant transportation, lodging, food, and medical assistance. In the spring of that year DeAnna and I had taken a military bus on our first trip across the Iraqi border. As we passed beneath the huge stone arch I had this strange realization, *"I am taking my wife into Iraq and I have no idea where we are going, where we will stay, or what we will do."* And yet I knew it was the right thing to do. I can only say that we went by faith.

The military also gave us MRE's (Meals Ready to Eat.) In fact we had Italian, French, British, and American MRE's. There was an entire warehouse just outside of town, filled with bottled water, and another one with toilet paper. It was all for our disposal (pun intended). We had received other types of help from the military on various trips. We had been transported in a German Air Force Mosquito helicopter along the border on a trip to Silopi. And we'd taken multiple trips in the huge bus-like American Chinook choppers. DeAnna is an RN and served at first in a makeshift clinic on a hillside near the Iraqi border and later in a dispensary in a transit camp in Zakho, Iraq. Another time a British Humvee took us to a small town, Begova, where we rebuilt a hospital clinic the Iraqi army had destroyed. They mounted machine guns on the roof of the hospital to protect us while we worked, and strung razor wire around our encampment as protection.

"Stay within the razor wire," we were instructed. "We have removed the mines from the area inside the wire, but not outside it." Enough said! We were grateful for all the help and logistics the military provided. We could not have accomplished our work without their help.

It looked like I was going to need some help again. I explained to Hans that I thought I had pancreatitis. I told him about my experience in Santa Barbara many years earlier. I immediately stopped eating and drinking. I explained to him that I had to get out of Iraq and back to Germany as quickly as possible. It had taken us three days of travel to reach Zahko, Iraq from Germany. That night Hans drove the team's Land Rover across town and stopped at the house where the US military officers were living to ask for evacuation assistance. Without a medi-vac from the middle of that dessert-heat I would never make it to a hospital in time.

I was instructed to meet in a certain clearing at, "Oh eight hundred." I was doubled over in pain as I waited for the "all clear" to climb into the chopper. It was an Apache, outfitted for transport (rather than assault). It took thirty minutes for the pilot to go through all the instrument checks. It was just the pilot and myself. He flew south down the country to a large landing field in an Iraqi village called Ser Sinc [sir SINK]. The airstrip there was capable of

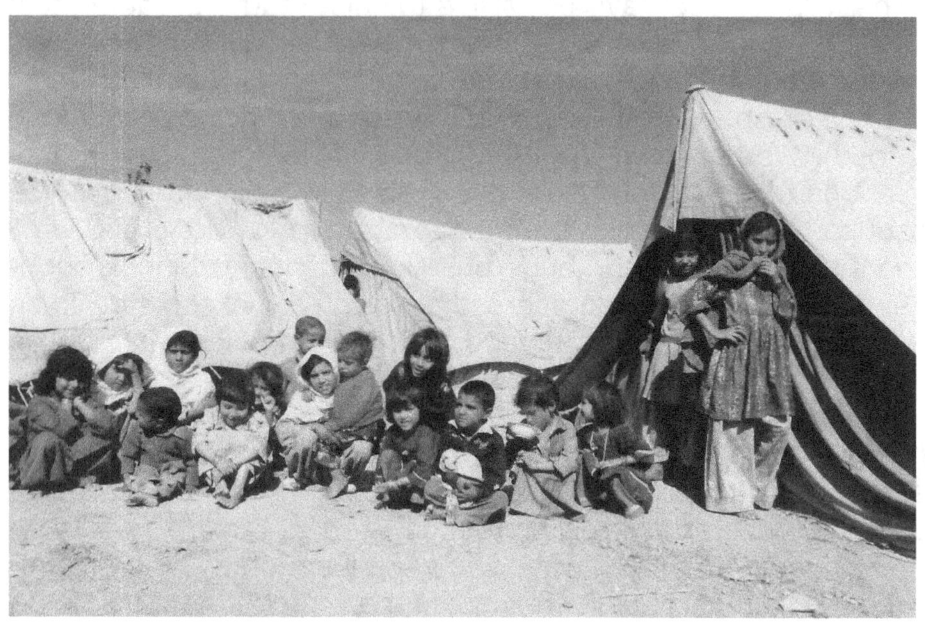

5000 REFUGEES WERE HOUSED HERE IN SILOPI, TURKEY. OUR WORK HERE WAS TO INTERVIEW EACH FAMILY TO ESTABLISH THEIR NEED FOR RESETTLEMENT.

handling a C130 transport. The US had bombed the airfield during the air campaign that began January 17, 1991. Then at the conclusion of hostilities, the craters had been filled and the runway patched to make it useful for US planes.

I was surprised how simple everything at the "airport" seemed. Desks were made from two by fours. Sandbags stacked high established walls. Modified army tents had become offices. I was grateful, very grateful, to be transported. I climbed up the drop-ramp inside the aircraft. The C130 was completely empty inside. Along each wall were simple canvas jump seats. I sat down and began to strap myself in.

"The cabin is going to get really cold," the pilot cautioned me. I could see there was no insulation at all, just tubes and cables running along the inside of the fuselage.

"Why don't you come up and sit in the cockpit?" he invited.

And so I made the flight north to Incirlik [IN jer lick] Air Base in Turkey seated right behind the pilot. It was just me, the pilot, the copilot, and the mail. I was on an elevated bench up behind the captain, with a magnificent view of the clouds and landscape. At the US base in Incirlik I went inside to ask about further transport to Germany. I was instructed to take a Turkish taxi to the city of Adana where there is a public air terminal and buy a ticket. *"Doesn't hurt to ask,"* I thought. By now it was evening.

At the Adana airport I learned that the next flight to Berlin was not until the following morning. I felt very alone. I had nowhere to go, no one that I knew in Adana, and no desire to go find a hotel. So I spent the night laying on the marble floor in the air terminal. The abdominal pain was not getting any worse, nor any better.

After a lot of Tylenol and a very restless night on the hard floor I caught the morning flight to Berlin, and took a taxi to my familiar hospital in the southern district of the city, in Zehlendorf. It was good to be "home."

After a two week stay in the children's ward I was ready to go back to work.

Chapter 18

Hepatitis A

t is easy to think that life is all about us individually. Especially when you are chronically sick or injured. Everyone asks you how you are doing, like you are something special. In fact, because I have cystic fibrosis I got really sick of the attention. No pun intended.

"How are you?" people routinely asked. I would wonder, *"How do I tell them I feel awful? They really don't want to know. They are just being polite. But maybe I should be honest and say, 'Oh, I'm dying. How are you?"*

It is also hard for the spouse (or siblings) of a CF person. All the attention is given to the terminally ill patient. Yet most of the actual work in life falls to the spouse or parent.

I recall the time in 1993 when I flew to Turkey for six weeks. We planned for DeAnna to take our two small daughters (that we had adopted from Iraq) back to the US and stay with her parents. That meant she had to do all the parenting during my absence. And she only got three phone calls from me during the six weeks. There was a good reason for this. First of all we were driving on little country roads day after day and there were no pay phones. And when we did find a yellow phone box in some village and dial up San Jose the calls were very short because it was impossible to shove enough Turkish Lira coins into a PTT phone box to keep the long distance phone call going. Such an absence from one another was really difficult.

On that trip I traveled with my colleague Marcus who also left his wife Irina with their two little daughters. They stayed the same six weeks with Irina's mom in Mosbach, Germany.

Marcus was my neighbor and colleague in Berlin. He drove an old brown VW Transit bus. He thought it was a great machine, not for its horsepower obviously, but for its efficiency. Never mind the bits of rust in the corners. (It snows in Berlin.) For Marcus, as with most Germans, efficiency matters. I had to agree the van had lots of room inside. Over the years we had hauled lots of stuff in it.

Our work in Berlin involved visiting many Kurdish/Turkish apartments and Turkish markets. Marcus spoke fluent Turkish, and I struggled along with Kurdish. Together we'd climb five stories and knock on the door of a Kurd or Turk so we could sit and drink tea and talk about life. When fresh fruit was served we knew that was the cultural signal that it was time to leave. But our talks could easily go on for three hours. We consumed buckets full of pistachios.

It was during one of those times spent together traipsing around the ghetto that we dreamt up a great plan. We decided to drive Marcus' VW Transit from Berlin all the way to the border of Iraq. Our purpose was to spend the time visiting Kurds who had written in to a Bible radio program located in West Germany. These men lived in villages scattered all over the east of Turkey. Seldom will a foreigner ever go to these villages. But various people from across eastern Turkey had heard radio shows and had written to Europe and expressed an interest in learning more about the *Injil*, or Gospels. The Koran commends Muslims to read the *Injil,* yet most have never held one, less read any part of it. We decided we would take a road trip through eastern Turkey to visit these men, give them their own copy of the Turkish *Injil* and show them a video about the life of Christ.

Turkey has a very tight censorship system. Only books or videotapes that were approved by the central government could be transported, sold, or even owned by the general population. Recently the Jesus video had been approved by the Turkish government so we purchased some in Berlin to share with people. These had actual approval stamps from the Turkish government that were affixed to the video cassettes. This showed that they were legal in the country. Of course no video tapes in Kermanji were allowed - even the identical video of the story of the life of

Christ. That would be considered seditious. Kurdish was still an illegal language.

Our plan was to bring legal copies (Turkish) of the Jesus story and legal copies of the *Injil* (also in Turkish) to people who were way outside the cities - who could never get hold of such items. These people had no cars and they lived hundreds of miles from a big city. In the Kurdish region it was even more difficult to travel as Turkish military were always stopping people and checking baggage, asking questions, etc. People didn't want to endure such harassment. Their is an old Turkish proverb that says, "Travel is a foretaste of hell." I think Travel through Turkey is still pretty much the same as when the proverb was written. However, we were willing to drive four thousand kilometers from Berlin so they could get these materials. It would be a great excursion. And there is nothing so important as the Word of God. Every people should have the opportunity to read the Word of God if they want.

We left with high expectations. Marcus had designed a special platform bed from a piece of plywood so that he could sleep crossways over the driver's and front passenger seats. I could sleep in the back. We strapped a five gallon jug to the back of the front seat; that would be our water storage. He assured me we could fill this jug up at every village. These villages had been established hundreds (or even thousands) of years ago precisely because there was a spring flowing out of the ground or a river nearby. All we had to do was drive up to any of these springs and fill our jug. Free spring water! We packed a few pots and pans, a pathetic little stove, our clothes and sleeping bags; and we were all set. He had also created a velcro system of mosquito netting that covered the open slider door, so the bugs wouldn't eat us at night and we'd still get some air in the van. I had purchased a portable VCR player that was pretty small, so we could store it safely. Our desire was to show the videotape every chance we got.

We had to be discrete about the VCR, and even about the tapes, because although everything we were doing was perfectly legal, there is a different sort of law that rules in the countryside. Turks are Sunni Muslims and in the countryside they are highly suspicious of foreigners in general. We were going to some really out-of-the way places, where no foreigners visit. When we drove the brown van up some dusty road in the mountains the first thing people did was notice the foreign vehicle. First of all nobody drove VW vans in Turkey. They simply weren't available for purchase there. And then they saw the license plate. European license plates begin with a single letter denoting the city where the vehicle has been registered. "B" announced to everyone that the van coming across the open field was from Berlin. *"Why on earth is a van coming to our village all the way from Berlin?"* was on everyone's mind. And the next thought was, *"Who invited these people here?"*

The first to see us roll up through the dust was usually boys playing in the roadway. They'd run ahead and cut through the poplar trees and grape fields to announce our arrival. By the time we pulled into the middle of town pretty much the whole village had come out to see us. We did not want to get the poor fellow who'd secretly corresponded with Germany into trouble, for we knew the price could be his life. So we had to meet and greet people, play some music on the *saz* (local Turkish stringed instrument) and drink lots of tea. Generally, the person who had corresponded would choose a discreet time to approach Marcus and talk about his desire for an *Injil*.

In many cases it was the village elder or chief who invited us into his home. Culturally it is the host who is honored by having a guest. Hosting a foreign guest is even more prestigious. So the elder in the village wanted the honor of hosting the guests from Europe. Often times he would also want to watch the video, as his interest was also great about the man Jesus, of whom the Koran speaks highly (such as "He is the Messiah.") After the movie there would be more tea, and lots of talk, sometimes till two in the morning. Then they would roll out the bedding so we could sleep in the main room of the simple home. Although these men were Kurds, they understood Turkish perfectly since it is the national language and is used exclusively in schools.

In one poor village we visited the home owners had just one drinking glass. It is always necessary for somebody who has traveled a long way to be offered a glass of water. And to show acceptance it seems right we should drink it. Marcus or I were always offered a drink of water ahead of everyone else. I would look at that glass, say a quick silent prayer, and drink the water. I had no idea where the water had come from or if the glass was ever washed. After I had drunk from the glass it would be filled again, until everyone in the room had been refreshed with a drink.[28]

Generally while the men were seated cross legged on the Turkish carpet with backs against the clay walls it was the women who were at work in the kitchen. They would gather the very best produce and meat and prepare a delicious soup. It might take them two hours as everything was done by hand. Then a young girl would bring in a platter heaped with rice and chicken or lamb. She'd deliver plenty of flat bread, *nan* [Nahn], which was not only food but the main utensil. We'd tear off a piece and pinch a bit of rice and veggies from the platter with the *nan* and then put the whole assembly into our mouths. Often the soup was in just one large bowl and each person reached forward with their own spoon and took their spoonful from the nearest side of the common bowl. These people lived very simply, but entertained lavishly.

In one home we rose early and prepared to move on, only to discover that our bodies were covered with little red bumps (bedbug bites). In another I went to use the "toilet" and found a straw structure like an Indian teepee that was about four feet high. On one side was an opening. I looked inside and could see a round hole in the dirt. I wondered how I'd manage to squeeze my backside into the low straw roof opening (I am six feet tall) and still get a good aim at that four inch hole in the ground. Enough said.

The hospitality of those who had so little never ceased to amaze us. We had come to bring them a message of hope, and they had given us acceptance, generosity and true hospitality.

One morning we stopped the VW to admire a steep hillside covered in full blooms. Set among the flowers were a hundred or so boxes, bee hives. No sooner had we stopped the van than a Kurd appeared and invited us to climb the slope for a breakfast of

---

[28] Here's an interesting tidbit: Up to 50% of the deaths on the Oregon Trail are attributed to cholera - which is a water born illness. I was very aware of the risks of illness from dirty water or dishes. https://en.wikipedia.org/wiki/California_Trail#Deaths

tea, bread and fresh honey. He opened a hive, brought out a chunk dripping with honey and served us like royalty, as we sat on crates looking at the early morning sunrise. On another occasion we parked our bus at the side of a lake for the night. Some fishermen invited us out on their boat and we spent the afternoon pulling in nets.

One man met us in a small town and invited us up to his village in the mountains. We drove for an hour, well beyond the reach of the Turkish military garrison. These garrisons are placed along major roads to keep an eye on the Kurds. At night all the soldiers return in their armored personnel carriers and park behind stone walls and inside the barbed wire. When we reached the home of this man we were surprised to see he had an entire wall of his home decorated with a tapestry depicting Christ praying in the garden of Gethsemane. He joyfully watched the Jesus video with fascination and we left him a copy.

On the way back down the mountain track we were met by two Turkish police standing in the narrow dirt roadway. We stopped and Marcus rolled down his window.

"May we see your passports?" they said in Turkish. We handed them Marcus' German passport and my US one.

"Follow us," they abruptly stated, and they pocketed our passports. We realized that we had just been placed under arrest.

Naturally we followed their tiny white sedan down the rest of the hill and to the main police station. We were immediately separated and led to private rooms by an officer. For over two hours they interrogated us individually. I had been filming things on our trip with a camcorder and they insisted on watching every minute of it. Then they searched our vehicle. They did not find the VCR nor the videotapes of the Jesus Film. We knew that even though they were legal they would be confiscated. We did not drive four thousand kilometers so we could give our six video tapes to the police in Erzincan [err zinn JOHN]. On our long trip down from Berlin we had given careful thought about storing the videotapes. Before we boarded the ferry to cross from Italy to Greece Marcus had removed the large boxy taillight housings on the VW bus and stashed all the tapes in the big vacant holes of the rear quarter panels.

After the interrogation at the police station we were released and we continued on our journey. In our rear view mirror a little white police car followed us wherever we went. The police proceeded to take telephoto photos (quite flagrantly) of everybody we talked to. People avoided us like the plague. Marcus couldn't even go into the barber shop for a haircut without the employees getting captured on film. People were clearly intimidated. That night we again slept at somebody's home who welcomed us eagerly. But the police arrived early in the morning and interrogated the terrified family members. Then they confiscated the gospels we'd given them and the video story of the life of Jesus.

We knew we had to change our plans.

Marcus had lived in Turkey and knew that each province had its own police force. Telephone communication was very sketchy and it was unlikely the Erzincan police would call the next province if we left Erzincan entirely. (There are 81 provinces in Turkey.) We hoped they would stop harassing us and photographing our friends if we left their province. We decided that we first needed to lose our tail.

Late in the afternoon, when most Turkish men want to take a nap, we drove up a narrow mountain road to a magnificent waterfall park. This was a unique park because an enormous amount of water gushed right out of giant rocks in the hillside. There was no (above ground) river that fed the waterfall, just a hillside covered with stones. Because it was so unique and quite beautiful it had been made into a park. The waterfall was at the end and top of a long road. The police were satisfied that we wanted to have a picnic so they parked their car at the bottom of the road and waited for us to come back down to get back out onto the two-lane highway.

An hour later, after we had taken a good bath in the icy stream, we climbed back into our bus, released the brake, and rolled quietly all the way down the hill past the police, who were fast asleep in their car. As soon as we hit the bottom of the hill Marcus started the engine, turned right and we continued driving until we'd reached the next province, Tunjeli [toon JELL ee].

It's important to note that during this period Kurdish separatists in eastern Turkey were taking European tourists hostage and holding them for ransom, to fund their Marxist revolution. We knew about this risk when we started our journey. However, we did not know that Tunjeli province was the center for these activities.

For almost an hour we climbed a very dusty dirt road that ran along the edge of a cliff and stream outside the city of Tunjeli. Finally we could see the summit up ahead. The mountains around us were not just gorgeous they were formidable. At the summit we were stopped at a checkpoint by armed Turkish soldiers. We stopped and greeted them in German. If Marcus had spoken to them in Turkish there would have been a long discussion about why he, a foreigner, could speak their language so well. It was not a dialogue we wished to have. In broken German they asked us where we were going. (Some two million Turks live in Germany and many return to Turkey to do their military service, so for many Turks, German is a second language.) We explained we were heading down into the valley to visit the headwaters of the Munzur river. It is a beautiful landmark that is visited by many tourists. We also would be passing through Ovacik [OH vah jick], which is where a man named Jamal[29] lived. He had written to Marcus after hearing a radio message, but of course we didn't tell this to the guards at the checkpoint. It would only have caused Jamal grief.

"Es ist geschlossen!" he announced, referring to the roadway. (It is closed.) We asked him why he hadn't closed the road at the bottom of the forty five minute dusty climb, rather than at the top. He provided no answer, as if we'd expected one. We begged him to let us past so we could see this amazing Turkish waterfall and natural wonder. It was to no avail. He told us we had to turn around.

Forty five minutes later, after eating more dirt sucked in through the open windows, we rolled back into the main capital of Tunceli province, a city bearing the same name. We stopped at the market to buy some fruit and consulted our map.

"Look, Marcus. If we drive all the way around this mountain range there is one more skinny road that goes down into the Tunceli valley. Maybe we could get in to see Ovacik that way." He

---

[29] Name changed for security

was skeptical, as was I. It would probably be just another closed road. But we knew that the fellow who'd written Marcus was sincere about knowing Christ, the Messiah. Many Muslims have had visions and dreams of Jesus, who calls to them to "Come," or "Follow Me." Muslims put much greater emphasis on dreams and their meanings, than westerners. When a Muslim decides to seek the Messiah, they are intensely certain He is the Way, the Truth, and the Life[30].

So we decided to give the long detour a try, even though it meant an extra eight-hour drive. Toward dusk, just about ten kilometers before the "little road" we'd seen on the map, we saw a line of Turkish tanks doing target practice. It was a grim reminder of the intensity and seriousness of this conflict between Kurds and Turks, a battle that has raged on and off since 1903. We were slowly climbing a steep hill when off to the right a group of Turkish soldiers on foot appeared out of some bushes. They pulled us over.

"Now what?" we thought. To our pleasant surprise they just wanted a lift.

It is not uncommon for people who are rich enough to own cars to give other folks free rides in Turkey, especially when they are way out in the country. Otherwise the people might walk all day on foot in the blazing heat just to get to town. So Marcus was happy to help them out. After all, we had a great big van. These four soldiers happened to be going to their barracks and they had a fifty kilo sack of rice with them. They did not relish the thought of hefting it up the hill the last four kilometers to their barracks. They flopped it on the floor inside our van. We kept driving.

Around the next bend was another checkpoint. *"Dear God,"* I silently prayed. *"If we get turned back here, there will be no way at all to get to the town of Ovacik."* It was a serious prayer. Our Turkish passengers then shouted something to the guards and the guards lifted the gate. I realized in a flash that the soldiers did not want to haul their rice sack to their barracks, so they had allowed us to enter onto their base. We were on that skinny little road that went into the valley of Tunceli. We were in!

---

[30] John 14:6

A short distance further the soldiers stopped us and they off loaded their cargo. They wished us well. If they only knew! We continued on down the one lane road thinking at any moment they might come and fetch us back, but they never did. We honestly felt the presence of God in a special way. It seemed like his angels had cleared the way for us to travel right past the guards. It was like he had shut the mouth of the lions.[31]

It was a very windy and rutted mountain one lane track that led us down into the valley. The cliff dropped straight off to the left of the van. There were no guardrails. We made one stop at a village that had been carved into the mountain side. Goats wandered in an open courtyard. We could see the flat mud roofs as we descended down the dusty path, the VW bouncing along.

"Glad we put new shocks on in Thessaloniki, (in Greece)" Marcus said. I was more concerned about the brakes.

We were greeted with a cautious hello by the herdsman. When they understood we were just passing through they insisted we pause and come into their humble abode. A blackened fire pot was propped on three stones in front of an open wall. The roof and wall were covered in soot. This was where the lady of the house did all her food preparation, and no doubt where they heated water if they wanted a warm bath. The floor was dirt, the walls carefully fitted stones. The ceiling was poplar poles set about sixteen inches apart, covered with split wood, which was then covered with dirt. On the flat roof, where fruit and vegetables were dried in the summer and where their goats wandered at other times, was a long concrete cylinder with a bowed handle. When it rained this concrete roller was used to press the water out of the muddy roof to minimize leakage inside.

Turkey does not invest as much in infrastructure in the eastern part of their country. Istanbul has seen an influx of Kurds recently, as their villages in the east have been systematically destroyed and people re-located. Diyarbakir, the largest city in the east, has seen an explosion of growth as apartment buildings spring up like summer wheat. Entire village populations are moved into the cities and former farmers and shepherds have to take menial jobs.

---

[31] Daniel 6:22

Most Kurdish girls in the east had not been to school; instead staying at home to help their mothers in household chores. Life in the village is hard.

"I need a haircut," I said to Marcus as we finally rolled into Ovacik.

"First let's get a bite to eat," he countered. So we drove down the valley towards the famous falls and found a very nice restaurant overlooking the rushing river. The water was almost milky white. We found a table outside on the open deck. I greeted the men we saw around us in Kurdish, which caught them by surprise. There were no Americans who spoke their forbidden language. Most of the men had been to school and learned Turkish, but Kermanji was still their heart language.

"*Tu Kurd i,*" they would say to me, ("You are a Kurd.")

"*Ne, Ez Amerikî me,*" I replied. (No, I am an American.") Then there followed a dialogue I'd heard repeatedly.

"How come you know our language?" they'd ask.

"I studied it in school."

"No" they'd say, "There are no schools that teach Kurdish."

"Yes, there is. I went to one."

"Where?"

"In Berlin. At the Free University." They would look at me with amazement and delight. A single Kurdish language class had been added at the University during our fourth year in Berlin.

And so it went. They absolutely loved it. Speaking their language was a way of showing them dignity. It demonstrated that their culture had value, that they were not a worthless people. They have a rich tradition dating all the way back to at least 500 BC. In the book of Daniel the reign of the Medes and Persians is described. Kurds are considered to be the descendants of the Medes.

Marcus pulled out his *saz* in the restaurant and began to play in the old traditional style of Turkish musicians. Music can cross a thousand barriers and this day was no different. In no time there were eight or ten Kurds who had pulled up chairs and were listening to the melodies he plucked on his five string *saz* (which he had made himself). He did not have the greatest voice, but his heart was sincere and his smile winsome. They had not heard such lyrics or melodies before. But it was a distinctly Turkish in-strument and they loved it.

In Islam there is no singing during Friday morning prayers. Muslims love music, but they have never heard anyone sing praises to God. They do believe in the Zebura, (the Psalms), but have not read them, nor do they realize they were originally penned as words to melodies meant to be sung.

Some years before our visit, a Turk had become a follower of Jesus, and he was moved to pen some poetry, which was later put to the local style of traditional Turkish music. Marcus began to play some of those tunes and began to sing in Turkish. The men were transfixed.

Turning to me one of them said, "You know it is good you are a Kurd. Because if you weren't you'd make a good hostage." I didn't ask if he was serious. I was just glad I'd done my home-work.

Later that evening, while getting my haircut in the local barber shop Marcus casually asked if the barber knew Jamal (the one whom we'd come to visit.)

"Oh yes," the man answered. "He has started a 'Jesus Club." We were taken aback. First we had never heard of anything like a Jesus club, and the second thing that amazed us was this man spoke so openly. It seemed like the Kurds were far more open minded and religiously tolerant than their Turkish masters.

Later that evening we met Jamal and talked with him late into the night. His family hosted us, and he watched the Jesus video with his entire family - twice. I fell asleep long before it was done the first time.

I had seen it dozens of times already, even in gas stations. We often camped under the bright and secure lights of a filling station when we were out in the boonies (for safety), and the attendant who was sitting there all night (surely bored-to-death) keeping the station open, was more than willing to watch a video. But our copies were in Turkish, which I do not understand. Marcus would discuss finer points with them, answer questions, and leave them with an Injil (the New Testament) if they wanted one.

As we loaded our few things into the van the next morning Jamal came to us and asked if he could join us on our journey. He said he could always find his way home when we had to leave Turkey. He wanted so much to learn more, to become a student of the Gospel. It would be a great opportunity to teach him so much more. Then we thought about the challenges that we would have to face as we crossed the many Turkish checkpoints. It would be even more suspicious if a German, an American and a Kurd were traveling through the countryside. We also thought about his town and how much his friends and family needed him. We did not want him to get drawn to the west, but rather drawn to Jesus. Christianity was born in the Middle East. It is not a western religion. Jamal should stay in his town and be a witness. We had to turn his offer down and regretfully travel on without him.

The next province we drove through was Elazig.[32] While staying in a vacant campground on the edge of a lake outside of the town we noticed there were lots of frogs.

"Hey, Marcus, have you ever eaten frogs?" I should have known his answer. Germans are not French. "You catch 'em and I'll cook 'em," I told him. This was too much of a challenge for him to just let it go. He developed a plan.

"I can catch these things, just watch!" he proclaimed. With a long reed of grass in his right hand, and a white five gallon bucket in his left hand, he made his way down to the murky water's edge. We were all alone at the campground, having parked the VW bus right down by the water so we could give it a bath. Thus, nobody saw our ridiculous antics. He wiggled the end of the reed. The frog saw the movement and began to hop toward the reed. I noticed that Marcus was wearing a nice long sleeve white dress shirt. He continued to stretch out over the green muck in pursuit of the frog. He held his bucket down low near the water's edge. Wham! He grabbed the frog in his left hand, threw it in the bucket, and covered it with a rag.

With a big smile on his face, and the look of a proud third grader on his face he said, "I told you I could do it!"

I realized I was going to have to keep my end of the bargain. So I got our stove and frying pan out. I had no idea how to cook a

---

[32] https://www.mapsofworld.com/turkey/turkey-political-map.html

frog, and had certainly never eaten one. But a challenge is a challenge. Marcus caught several more in no time at all.

"Who's going to kill 'em?" he asked. "Seems to me it ought to be the cook." I reluctantly volunteered to do the grisly deed.

"Where's your axe?" I asked. We then located a tree stump and I quickly dispatched the frogs and let their legs fall into the fry pan. I figured a bit of butter was called for; the French put butter on everything.

What I didn't know was I should have skinned the legs before frying them. This may have been a critical step. We also had no flour nor garlic. We did have salt. After frying them for a bit we each ate one. We decided there must be more to the preparation than what we'd done. We tossed the rest.

Our journey continued and was filled with many interesting characters. One night we pulled into a town and stopped to grab a bite to eat. The "cafe" was an open air make-shift shelter. We ordered eggs. I noted a creek ran behind the cafe in a shallow ditch. I wondered if this was where the dishes were rinsed and maybe washed.

Stay with me, I'm coming to my point.

A highlight was our climb up the manmade hill at Nemrut [nehm Root]. It was built by Antiochus I (69-34 BC). At the top of this seven thousand foot mountain were enormous statues, erected by the king, probably in honor of himself. Each statue was thirty feet tall and some of the stones used weigh an estimated nine tons. This place was usually inundated with tourists; it even had a helicopter pad for visiting dignitaries. But we were all alone, since some tourists had been taken hostage and the remainder changed their travel plans. We walked around for a bit and took pictures. During our descent down the steep rocky incline my stomach began feeling queazy.

"Marcus, do you have anything for an upset stomach?" I asked. We stopped eventually at a shop and bought some pills and some Pepto Bismo. It really didn't help. I wondered what was happening inside me. The word "upset" does't really begin to describe my digestive nightmare.

Turkey's roadways were not peppered with attractive rest stops. Restrooms along the wide expanse of roads between towns were non-existent. I was reduced to near instant requests that we stop our bus, at which point I'd launch myself from the vehicle to locate some bush or rock behind which to "rest." It was not pretty at all.

We made a few more stops to sleep, like in Adana, where a couple years earlier I had passed through with pancreatitis and spent the night on the airport floor. Only this time we stayed with a Kurdish family and watched the Jesus film together. Finally we reached the Marmara Sea and then after a night we crossed the Bosphorus bridge to reach the European side of Istanbul. I was feeling really poorly. We pulled into a Turkish hospital to run a test. I was shocked when they gave me a paper pill-container about one inch in diameter for my fecal sample. That was all. *"What are they thinking anyway?"* I will spare you the details. The sample indicated I did not have amoebic dysentery. That was all they tested it for.

Marcus was doing most of the driving now, since I felt so lousy. He drove straight through as long as he could. When we reached southern Germany I knew I needed to go to a hospital immediately, but preferred my hospital in Berlin - where I had a medical chart, a history and a chance of recovery. It is easier to battle a chronic illness in familiar surroundings with physicians who know the patient's history. So Marcus took me to the airport in Freiburg and I said goodbye to my dear friend and his VW Transit. I then flew into Templehof, Berlin's domestic airport built in 1927.[33] From there it was a familiar ride to the hospital in Zehlendorf - where I was nurtured back from the edge. I was diagnosed with hepatitis A.

To this day I do not know if I got sick from eating frog legs with their skin, or whether it was the unwashed dishes from which we'd eaten the eggs, the many glasses we'd shared, the plastic water jug that carried our spring water in the hundred degree heat, or if it was something else. Certainly we were exposed to all sorts of things on that journey. Sometimes illness is a price peo-

---

[33] This was the airport used during the famous 1948-1949 airlift. The Soviets had blockaded the city for 15 months, preventing any food or supplies into West Berlin. The allies fed the city by continuous flights into Templehof.

ple pay who go to the tough places. While I was in the hospital DeAnna returned from the US to Berlin with our girls. After my discharge she began a lengthy period of caring for me in our apartment.

She said to me recently, in a serious no-nonsense tone, "You have no idea what it was like; you were asleep all the time!" For a full six months, I mostly slept. I was a jaundiced figure, skin and bones hanging on to a frail frame. My wife had to struggle just to wake me, and then force me to eat something, while at the same time caring for our two energetic girls, ages three and four. She did not know if I would ever come back from the precipice. I was of no help around the apartment at all. She went out to buy groceries, took our oldest to preschool, handled the finances. I was pretty much oblivious of life. I can honestly say I have no recollection of those six months of life. She did it all, for me. I could get myself up and eat, go to the bathroom, and then go back to bed. That was pretty much it.

I cannot imagine what it was like for her to return from abroad and find her husband hanging on to life, all the time wondering, *"What will become of me now? What will happen to our daughters?"*

I salute her. I simply cannot repay her for her devotion or faithfulness. To me she is a saint. Without her I would not be here; I owe her my life. She is like the, "Friend that is closer than a brother."[34] The Scripture also says, "Greater love has no one than this: to lay down one's life for one's friends."[35] She truly laid down all the desires for herself and spent her life for me.

Surviving hepatitis A or any illnesses, requires a commitment to the truths of faith, hope, and love. And as the apostle Paul says in his letter to Corinth, "The greatest of these is love."[36] A loving support network when facing any major illness is key. It is not a struggle that can be fought alone.

---

[34] Proverbs 18:24b

[35] John 15:13

[36] 1 Corinthians 13:13

Chapter 19

Good People

Across the inside of my left forearm is a three inch scar that runs at a right angle to the arm. This scar has a special story. It lies across the brachioradialis muscle, if you know muscles. It runs right across the direction of the arm's veins. It was in the spring of 1993 that I was given that scar, and it never served any purpose. It was not an accident; it was a calculated attempt by surgeons in an excellent German hospital in Freiburg, southern Germany. They were doing something called a "cut down."

I have, as I have mentioned numerous times, difficult-to-find veins. That is primarily because they are no longer there. A nurse, or in some countries it's a doctor, does their absolute best *not* to inflict pain when starting an intravenous line. (Sometimes, when the tape is removed from my skin they seem to lack that sensitivity. Ouch!) The needle is poised above the skin, as he or she gently palpates the skin with the hope that the targeted vein will jump up and say, "Here; stick me here!" It never happens of course. A really good phlebotomist can feel the vein with the most delicate touch. I liken it to the sensitivity I can feel in my palm when I gently swipe my hand across a sanded piece of body work on the car that I restored. I can feel the highs and lows of the surface - even when they are completely invisible to the naked eye. I really admire phlebotomists who have that touch.

So many medical professionals have tried to start IV's on me, or draw blood from my pathetic skinny limbs, that I sometimes just count their failed attempts to pass the time.

A lot of preparation goes in to prepping a patient before the cannula is unsheathed and the steel is prodded through the flesh.

There is an IV pole, a bag of saline, tubing that is hung and primed, sometimes an IV pump that's in place, the requisite strips of tape that are ready to be slapped on my hairy forearm, alcohol squares known simple as two by two's and the latex gloves.

"Are you allergic to latex?" I am asked.

"No, I am just allergic to new nurses."

The top count for IV attempts on me was actually in Germany, in a very modern and well equipped hospital, and in the children's ward no less, where physicians are used to tiny arms and tiny veins. I was stuck twenty-two times! I was dehydrated because I had a raging fever. The body sweats fluid to try and cool itself down, hence the dehydration. A nurse reading this would say, *"Well of course!"* When someone is dehydrated their veins go flat and it is difficult for the nurse to see if the needle is in the vein. If you are a patient and on the way to a hospital and you have bad veins, take this advice, "Drink plenty of water before you get there." Once you are in emergency they won't let you drink anything anyway until you've been examined, which might take six hours.

I felt sad for the poor German doctors; they kept fetching a new doc because nobody was willing to undergo the continuous agony of afflicting pain on me. They tried for two hours to get the IV going. At many US hospitals, particularly where nurses have to start the IV's, they have a "two sticks only" policy. Then they go fetch another nurse to try some more. That means that everything the first nurse has learned during those two failed attempts is lost knowledge, as the new nurse approaches my bedside and starts tapping my ante cubital site again.

"I have not had a vein at that site in forty years," I say. "I have no veins there," I tell her. She keeps tapping. *"Oh well,"* I think. *"Let her figure it out for herself."* Two hefty bruises later from blown veins she apologizes and traipses off to pass the baton. Blessed be the nurse who actually listens to the patient when he/she says, "Here is my best vein. Try here."

If I sound cynical it is because I am. Most medical professionals assume that since I am the patient and they are the practitioner I must know next to nothing about medicine. They don't understand that I have had more than a thousand IV's. And when I tell them this I know they are trying hard not to roll their eyes. It is the same if I tell them I've been an inpatient in hospitals over a hundred times. So I continue to endure their learning curve.

But back to the story about the cut down. After many failed attempts as an impatient at the *Universitaetsklinikum Freiburg* (University Medical Center in Freiburg) the doctors decided to send me to surgery and put in a lengthy catheter into a major vein. The plan was to place a "port" in my forearm, which would perform just like it sounds, as a docking place for future veinous access. Placed under the flesh, which is sewed up over the device, the port allows a needle to be pushed straight down through the surface flesh. The port has a rubber surface on top and a steel plate on the bottom. The special access needle stops when it hits the metal plate. Attached to the port inside the arm is a long catheter, maybe eighteen to twenty-four inches long and it runs to the heart. This allows for a full two week course of antibiotics without getting stuck a bunch of times every three days. Another beauty of this invention is that when I am discharged the port remains in me, and is ready for use in the future.

Normally I'm given a short one to two inch catheter that lasts just three days (if one is lucky.) To find a big vein for use with a port the doctor was going to have to cut down through the flesh in my arm. The procedure couldn't be done in the patient's hospital room; it had to be done in surgery. So I signed the papers and was transported down to the surgical suite. I am not sure why they call it a suite, because there are no couches or wide screen televisions or a kitchenette.

This hospital, unlike the other fifty that I had seen, had the most unique means of moving the patient from the gurney into the operating theatre. (Again there are no TV's in this theatre.) My gurney was rolled up alongside a "window" that was maybe eight feet long. Extending out over the window was a ledge that was wrapped with a rubber mat, similar to those people-movers you stand on at some airports. The gurney was brought up to the height of the ledge and I was pushed, lifted, and nudged over until my body lay on this rubber mat. The mat began moving and before I knew it I was transported through the wall and was on the inside of the operating room. The rotation stopped and I was then moved onto the operating table/gurney. That was how the room was kept sterile; there were no swinging doors to the outside nor gurneys that had been in hospital corridors rolling in and out of the sterile room. Pretty cool.

The surgeon talked to me as he did his procedure (in German of course.) I will spare you the details. After an injection of lidocaine (the most amazing drug of all time - in my book) he explained he would be making a small cut and probing to find a nice straight vein. He began with a cut, perhaps one inch long. I don't know how deep, but he had to go pretty far down to find something worthy. Then he opened the innocent vein with the scalpel and inserted the catheter. These catheters are sheathed in a long skinny plastic bag so they stay sterile until the actual part that is to be inserted can be unveiled. He met with resistance.

"It seems there is an obstruction in this vein," he said. "Perhaps a scar from a previous IV, or maybe it's a junction." He decided to probe around a bit more. This continued and continued. After a while he would enlarge the cut at the surface so he could probe for more veins. He found a second vein but couldn't thread the catheter in for more than a couple inches. There was no way he could put the port in at that point; he needed to thread the whole catheter up inside my arm to get close to my heart.

So he opened up the arm a bit more in search of another vein. He did this over and over for a span of about two and a half hours. Pity the poor people who were waiting to use the operating room after our scheduled thirty minutes. He found a third vein and then a fourth, each time meeting resistance when inserting the catheter.

In the end he expressed profound apologies and stitched my arm up. I expressed my thanks for his efforts (I knew he had to be very discouraged) and was placed up on the shelf for my journey through the window and onto my waiting gurney. At the end of the day all I could show for the day's agony was a nice bandage on my arm. At least I still had a tiny IV in my right arm to keep antibiotics flowing until plan B was formulated.

In this experience and in countless others I have learned not to be bitter or hold grudges against medical professionals (though it is still a challenge). They have saved my life innumerable times. It is also true that I almost lost my life numerable times through failures in pharmacology, surgery, and patient care. However, there is nothing to be gained by reciting all these failures, although it would make for some great stories. In each case I notified the appropriate person, i.e. head nurse, transplant coordinator, even the hospital CEO. But I have never ever had the desire to sue somebody for a screw up. Even when my seventy-eight year old father died from a medical oversight.

Colossians 3:13 says, Bear with each other and forgive one another if any of you has a grievance against someone. Forgive as the Lord forgave you." I know that God has forgiven me of all my wrongdoings. How, if I am to live like Jesus and if I invite Him to fill my whole life, can I not forgive others? Forgiveness is at the core of the Gospel of Jesus Christ. It is unique to the Christian faith. So I press on.

Plan B was to put the port device in my chest, on the right side. This time the surgery was successful, those veins had never had short peripheral IV's that caused scarring. For the next five years I was able to use this port for all my IV treatments. I was given a box of Huber needles to take home with me. When my German house doctor (yes they still have those!) ordered a course of IV antibiotics I would access the site myself with a Huber needle, fill an extension line with saline, connect the tubing, mix the powdered antibiotics with sterile water, fill the portable battery powered pump syringe, program it, and carry the whole kit with me wherever I need to go. Germans are more flexible than Americans with some things. Every country and hospital has its own protocols.

I had the most wonderful *Hausartzt* (private doctor), who lived in our village of Kandern, in southern Germany. We had moved there from Berlin in 1994. Dr. Joachim Gieringer would even come to my home if I was too weak to make the trip down the hill and across town to his office. It always felt funny when he'd come in with his black bag to take my temperature, listen to my lungs, and ask me questions about my health. It felt something like being royalty and living in the 1800's. But one night his personal attention saved my life.

I woke around two am and could not breathe. I was connected to oxygen via an oxygen concentrator, which I used at night. It was a large box parked beside my pillow on the floor. This is a machine that takes room air and removes the 78% nitrogen from the air, leaving just oxygen. When I woke that night, struggling for each breath, I knew my lungs were failing me.

I had noticed a decline for months. As my lung capacity fell below twenty-five percent I had begun taking a new medicine manufactured by Genentech. It worked by loosening the secretions in my lungs. This helped me clear some of the gunk that built up from infections. The medicine was put in my nebulizer and inhaled twice a day. Called Pulmozyme it had increased my breathing capacity to thirty-five percent, which was a huge improvement for me. It was not available in Germany, but as a US citizen I was able to fill prescriptions from American doctors. I had the best of both worlds: a private doctor and American meds! The difference between twenty-five and thirty-five percent meant I could walk and visit people instead of sitting on a couch all day. I could work.

But in the middle of that fateful night no medication was going to help me. I called Dr. Gieringer. I felt bad for calling him in the middle of the night. He came immediately to our apartment to check on me. He saw my blue lips, my hunched over torso fighting for each breath, and noted my elevated temperature. He called an ambulance. Soon I could hear the whaa-aah, whaa-ahh as it came up the hill in our peaceful neighborhood. I knew the hospital was four hours away in Freiburg and I expected a long ride - strapped down laying on my back of all things, the position which meant even more struggle to breathe. Then I would be admitted. One of the worst things about being checked into a hospital, especially one where you've never been a patient, is the time-consuming medical history that is taken. And I have something of a history. Then there are the battery of tests. It seems forever before one is actually in a patient room.

But I was amazed and blessed by Dr. Gieringer. He rode in the ambulance all the way to Freiburg. (I don't know how he got back home.) He gave great attention to my care during that journey. When we arrived he talked to the admitting staff and answered all their questions. Because I was gasping for air talking was extremely difficult. Having to answer questions deprived me of needed oxygen. Dr. Gieringer knew my medical history and knew the course of treatment I should be given. He also, as a doctor, could speak eye-to-eye with the admitting physician. He remained at the University Medical Center of Freiburg until I was given a bed and had an IV. He was a life saver.

I have had some great physicians on my health journey. If I began to list them all here it would take many pages. I have also had some friends who have gone above and beyond. One of them called me about the time I was coming out of the hospital in Freiburg.

"Dan, did you know it is now possible to do a lung transplant?" Chris Crossan asked me. It was very hard for me to think, when oxygen deprived, and even harder to make life or death decisions. I was more inclined to just sink lower and lower. In fact about the time Chris called me all I wanted was to live until spring so I could see the flowers bloom one more time in my little garden. I was that bad off.

Chris continued, "Look Dan, I want you to look in to this. You don't have to decide about surgery, just find out about it, okay?" Chris was such a nice guy it was hard to refuse him.

I told him, "I was shown an article about it in 1992 by Dr. Wahn in Berlin. He explained that although the surgery does sometimes work, there are precious few organs available in Germany. Especially lungs. The German public just isn't comfortable with the idea of donating parts of a loved one yet."

Chris wouldn't give up, "Well you need to try in America then."

"You mean fly all the way home just for a surgery?" (It sounds rather lame as I write this, but that's what I said.)

"Hey," he continued, "This is your *life* we're talking about!"

I had met Chris in the most unlikely places, in a twelve man army tent in Zakho, Iraq. He was the first person DeAnna and I met after we disembarked the bus with our two bags and looked at the NGO (Non Governmental Organization) relief encampment. We were shown his tent and he invited us to share it. Over the years, as Chris and I worked together in our shared interest of serving Kurds, we had become very close colleagues.

He called me again from his home in Frankfurt a few days later. "Listen Dan," he said. "I have put five hundred dollars in a special fund to pay for all the phone calls and faxes you will need to pay for, as you research hospitals in the United States. I really want you to look into this." I was dumfounded. I could see that he was really serious about this pursuit. So I began to do some research.

The first thing I learned was about UNOS. The United Network for Organ Sharing was a new agency that was intended to make organ availability somewhat "fair" for all the various hospitals and states who had need of them. It would also establish priorities to determine who would get an organ and when. After requesting the information, I received a fax with a list of fifty-five US hospitals that did double lung transplants.[37] UNOS said they would send me the survival statistics for any ten of these hospitals. I looked at the list of fifty-five. *"How do you make such a decision?"* I wondered. In the current day we could do an internet search, and gather more data in five minutes than I could have gathered in five months.

I selected ten hospitals that were near my home or near relatives' homes. I began faxing requests for information. It was important to have a support network and a suitable residence, both while waiting and also after the transplant. I didn't want to be in Pittsburgh, for example, even if they had a great center, because I have never even been there and don't have any kind of link with that area. It was easy for me to choose Stanford University Medical Center; it was just forty-five minutes from my home. It also had a 95% survival rate at the time and 50% of their patients were alive three years after the transplant. That might not seem like much to the reader, but to a guy whose dying it seemed awesome. Another three years of life sounded amazing. University of San Diego was also not too far if push came to shove. I selected some others too.

---

[37] At the time of this writing there were 74 US lung transplant centers. https://www.srtr.org/transplant-centers/?query=&distance=750&location=&state=&recipientType=adult&organ=lung&sort=rating

When I received the flood of faxes with all the material it took some time to sort through it all. The survival statistics were helpful, but also could be misleading. If a hospital boasts that fifty percent of its patients were alive after five years that might just be because they never attempt any surgeries unless the potential outcomes look really good. Other hospitals might be willing to take on really risky patients out of compassion, which could make their statistics not look too good.

As I weighed all the pros and cons Chris called again. "What have you discovered?" he asked. I told him I had chosen Stanford as my number one choice and San Diego as my second. "That's great," he said optimistically. "Listen Dan," he began in a somber tone, "Karen (his wife) and I have prayed about this a lot and decided that I'd like to donate one of my lungs." I couldn't believe it. Here was a guy with four young daughters, a demanding job, an exciting future, and he was offering to risk his very life for me! I was speechless. There was a silence as I digested what he was offering.

"Chris," I began. "I cannot even fathom such a decision. It overwhelms me." I swallowed. "I really, really appreciate you, brother. You have the biggest heart of anybody I have ever known. I am deeply moved that you would take such a huge risk for me. I don't know what to say."

"You don't have to say anything," he said. "Just get on a list and get that transplant!"

Later I learned that I would have to have two lungs from the same donor. I appreciated his enormous sacrifice but it wouldn't work. It wasn't like a kidney transplant. They could not replace just one lung because if they did, the remaining bad lung would quickly infect the new one. I didn't even mention that there was the issue of blood type and lung size because there was no point in it. Quietly inside I was glad there was no way it could happen; it would have been too much for me to think of the risks to him and his family.

But in that moment I realized that this man was more of an expression of the true sacrificial love of Christ than I would probably ever witness. Chris was willing to risk death that a friend might live. Friends like that are not easy to find. Chris is a friend like no other.

Good doctors. Good nurses. Good friends. A God who cares. I have been blessed beyond my writing ability to express it.

Chapter 20

125 Pounds

The evaluation (to be put on the waiting list to receive a transplant) was as confusing as it was lengthy. The extent of preparation is understandable as I look back. But for the person entering this new reality it seemed like an insurmountable list of tests and requirements. It began with my introduction to Dr. Theodore. He struck me immediately as rather distant and almost unfriendly. For those who knew him well this was not true, but for the new patient it sure seemed this way. I later learned from his nurse that he acted that way toward his new patients to protect himself from grief. Many of his patients died before receiving a transplant. She assured me that he was warm and friendly once it became apparent that I would survive. Somehow I didn't find this very reassuring. Besides the X-ray, the lung function test, the blood work, the heart echo, the EKG, the full medical history, a stress echo, and much more, there was a minimum weight requirement.

I only weighed one hundred twenty-five pounds. Ever since I was about sixteen I had weighed that much. I had grown to be six feet tall but hadn't gained weight. I know most readers are thinking how wonderful it would be to have a free pass to eat as much ice cream and chocolate as one wanted, but for those afflicted with the inability to gain weight it is no laughing matter. Some fat is important to maintain health. In many countries an attractive woman is a fat one. That's not true in America, but then neither are malnutrition, malaria, and starvation national health concerns.

For me the lack of weight meant I got sick quicker, I became dehydrated faster, and I did not recover as soon after being bed ridden. Perhaps the only advantage of being a light weight meant less physical work for me to walk and also to breathe.

"You have to weigh at least one hundred forty pounds," Dr. James Theodore (1935-2003) explained to me during my lung transplant evaluation. He was the medical physician at Stanford University Medical Center that was responsible for conducting all the pre-transplant evaluations. This was one of the many criteria the hospital had determined would give the patient the best chance of survival. This was the bottom threshold. I looked at him with amazement, as if it was some sort of joke.

"I have weighed one hundred twenty-five pounds for the last twenty-two years," I told him. "There is simply no way for me to gain weight. I have tried supplements, exercise programs, and have eaten everything I can to gain just one pound. But I can't gain weight!" He was not impressed. "I even put special oils and fatty acids in my diet. Still I cannot gain an ounce." Ensure Plus, high protein shakes, taking enzymes with every meal and every snack - nothing helped. I told him there was no hope for me to gain weight.

Dr. Theodore replied, "Mr. Lagasse, that is the requirement." I was afraid this could be a deal breaker.

"Well what should I do?" I asked.

"We can put a stomach tube in," he said casually. That sounded ghastly to me, not to mention uncomfortable.

"What do you mean?"

He then explained it as if it were as easy as putting a bandage on a finger, "We just put a hole through your abdomen and put a plug in. To give you nutrition we connect up a feeding tube with a pump and you plug the tube into the port that goes into your stomach." I could not begin to imagine what on earth he was talking about. It sounded awful.

"Let me try on my own to gain weight this month," I said, not believing I could really do it. I just knew I didn't want a hole poked through my abdomen.

That month I ate as much as I could all day long. The problem with stuffing my stomach, however, was that it pushed up on my diaphragm. That in turn made breathing much more difficult. And it was breathing - or the lack of it - that was my main problem. I realized I was not going to move that hundred twenty-five ceiling any higher, no matter how hard I tried. I finally relented and was scheduled for surgery.

I asked later how the surgery was performed, since I was anesthetized the whole time and missed the action.

"Oh, it's not hard," the gastroenterologist said. In order to insert a Percutaneous Endoscopic Gastrostomy (PEG) we first inflate the abdomen. In my mind I was picturing a peg, like the kind that's put into a wine barrel. I looked down at my belly at the plastic plug with a hinged cap on it. Indeed it looked and functioned just like a plastic peg. He continued, "Once the gut is inflated we illuminate it on the inside with an endoscopic light. The spot on the abdomen that shows the brightest is where the stomach is closest to the surface. That's where I insert the scalpel."

"So basically I was stabbed in the stomach," I thought. Okay, so it was a very small stab. I guess any surgery is rather crude when you come right down to it.

"When I have a small incision made I quickly insert the peg," he concluded. It turns out that the stomach has an incredibly fast healing time. The hole that is made on the inside of the stomach heals in around thirty minutes. This is a good thing, since the stomach contains some really harsh acid.

"The entire procedure takes from fifteen to twenty minutes," he said. With my new belly button in place, I was sent home to begin my new life getting fed at night.

The outside skin where the incision was made takes longer to heal, but the peg can last for a year. It is held in place by a small balloon that's part of the device. It is inflated inside the stomach. The balloon has an access point on the outside where a physician can take a regular syringe and push air in to inflate the balloon. The plug itself opens and closes, similar to a valve on on an air mattress. *"This is pretty clever,"* I thought and I began to use it.

Every night DeAnna would role the IV pole with a special pump hooked onto it into our bedroom. We were living with her parents in their former dining room. (Bless their hearts!) They had built a wall and installed a door and it had become our bedroom. Hanging from the pole was a bag, not unlike a standard saline bag. Only this bag was opened at the top and two cans of high calorie nutritional formula were poured in. This is not something you would want to drink; it even said so on the can. I am sure it would have tasted nasty. Each eight ounce can contained five hundred calories of stuff my body needed. It was a light brown color.

During the day I ate huge meals, taking in an estimated three thousand to thirty-five hundred calories. At night, while the pump made its rhythmic thump-thump thump-thump, I received another one thousand calories. That's a lot of calories. It's also a lot of volume. My stomach was full all of the time. I was miserable.

Getting into bed was a trick. I had an IV pole with a standard intravenous line giving me antibiotics. Then there was the oxygen tube that hung in my nostrils at one end and was connected to the oxygen concentrator on the other. And now I had the feeding pump and its plastic line that went under the covers and into my abdomen. Attaching it was rather simple. Just unplug the PEG and insert the tip of the feeding tube into the device. I hoped I didn't have to get up to use the bathroom.

I had to lay on my back, which made breathing difficult. But gaining weight was essential. I had to somehow reach that magical one hundred forty pound required weight! It seemed impossible. But I endured the discomfort of all the plastic lines laced about me. During the day, when the feeding pump was disconnected, and I was in between my IV antibiotic infusions, I just had the O2 line to deal with. I could walk across to the family room, get on the exercise bike, set the level to 0, lean forward to rest my upper body weight on the handle bars, then pedal for 30 minutes while I watched, "The Price is Right." The television show was just enough distraction to break the boredom. My body needed to keep moving if I was to be in any kind of shape to survive the transplant.

It was in the middle of the night when disaster struck. DeAnna had rolled over toward me on our king size mattress. She felt something wet and sticky on her arm. She instantly moved. There was more wet and sticky. She was awake immediately and she got up and turned the light on. Sixteen ounces of nutritional supplement had been pumped out onto our mattress instead of into my stomach. But that wasn't the worst part. The line had not just become "unplugged," rather the whole PEG had come entirely out of my abdomen. She looked at the mess in the bed. The clean-up would have to wait. Dan had to get to the hospital.

Quickly she got dressed and I tried to pull myself together. My pajamas were soaked in the stuff; my chest and belly covered in the mess. What a nightmare. The worst part was the knowledge that the inside of the stomach would heal closed within thirty minutes. We notified Stanford that we were on our way into emergency.

It is normally a thirty-five minute drive from Almaden Valley in San Jose to Stanford in Palo Alto (when there's no traffic). I am sure we made it in record time. Once at Stanford the Gastroenterologist met me in the Emergency Department and took a quick look at the situation. He held the tube and device in his hand and pushed it back through my abdomen. Then he connected a regular syringe and re-inflated the balloon inside to hold it in place. It was that simple. We felt both relief but also a bit annoyed. If we'd known all we had to do was push the device back in we could have done it at home and saved a lot of agony.

Much of medicine is just knowing the right little tricks to use in the right situation. I learned this from watching umpteen IV's started. I put my IV starting education to use one year while we were living in a tent on the border with Iraq. (That's a story in itself.) We had a dehydrated woman on our team who had an infection. And I started an IV in her forearm. There are important steps to follow, sterile procedure to observe, and an amount of skill and knowledge to possess. But with that PEG it was as simple as grabbing it and pushing it back in the hole.

For the next eighteen months I used that feeding device. On the average I gained almost a pound a month. When I was wheeled in for my transplant surgery I weighed exactly one hundred forty pounds. I was very pleased, as was Doctor Theodore, though he tried not to show it. The PEG never fell out again, but we would have many more lessons to learn, both in medicine, in patience, and in courage. The PEG was to prove invaluable to me, even after my transplant.

Chapter 21

Gall Bladder Surgery

"Faith Is Being Sure of What You Hope For"[38]

It was November of 1995 in San Jose.

"Man my stomach hurts," I said to DeAnna. I normally didn't get stomach aches. Except for the two times I had pancreatitis, when my pancreas was blocked and the enzymes were actually digesting the organ itself. Oh, and then there was hepatitis A. Other than that I could not remember having had stomach pains. This pain was a little more toward the middle of my stomach, near the navel. And it didn't hurt nearly as bad. I tried to ignore it.

But as the day wore on and the pain persisted into the next day I decided it was time to see a doctor. I never liked succumbing to a doctor's visit, because it meant possibly giving up my freedom. Nobody likes to be admitted to a hospital and told what to do. And of course doctors are used to telling people what to do and hopefully patients comply. I usually followed orders, but generally only after I got a lot of information and some questions answered. Knowing *why* makes compliance easier. This time was no different.

The doctor asked where the pain was. He poked around my abdomen which seemed pretty unnecessary to me as it was creating a lot of discomfort. Then he ordered some lab work and radiology reports. Finally he had some results.

---

[38] <u>Hebrews 11:1</u>

He announced, "I think you have an infected gallbladder." At first he used a fancy term (which I have forgotten) and so I had to ask what it was. This gave him a psychological advantage. I wasn't even sure what the gallbladder was used for, and was even less sure where it was located. Although by the pain in my belly I could make a good guess.

"What do you do for that," I asked? It's funny how men think. There has to be a "fix" for every problem. So I asked him what he did for a gall bladder infection.

"We take it out," was his simple answer. I looked a little shocked. I imagined one of those long scars in my side that you read about in magazines where people in India have their organs stolen. "We do it laparoscopically," he said. He then explained what that was. In 1995 it was a fairly new technology. "We make three small incisions about a centimeter long each. A "centimeter" still sounded like a lot, as I thought about a cut in my stomach. But he continued. "We insert a catheter into each incision, one for a camera, one for the scalpel, and one for a grabbing tool." I can't remember his actual words but that was the gist of it. It sounded pretty simple. They would just cut out the source of the nasty pain in my gut and pull it (deflated of course) out one of the tiny incisions. I was "all in," as they say.

I simply said, "Go for it."

So a while later, I answered the perfunctory insurance questions, completed the admission procedure, responded to the sobering questions about the advanced directive, and got my two armbands. (In case one arm falls off and they can't find it?) Then I checked in at the correct department, and heard the familiar instructions, "Disrobe completely and put this gown on, with the ties in the back," (as if I had no idea how to put a gown on). I was now ready for pre-op. I lay on the gurney lined up next to a row of other people – all who looked *much* older than I, and waited for the inevitable: the insertion of the IV. They always need the intravenous line so they can, "make you comfortable." That is a euphemism for "keep you from making a fuss." Plus they need to give you fluids, which means plenty of saline. This helps relieve some of the stress put on the heart. Of course they don't say that, rather one's told, "We need to give you some fluids."

Then the nurse sits down in a chair next to and below your gurney, while you are trying unsuccessfully to keep your body parts covered with a tiny gown, and she takes a complete medical history.

"May I have a warm blanket please?" I have learned to ask. This accomplishes two things. First it helps give you a sense of actually being covered up, and second it mitigates the freezing temperature in which they always keep the pre-op rooms. Then come a litany of inquiries about one's health history and allergies. I will never forget my brother's response after he had submitted to his umpteenth similar interrogation.

"Look," he said while in pain, "Please read my chart yourself. You'll see that I have already answered these same questions *three* times." Well, he may not have been that irritated or rude to the nurse, but the sentiment certainly expresses how I often felt. I thought, *"Here I am about to be put to sleep for what could be the last time in my life, and I am kissing my wife for what could be her last kiss from me, and you are asking me for the sixteenth time if I am allergic to latex!"*

I am always a bit groggy when I wake up in the post-op room. It usually takes about an hour to recover my senses – so to speak. I guess I was taking so long to wake up they decided to just send me back to my room I had been given on the ward. It has never been explained to me why I was not kept in the recovery room until I was lucid (as is protocol), but not being one to initiate law suits I never found out. Instead I was sent to recover from the surgery on the "floor", rather than being sent home right away. The floor is hospital-speak for a regular ward; it is not actually the linoleum floor. Since I was so compromised with my lungs being perpetually filled with "gunk" as they politely say, they had sent me to the children's hospital, where people with cystic fibrosis were (at that time) being cared for. Nowadays it is recognized that although cystic fibrosis is a children's disease, advances in health care has made it possible for children to grow into adults. So places like Stanford University Hospital now have a clinic for adults with CF. But in 1995 (at age 37) I was still in the pediatric ward.

So I lay on a normal hospital bed. My beloved wife – who so faithfully sat beside me on countless plastic chairs in countless strange hospitals – waited for me to awaken. I am told I was a bit groggy and was unaware of what I did or said at the time. At least I take no responsibility for it. My dad and some others were in the room with DeAnna. I guess I was very happy to see my wife.

I leaned way over the side of the side of the bed, said, "I love you honey," and then gave her a big sloppy kiss or two and tried to grab her in some way. She hesitatingly told me about this quite later, (after the initial embarrassment had worn off). I then drifted back to sleep, no doubt with a grin on my face.

DeAnna is accustomed to surgical procedures and as an educated RN she has some concept of the way things are supposed to go. A regular floor nurse came in at intervals after the surgery and took my blood pressure. DeAnna assumed the young lady had everything under control. She waited an hour, then two, then four, and when after five hours I still had not woken, she called the charge nurse. They call her the charge nurse because she is "in charge" not because she runs your credit card each time you are given an aspirin.

"You mean he hasn't woken up?" the incredulous nurse asked. She looked at the sheet showing my recorded blood pressure readings. The floor nurse had neglected to report to anybody that my blood pressure was falling dramatically (which indicates internal bleeding). Her face turned a different color and then she pressed a button on the wall. It sent an alarm out to their staff. The look on the nurse's face did not cheer my wife up at all.

DeAnna said, "He fell asleep after they brought him from surgery and never woke back up." A different nurse quickly took my blood pressure, as doctors and other nurses flooded the tiny room. Apparently my blood pressure was very *very* low. I don't know how low, but I do know that I was rushed out of the room and taken back to the operating room. I was of course still "asleep". The charge nurse explained to DeAnna that the floor nurse was new and did not understand that falling blood pressures post-op indicated internal bleeding. As I lay in ER I lost a very decent shirt to a pair of scissors and a nasty long needle was inserted into a nice decent smooth piece of my chest.

They re-intubated me and then somehow ran tubes through the same tiny holes near my naval which they had stitched up, found the source of bleeding and somehow patched up my cystic artery. That is the artery which pumps blood (under high pressure) down into the lower extremities. I was later told that this artery is sometimes in an unusual location – about two percent of the time, which can lead to it being "nicked" during the operation. I was not really pleased to be among the special two percent.

Of course I only know all of this from my wife's narration. And she typically understates things. I *do* know that when I was medicinally awakened from the surgical repair after being extubated *I could not breathe*. There was a doctor leaning over me saying, "Breathe deeply." This is a ludicrous thing to say to someone who has been fighting a lung disease all of his life. There is no such thing as a deep breath. I had only known shallow breaths for the past ten years or so of my life. I had been on oxygen for a good part of the past five years. The doctor pointed to one of those computer screens you see in movies that show various bumpy lines and colorful numbers. I could see the O2 number, which should be in the high 90's but was around 72, and the CO2 number which should be low, indicating that your breath is effectively eliminating the carbon dioxide from your blood. I think I have this right. Anyway, my CO2 was way off as well. I knew this was very bad.

The doctor explained that normally they would intubate someone who had these kind of numbers. Intubation is when they pry your teeth apart with a special tool (after they have made you "comfortable") and then they stick a pipe which can be bent to "fit" your airway down your airway so a machine can take over the inhalation and exhalation that your body normally does without you thinking about it. Sorry to get so graphic about it, but you have to understand that being in the hospital and submitting your flesh to other people *is* a very graphic experience. I had already been intubated and subsequently extubated earlier that same day for the removal of my gall bladder. In the interim ten hours I had had no chance to clear my lungs of the build-up of bacteria-laden mucus. Prior to my surgery I had been doing lung clearance therapy four times a day, otherwise I could not breathe. On this day I had been lying prone for an entire day without clearing my lungs of the mucus that had been collecting. Plus I had just come out of two major surgeries and lacked the huge amount of strength it took to force myself to hack and cough the phlegm out.

"Normally we would intubate someone who has levels of carbon dioxide levels like yours," the doctor continued as he pointed to the monitor. "But in my experience if we intubate a cystic fibrosis patient in your condition, the patient is never able to be extubated." I knew he was being polite for saying the patient eventually died. Extubated is the wonderful experience when the tube is removed, the machine turned off, and you breathe on your own again. You have a terrible sore throat of course, but you are wide awake and you are *breathing on your own*. This is normally so wonderful it's like waking up from the dead.

Plus there was the fact that my abdomen had been cut up inside and that made coughing, which was primarily an abdominal exercise, very painful. I did my best, but it wasn't good enough. I understood what the doctor was saying, even if I didn't fully understand the numbers on the screen. He was saying that if he intubated me again I would indeed be seeing heaven pretty soon. I wasn't quite ready for that yet. I imagined myself in such a state. I would lay in a bed for a time with my family gathered around me listening to the drumming rhythm of the machinery that was breathing for me. But I would never breathe on my own again. My lungs would continue to fill with mucus, at an ever increasing rate, until there was no more room for any oxygen transfer. At the rate I fought for breath each day, coughing up crud to make room for air, I knew I might last for at most a day or two, maybe just a few hours.

The sedation I'd been given continued to wear off. I tried to cough. It was taking all my energy. I concentrated as hard as I could on my breathing. They were giving the maximum amount of oxygen they could through the nasal cannula but my oxygen saturation levels kept falling and falling.

My dad came in to see me. I was in the intensive care unit, although I have little recollection of anything in the room. I remember seeing the monitor and hearing the continual beeping. I can still see the bed in front of me. At some point I had gotten out of bed, because for a lung sick patient the most difficult place to be was on my back.

I sat in a chair (it is easier to breathe that way.) While facing the bed I rested my forehead on the edge of the bed and put my arms up on the bed as well. This opened my chest as much as possible and reduced my body weight from my chest area. Still I could not get enough air. I coughed and spit repeatedly. Then I would fight to get some air into my lungs again. My dad and my wife took turns coming into the intensive care unit to cheer me on, to love me, to pray for me, to hope I'd make it. But I felt I wasn't going to make it.

I could feel the energy leaving me. Most of us don't realize what drains us of energy. Our muscles work a lot to hold our head up straight. When we wash our hair it takes a lot of energy to hold our hands up to the height of our head. When we stand up it takes energy. It is so much easier to sit. Walking takes a lot of energy. To those of us who are healthy we are oblivious of this. But to those of us who are "over-the-hill" it becomes increasingly apparent. At age thirty-seven I was way over-the-hill.

I didn't think I could make it. I sensed the end was near. I was getting shorter and shorter of breath. Every time I worked up the energy to cough I was getting weaker. All I could think about was the next breath of air. I felt I was drifting away. I was feeling light headed. My wife was allowed in to see me. She kissed me and said some encouraging words. She is very good at this; she is the personification of sweetness. It is why I married her.

An hour went by while I struggled to breathe. My saturation figures still looked very bad. My dad came in to see me. (I think I was only allowed one visitor for ten minutes every hour). This meant my wife had to usually wait two hours to see me, as did my dad, since they were swapping their ten minute time slots. He put his head down near mine.

I held his hand on the bed and whispered to him, "I'm not..." shallow breath, shallow breath, "...going," shallow breath, shallow breath, then a deep rugged cough, "...to make it." DeAnna had somehow joined us. Her eyes filled with tears.

"Stay with us, Dan. We need you. We love you," she said. I cannot begin to imagine how this must have felt for my dear wife, the mother of our two energetic girls. Or what it felt like for my father. He had already stood beside the bed of my older brother, who at fifteen had died from CF. I could not begin to wonder what he was thinking; all I could focus on was if I had the strength for one more breath.

"Goodbye, dad…" shallow breath, shallow breath, "…I love you both." He squeezed my hand firmly.

"Hang on, honey," my wife repeated. I cannot honestly say I remember what my dad said. The tears welled in his eyes. He encouraged me to hang on.

The doctor was present, wrapped up in the emotional scene before him.

"Hang on Dan. You are on the transplant waiting list. You've got to hang on."

At some point my attention was diverted to a football game that was playing on the television in the ICU. It was the 49er game in a year that saw the team become NFC west division champions. It was a game that interested me.

It would be far more dramatic to say that I saw a great white light and a man standing there in the midst with a flowing white robe saying, "Stay there, Dan; be with your loved ones; they need you." But in all reality I think it was the football game that actually brought me down to earth. Sure I continued to cough and spit and fight for every breath. But I was also conscious of the fact that my attention was slowly drawn away from my fight for breath and from the tension of life slipping away from me, and it was slowly focused on the yardage and the first-down potential. Medically speaking I was no longer as anxious or tense, which is a result of hypoxemeia. That is how doctors would explain it. Slowly it became clear that I was going to recover. I see the hand of God in it. He used the distraction of a football game to ease my anxiety. The passing of time allowed the sedation to wear off too.

Sometimes we have this illusion that God's miracles are always done with dramatic flair and hyperbole. We learn how the seas were calmed amidst a ferocious storm. We read about five thousand hungry families fed with a few loaves of bread and a couple of little fish. And we look for such drama from our Lord. We feel we don't have his hand in our lives if it can be easily explained in natural terms. But other times Jesus meets people at a wedding and provides some excellent wine and nobody knows where it came from. He gets no credit or praise from the wedding revelers.

Somebody says, "Hey this guy saved the best wine for last!" Then the wedding host gets the praise, perhaps like doctors who perform surgeries. But behind the scalpel, behind the anesthesiologist and the fancy drugs and the technicians with their slick new devices is the hand of God quietly at work.

In the hours and days that followed I continued my battle to breathe and the daily regimen of chest percussion therapy and autogenic drainage. I also noted that I had a bruise that began at my naval and went all the way down to my knees on both legs. It was just one huge black mass. It was the internal bleeding. I was told that when the surgeon had completed the simple removal of my gall bladder through one of the tiny incisions, they had removed the little light from the second incision and the scalpel from the third incision. On the way out of my abdomen the scalpel had nicked the cystic artery. The effect was somewhat like if you accidentally cut a garden hose - just a little bit of course - when the hose was turned all the way on. Arteries are under high pressure, having come directly from the heart, and they are designed to forcefully pump your blood all the way to your extremities so it can make its way all the way back up to the opposite chamber of your heart. So this had been a pretty serious "leak." I was fortunate they were able to fix it, I was told. I tend to think I would have been fortunate not to have had it cut.

But that is looking at life entirely from the wrong perspective. It is easy to look at life as if the absence of problems is the equivalent of good fortune. I was soon to learn that coming face to face with death can be one of the best things in life.

I have a praying wife. And I don't mean a wife who gets on her knees for twenty minutes every morning and says her prayers. I mean that the two of us have learned to walk with Jesus and be conscious of His very presence every moment of the day. He is always watching us, He knows our thoughts, and He knows our every need. This does not mean that we don't take time every day to quietly share our needs audibly with Him and intercede on behalf of our friends and family in need. We do that too.

But we also have times when we cry out in desperation to Him because we are hopelessly up to our necks in a problem. The Lord knew during this crisis that DeAnna needed to hear something special from Him. The night I was in ICU fighting for breath she drove home and went upstairs to where our daughters slept. She laid on the floor between their beds. She was weeping inside and perhaps actually crying out loud because she needed to know in her heart of hearts that God was listening. She related to me later that as she cried out to Him she had an overwhelming sense of His presence. This was much more real even than when she asked Him to be her savior as a young girl of six. And it was more significant than when she committed her life to go anywhere and to be anything He wanted, which led her to Peru, to the Philippines, to a ghetto in East San Jose, to West Berlin, to eastern Turkey and to northern Iraq. This was beyond all that. It was about her husband, who seemed to be always dying. There is only so much of that kind of thing a wife can handle. And the Lord, who knows all things, knew she was going to need a lot more special strength to make it through the years ahead. So He met with her in a very special way.

As she met with Him on her knees on the mauve carpet in her parent's home she felt His presence. She did not hear an audible voice, she tells me, she just knew God wanted to assure her of something. She sensed the Lord affirming to her that, "Dan is going to make it. He is going to live. You will one day see him holding his grandchild." A tremendous peace overwhelmed her when that picture filled her mind. No longer would she fear the death of her husband. She would at times grieve as she thought about my passing away - one day down the road, but she would not have that imminent fear that I was going to slip from her presence during one of my recurring bouts of illness.

Now to anyone who heard her tell that story in 1995 following my gallbladder incident it would have sounded laughable. I was a very sick man. But to those with whom she shared it thirteen months later in another surgery - after I'd been given 32 units of blood - it would be an incredible encouragement. It would turn the tables for those who were to pray with her in the following months and years. Instead of discouragement it was a rock of encouragement. It would become the assurance of what was hoped for. It was faith.

Most of us have some amount of faith. If we are true followers of Jesus, we have faith we will see Christ after we die. We prayed to receive Him. We committed our lives to follow Him and to do His will. Many have kept that commitment and can honestly say they have the assurance of salvation. When we eventually face death we will be at peace, even rejoicing for the moments ahead when we shall see Jesus. Perhaps we have never had a loved one come so close to death so many times that we needed that special word from the Lord that our loved one was, "going to make it." But the Lord knew that DeAnna needed it, and He gave her that assurance.

"Now faith is being sure of what we hope for and certain of what we do not see." Those are the opening words of chapter eleven in the book of Hebrews. The whole chapter is a history of famous people who were declared righteous because of their faith. Men like Abraham, Isaac, Jacob, Moses, etc. Hebrews 11:35 jumped out at me one day as I was reading the chapter for the umpteenth time. It says that, "Women received back their dead, raised to life again." I read it again and again. I realized I was reading the testimony of my wife.

I was teaching a Sunday school class years later and was trying to help the class (which is full of people who follow Jesus) to see that their own lives were full of acts of faith. They had just never articulated it in such a way. Each one had taken steps out into the unknown, trusting that God would provide, that He would bless, that He would meet their need, that He would heal, etc. I wanted them to recognize it and put it into words. I passed out paper. At the end of the class I assembled their papers and read it aloud.

"By faith Kim cried out to the Lord for healing from addiction and God freed her. By faith John bought an investment property and prayed to the Lord and it returned a profit of ten percent. By faith Steve adopted a son who turned out to have a disability and God blessed their family immeasurably because Jesus has been with them through every crisis and battle." Wow. By the end of the list all we could do was look to God with words of praise!

It was going to take a lot of faith to endure the next year, however. Surviving gall bladder surgery and a nicked cystic artery had been tough, but it was going to get rougher.

Chapter 22

Sinus Balloons

There is something about waking up at night and finding your bed soaked with blood that is significantly disquieting. Such was our experience when I woke up in our bed at home in January 1996. One requirement prior to a lung transplant for CF patients at Stanford was to get the sinuses cleared up as best as possible. The CF sinuses harbor the same nasty bacteria that destroy the lungs. So it makes good sense to make these big cavities in the head as accessible to antibiotics as possible. The solution? Cut some windows in the walls between these cavities.

It had been two months since my recovery from the botched gall bladder surgery. But it was very much fresh in my memory. On this day my ENT was talking to me about my sinuses. She explained that the sinuses of a person with CF often caused the most problems after a person had received new lungs. So it is better to fix them before the lung transplant. The sinus problems stem from the genetic defect in CF, which reside in every cell of the body. Of course the lungs are the primary organs damaged with CF. However, since the sinuses are involved in rinsing the nasal cavity of dirt, dust and infected crud, any thick secretions will create a home for infections. The best way to reduce this is to open up the sinus cavity. The open areas can then be flooded with topical antibiotics to combat the infections. The eight sinuses are separated by walls. In the 1990's a new procedure had been developed whereby windows were cut in the walls of the two maxillary sinuses. Hmmm. Sounded interesting.

Since I like construction I could picture this pretty well and it made sense to me. I asked a few questions and then basically said, "Let's do it." I was scheduled for rhino plastic surgery with Dr. Mary Lynn Moran. When I awoke following surgery I noted that my head was full of packing material. Dr. Moran had explained that this was special substances she'd placed in my sinuses that would reduce bleeding. Most of the matter would dissolve over time. She said I could go home and she gave me a special number to call if anything came up. I went home and DeAnna helped me navigate into bed with all my tubes and whatnot.

I had my IV pole with the feeding pump hanging on it as well as the IV antibiotic pump. The O2 hose from the concentrator was now attached to a mask to deliver O2 to my mouth That's because my nose was packed solid from the surgery. My room looked and felt like a hospital. I was lying on my back because of all the tubes, although sometimes I'd roll onto my side because it was easier to breathe that way.

Sometime during the night DeAnna awoke beside me. In horror she realized there was blood everywhere on my pillow and the bed sheets. She was awake in a flash and woke me too. Stanford's special number was called and we were on our way again to the hospital. Forty-five minutes later Dr. Moran was at my side in an operating room again working on my nose. Apparently I had sprung a leak. A big one. She removed the packing material and placed what I can only describe as customized balloons up my nose into the sinuses. They had a valve at the nostril end which enabled Dr. Moran to pump air into them. It sounds about as crude as it was. It also hurt like crazy. I soon had the worse headache I had ever experienced in life (to that point.)

They sent me to a regular hospital room to recover. Sleep was out of the question. It is normally out of the question anyway in a hospital, since one gets blood pressure, temperature, and oxygen levels taken at regular intervals. Then there is the respiratory therapist who visits four times a day. And nurses who are regularly in and out. Finally the doctors stop in each day and order blood tests, x-rays, and other tests, to check on your status and update your prognosis. That pretty much eliminates any sleep.

As I sat up in the hospital bed I had a device strapped around my chin so that a medicated-laden mist would flow up over my face. It caused my face to be constantly wet. Lovely. Of course I couldn't breathe through my nose. It was still packed with the balloons. I was still coughing constantly and getting physical therapy and respiratory therapy to clear the gathering mucus in my lungs. The mist also contained a high percentage of oxygen so my lungs wouldn't have to work so hard. My nose was out of commission for the time being. This simple window-cutting had gotten a bit out of hand. It was perhaps the most miserable four days I could ever remember.

After everything had stopped bleeding and the balloons were deflated I was sent home and began a slow recovery. The small windows in the wall of each maxillary sinus enabled catheters to be inserted up from the nostrils and through these windows for flushing with antibiotics. This seemed like a really great idea and did work to keep my sinuses pretty clear for several years.

Sometimes you have to suffer for a while before life gets better. If you refuse the suffering then life ends up a lot worse. One has to persevere. There is an excellent scripture that guides me in times like these. It's found in 2 Peter 1:6 and 7, "Now for this very reason also, applying all diligence, in your faith supply moral excellence, and in your moral excellence, knowledge, and in your knowledge, self-control, and in your self-control, perseverance, and in your perseverance, godliness, and in your godliness, brotherly kindness, and in your brotherly kindness, love...."

It is not just the self control and perseverance that is needed, it is the combination of those other character traits that provides the strength to endure such horrific treatment.

That was my first sinus surgery. I have had nine more since then. I can say (with gladness) that that was the worst. I am grateful to God and His gift to mankind of modern medicine that I can take each breath. Even through my nose.

I play trombone in a worship band regularly and there is a particular melody that really speaks to me. The beginning lyrics to Michael W. Smith's song *Breathe* can bring tears to my eyes:

This is the air I breathe
This is the air I breathe

Your holy presence living in me

This is my daily bread
This is my daily bread
Your very word spoken to me

And I I'm desperate for you
And I I'm I'm lost without you[39]

---

[39] https://www.azlyrics.com/lyrics/michaelwsmith/breathe.html You can listen to the song on Youtube here https://www.youtube.com/watch?v=Oad8ov10AjY

Chapter 23

"Wear the Beeper!"

The nurse emphasized, "Put this beeper on and wear it at all times. When the beeper goes off, call the hospital and come in immediately. It signifies that your time for a transplant has come." She repeated it again, "You must wear this at all times. Don't travel over two hours from Stanford. If you do, you must notify us and you will be taken off the transplant waiting list during your travel." I decided right then I wouldn't travel anywhere! I wore it everywhere hooked onto my belt.

Waiting is tough. Waiting for new lungs when you are dying is really tough. Not just for the hopeful recipient, but for his wife, his children, parents, friends, even the doctors and nurses. I was waiting in September 1995. I dutifully wore my beeper. I had been thoroughly evaluated for a transplant and found to be an eligible candidate. DeAnna and I also flew to San Diego and did all the testing for transplant evaluation at the University Hospital there.

About this time UNOS (United Network for Organ Sharing), decided that recipients could only be listed at one transplant center. So we dropped the San Diego option and put all our eggs in the Stanford basket. When I did the tests at Stanford, they found that my heart was healthy enough that it could be passed on to another recipient. This meant I was a candidate for either a double lung transplant, or for a heart/double lung transplant. I was able to be put on both lists: a double lung transplant list, and a heart/double lung transplant list. The second list had far fewer people waiting. One had to have a healthy heart to qualify for the second list.[40]

---

[40] This practice of double listing is no longer done.

This was called a "domino transplant." My good heart would be removed and passed along to another person, while I could receive a "block". A block was a heart and double lung that were all still attached together. This double organ transplant was pioneered by Dr. Bruce Reitz at Stanford with a team in 1985. His friend and colleague Dr. Bobby Robbins would be performing my surgery. While waiting for my transplant I tried to continue with my normal activities, which wasn't much.

One sunny afternoon, while living at the home of DeAnna's parents, we decided to go for a dip in their pool. I had a fifty foot oxygen hose, with a giant green torpedo tank in our bedroom. I figured out that if I took the screen off of their dining room window, I could pass the hose through the opening and it would reach the swimming pool. I was pretty exited about this. I didn't really plan to go swim, I just wanted to cool off in the pool and watch our children play.

It was always a careful dance for the family to navigate around my O2 hose, which snaked around on the floor.

"Don't step on it," was often heard. It pained me greatly when I was walking in the house and somebody put a foot on the hose, clamping it momentarily to the floor. My head would jerk back as if I was a horse with a bit in my nose. Almost as annoying was getting it wrapped around a piece of furniture. I was always retracing my steps to get untangled.

Our daughters Shirena and Jessica were like most kids and loved to play in the pool. It was a delight to watch them play. I unhooked the O2 hose from my face, passed it out the window, then made a calculated walk around and out the patio door and back to my O2 supply. I could tolerate short moments without the oxygen. I put it over my head and hooked it back in my nose.

Springtime in San Jose can be delightfully warm. Shorts and flip flops were standard attire. I stepped down into the warm water, tossed a ball to my daughters and began a playful exchange. Then I realized I had just submerged my beeper. I had this sudden thought that I might miss my transplant call. I quickly dried off and telephoned Stanford fearing they may have tried to beep me. No worries; they hadn't beeped. A few days later we received a new beeper in the mail.

We continued to wait and pray. My whole church had been praying for us. My daughter Jessica, age five, and Shirena age seven had prayed too. In kindergarten, Jessica came to her teacher and asked for special prayer for her daddy, who needed new lungs. This happened at recess time, which she told me was her favorite subject. So I knew it was a big sacrifice.

Then one night the real call came. A Stanford nurse rang us on the home landline and said we should come immediately. We had our transplant bag all packed and ready to go. It contained clothes and toiletries for both DeAnna and me. Driving the twenty-six miles up highway 85 and 280 took less time than usual. Our salvaged '85 Buick Century wagon was runny smoothly. We were both excited, but also felt a twinge of fear, wonderment, and anxiety. In a few hours I would be asleep and in surgery. My wife would be in the waiting room for six to ten hours. Our kids would be with grandparents. Friends and family would be praying. We had rehearsed these moments over and over in our imaginations, only now it was with a sense of *"can this be real? Is this really happening?"*

I was ushered into a prep room. I undressed so my chest could be shaved, washed and washed again. I think they used Betadine antiseptic. An IV was started in my right arm as I lay on my back. Laying on my back was still the worst position for me, as I struggled to get oxygen. My lower lobes had suffered the most from bacterial infections. Now I had both the O2 cannula and the IV tube hooked into me. I was set to be rolled into the surgical suite, put to sleep and receive a new chance at life. This is what we had prayed for. We had waited for this moment to come for eight months. It was going to change my life, our lives. Our hearts soared with hope and expectation. The moments passed by and we continued to wait. An hour. Two hours. DeAnna asked the nurse what was happening.

"We are waiting for the donor lungs to be evaluated for their health," the nurse explained. "They need to be in super condition." She explained that the donor's chest had been x-ray'd and the lungs appeared fine. We knew that organs sometimes come after there's been an accident. Injuries to a donated organ may not be readily apparent until they are actually removed from the donor.

I knew there is much more to a transplant of this magnitude than the layman like myself could ever understand. I knew that nobody was just hanging around doing nothing. Everyone was working at their peak. This was a big deal, not just for me but for every person involved. I was more than willing to wait as time went by, knowing that everyone had my best interests in mind. But doing nothing while you wait is sometimes very difficult. DeAnna and I prayed to Jesus for patience and peace. Our hearts were filled with calm.

The transplant nurse came back into the small room, pulling the curtain aside. She gently explained why we had been waiting so long.

"The lungs have been harvested," she began. We realized that some family had just lost a loved one that day. It is sobering to think about the dynamics involved in a transplant of this kind. There is grief, sadness, loss. Then there is sacrifice, understanding, and a spirit of giving. Finally, for the recipient there is hope and a future.

Our nurse continued, "The lungs were examined carefully. They discovered that they have had significant bruising. The doctors have determined that they are not good enough to use in a transplant. We don't want to compromise your chances by using damaged lungs." This had to be really hard for her to say to us. She tried to break this disheartening news as delicately as possible. "I am really, really sorry," she began. "I know this is a terrible thing to hear. I wish it were different."

I knew what this meant. Quite simply my chances for survival had just been greatly diminished. We were silent. We needed to accept this devastating news with grace.

"All things are allowed by God," we said to the UNOS lady. I groped for words but I felt a strange calm inside. "We are at peace with the outcome of our lives as they are in His hands." I continued, "It's OK." I did not know from whence the confidence came. "We understand the reasons, and It's OK," I repeated. "Our hearts are at peace. I'm sure the doctors made the right decision." The nurse had been expecting a much different response. Perhaps tears, or anger. But not peace.

John 14:27 quotes the words of Jesus, "Peace I leave with you; my peace I give you. I do not give to you as the world gives. Do not let your hearts be troubled and do not be afraid."

I can say with confidence that at that moment we both felt that peace, the supernatural peace that comes with knowing Jesus. There was a true feeling of disappointment. This was not going to be *our day*. But we were at peace.

The nurse removed the IV from my arm. I tried my best to get the brown betadine off my chest, to no avail. I got dressed. We thanked her and I put the beeper back on my belt. We called our families to let them know that we would again be in the waiting mode. We loaded my transplant bag back into the Buick and drove back to south San Jose. Neither of us knew at the time that it was going to be a very long wait before the next call would come.

The Jewish king David put it this way, "Great peace have those who love your law, and nothing can make them stumble. I wait for your salvation, Lord, and I follow your commands. I obey your statutes, for I love them greatly."[41] But would we continue to have that peace when the wait dragged on and on? How long is long?

DeAnna continued my daily regimen of chest percussion therapy four times a day and I continued doing autogenic drainage. I also did nebulizer therapies to inhale a variety of drugs designed to reduce inflammation in the lungs and to fight bacterial and fungal infections. Doctors prescribed regular two-week infusions of antibiotics. I plugged the feeding tube into my abdomen every night to get additional calories pumped into my system as I slept. I still had to reach that magical weight, 140 pounds. I ate voraciously during the day. I figured I needed at least 4000 calories a day to raise my weight one pound a month. I continued to ride the exercise bike for a half hour each day. My lips were perpetually blue. I talked in short gasps because it took so much energy. My family was seeing me slowly suffocate each day.

[41] Psalms 119:165-167

I should add that families like us who are involved in full time Christian work overseas often live by financial support from friends, families and churches who believe in them and their work. Since we were no longer working as missionaries overseas our two supporting churches felt they had to discontinue the substantial financial support they had been giving us. While we understood their rationale it made our lives financially difficult. That's one reason we had taken our two daughters and moved into the VanTuyl's home, into their former dining room. DeAnna's parents were super generous with us, and our occupation lasted over two years. We did get along with them very well; maybe it was because I didn't have the strength to argue with anyone. But without a doubt it was because of the generosity, the kindness, and the grace of Steve and Rena VanTuyl. They supported us like no one else.

Through this financial hardship we learned that as Christians we should not look to the institutional church as our support and strength. We should look to God alone. It is Jesus whom we worship, not the local church. And it was Jesus who carried us through.

This brings me to the big event. The following story is the reason many people know me. After people meet me they usually say, "Oh you're the guy who got the heart double lung transplant."

"Yup. That's me."

Chapter 24

Heart Double Lung Transplant

I was talking to a friend the other day. He was losing faith that God exists. He had read a lot of literature by atheists and was trying to figure out if everything he'd been taught as a child about God was just a lot of nonsense. I tried to show him that God had revealed himself in the wonders of nature. He also gave us a conscience and a sense of right and wrong. He gave us a desire to know Him. Then He revealed Himself to us in his Word, the Bible. My friend couldn't see it.

Then about a week later I was in a discussion with a fellow trombone player. He told me that he believed that God was everywhere, in everything, and that when he died he would just become part of God and part of everything. He said he had rejected the idea that God was distinct from man. He said he'd rejected dualism. I asked him where the world came from, where man came from, and why he had a heart with a conscience. He said he hadn't figured all that out yet.

Finally, in both cases, I told them a story about an encounter I'd had with God that defied reason. I wanted them to understand that God did indeed exist, and that he was separate from man, and finally that He wanted to have a relationship with us.

I began by telling him about my encounter with death while coming off the respirator after the gall bladder surgery. I told him briefly of the sinus surgery. And then I told him of the disappointing call for a lung transplant. Finally I told him an abbreviated version of this story:

January 26, 1997 was Super Bowl Sunday. This is a big day in America, bigger for many than Christmas, Easter, and the fourth of July. Stores run out of chips and soda. The streets are filled with people going to parties. The commercials get national attention as people vote on the best of the best. It is the quintessential holiday for the sport-addicted American citizen. Only that is not what it means to me. For me it is the day I got a new pair of lungs and a second chance at life.

The Christian life is about second chances. God is known as the God of second chances. He takes whatever garbage or filth that has been one's history and he creates a new person out of you. That is one reason the phrase, "born again" became popular. It connotes the whole idea that one is really dead in sin, in the rotten life of our present existence, but as we ask forgiveness for our wretchedness, Jesus come to us and cleanses us from all that and gives us a second chance. He creates us anew. That is very similar, in a physical sense, of what happened to me when I got new lungs. My old life of coughing up sputum, and trying to rid myself of the ugly foul smelling crud that slowly filled my body and killed my lungs - was gone. I received a new set of pink healthy lungs that efficiently processed fresh clean air. For me it is a perfect picture of getting the second chance of life.

When I was six I received that new life of knowing Jesus. I confessed my sinfulness. He changed me and gave me a new birth. That never went away and I knew that if I died on the operating table while the doctors attempted to put a new heart and lungs (actually they were used) into me – I would go to heaven in a flash.[42] I would be in the presence of the one who saved me. Jesus is my friend and companion. I know Him personally and relate with Him all the time. So death is no big deal for me. My death would be a big loss for my family, but that is part of what happens to us when anybody leaves this earth.

The adventure actually began on Jan 25th around midnight. Very briefly I was told on the phone that there was a pair of lungs

---

[42] 2 Corinthians 5:7-9: "But we live by faith, not by what we see. We should be cheerful, because we would rather leave these bodies and be at home with the Lord. But whether we are at home with the Lord or away from him, we still try our best to please him. (from the Contemporary English version.)

and a heart that was available. I should come to Stanford as quickly as possible. It was a cold stormy night as I dragged my oxygen bottle out to our old brown station wagon. I got sopping wet just walking from the front door to the car. DeAnna was going to drive. My hat came off in the wind and the car rolled over it. *"That was my favorite hat,"* I thought. But who knew if I'd live to wear it again? How ridiculous to cling to earthly things when one is on the verge of eternity. DeAnna drove us to Stanford Hospital.

I was placed in a room and prepped as before, only this time it became clear that the lungs were in great shape. The donor had died of a brain aneurysm, and had been declared brain dead. Her organs did not have to be instantly harvested, however. Lungs, once removed, are only viable for about four hours. We learned that the surgeon who would perform the operation was Doctor Bobby Robbins. But he had a problem.

He had been up most of the day doing another transplant surgery. It was very rare to have two transplant surgeries the same weekend. But that weekend there had actually been three. Two people had each received a lung from a single donor, and I was to receive a heart/double lung from another person. Dr. Robbins was exhausted. He decided to get a bit of sleep and then do my surgery in the morning. That seemed like a good idea so I did my best to sleep also. Surgery was scheduled for eight am.

I remember laying on the gurney and being wheeled down the hallway, watching the ceiling tiles go by. I chatted with the fellow pushing my bed along. He was an Arab. I asked him how he was enjoying his work at Stanford. Soon I was wheeled into the operating room and transferred from the gurney onto the operating table. Sedation medication was administered into my peripherally inserted central catheter and I went to sleep. The rest of this story was related to me later.

Naturally my family sat in the waiting room anticipating the outcome of the surgery. They gathered in prayer. They tried to eat. They took short walks, talked to visitors. They waited. Then they waited some more. After ten and a half hours Dr. Bobby Robbins came out with a dejected look on his face.

"We have tried everything we could. The bleeding just can't be stopped. His blood is not clotting like it should. He just keeps bleeding and bleeding. I'm sorry. We are losing him. There is nothing more I can do." We did not know until later that Dr. Robbins had kept working on me long after his colleagues had felt it was hopeless. He just wouldn't quit.

"Give it up, Bobby. We aren't going to save him," his fellow surgeons said. But he had kept working. Finally he had come to tell DeAnna that I was going to die. He left me on the table; the transplant operation was done. Dan Lagasse wasn't going to make it.

He sent for the chaplain and the social worker to comfort my wife. But she was on her knees with a group from the church. Her parents and my parents were all praying. Jesus can do miracles. And they asked for one.

A half hour later Dr. Robbins returned.

"My grandma used to pray for miracles," were his words. "One just happened. It has been a half hour and we haven't changed anything. But he's still alive. He has a long way to go and he is very, very sick, but he's alive." He continued to update them, "The bleeding has slowed considerably. His situation is still very unstable. I don't know what is going to happen."

DeAnna held that assurance (that I would live) from the previous year still in her heart. She knew I would live. She had no fear. That was a faith that was rooted in mercy, as she would say. God had heard her prayers, had seen her heart, and had seen her faith grow throughout many years of our journey together. He had answered her prayer and given her that faith to see me live. She remembered Hebrews 11:35 that said, "Women received back their dead, raised to life again." I firmly believe that God had given me life again because of the faith of many, in particular my wife. And certainly the skill and the refuse-to-give-up determination of Dr. Robbins.

It did not mean that my journey was not a difficult one. I woke in ICU with a tube down my throat. In the subsequent days my body became so swollen with fluid that my skin in my shoulder ripped when someone tried to roll me on my side. I had so many issues that I had thirteen subsequent surgeries. I remained in ICU for thirty-one days, the whole time on a respirator.

It was decided one night to give me a diuretic to reduce the amount of fluid my body had accumulated. In one night my body released four gallons of fluid through the foley catheter. That's thirty-two pounds! My fat torso, arms and legs lost much of their swelling.

Most of the time while in ICU I was sedated. Occasionally I would be awakened. I have a few memories of acting psychotic from the massive dosages of steroids I was given. For example I was certain some nefarious nurse had put frozen yogurt in my intravenous line to try and knock me off. When pastor and long time friend Kurt Jones from my church came to visit I grabbed his arm in fear.

"Kurt, you've got to get me out of here. They are trying to kill me! Somebody even unplugged my respirator!" My poor buddy was at a loss of what to do. His friend was loosing it.

I remember some visits from dear family and friends. No flowers that gave off scents were allowed in my room of course. Perfume binds with oxygen molecules in the air making it more difficult to breathe. But there were thoughtful cards reminding me of the hundreds of people who cared and prayed for my recovery. God heals. I needed a lot of healing.

There were also several failed attempts to extubate me. During these times I was brought out of an induced coma so I could attempt to make my lungs perform. But they were still too injured and I was too week.

Early on a clot formed somewhere in an artery blocking the blood flow from my head back to my body. Normally a blood thinner would be given a patient who is at risk of developing blood clots. But I had bled so profusely during my surgery they feared any blood thinner would be catastrophic. What should be done? The blockage had caused my head to swell creating intense pressure. My face was contorted out of all proportion making my head the size of a basketball. I was unrecognizable. My lips were so puffed out that my lower lip hung down below my chin. Research doctors took photos of my bizarre state. I had the worse headache one can imagine. I was certain I was going to die that night. I looked forward to waking in heaven and being free from the agony and suffering. Before they sedated me again to attempt a surgical procedure my wife came in to see me. She brought small photos of our two daughters. She hung them from the bar above my bed where I could look up and see them.

"Listen," she said firmly, "You can't leave us. You have work to do. Our two daughters need a father to raise them!"

Over the next couple of days two heart surgeries were performed to remove the clots. They were suctioned out via a catheter inserted in my femoral artery. The swelling in my head receded. Two stents were inserted to prevent the veins from collapsing.

While in ICU multiple bronchoscopies were done to assess the health of the new lungs. This is the insertion of a tube down into the bronchioles. DeAnna finally gave carte blanch consent to my doctors to perform whatever surgeries were necessary in the night, so she could get a little sleep. It was an impossible situation for her and my family, as they wanted to be at my side whenever possible, yet they still had real-life responsibilities to fulfill.

I recall hallucinating at one point, imagining there was another patient in the room, when in fact I was in a private ICU room. I was also sure there was a window across to my right (but I of course I could not turn my head to look out of it) when in fact there were no windows. And I stared for hours at what I imagined were a row of three overhead televisions all playing advertisements for steak and lobster. (There was just one TV.) I had been given liquid nutrition, pumped into my stomach tube for the entire month through my PEG, so solid food was always on my mind. (Two months later after my discharge my parents took us to the Red Lobster to enjoy their advertised special. I was disappointed to learn that the special offer had ended the previous day. I told the waiter about my ordeal and they made an exception. And that was not a hallucination!)

Conversation was impossible with the tube down my throat. I couldn't ask the doctor the many questions I had about my prognosis. He could of course ask me questions about how I felt, but my thumbs up or thumbs down was my only way of responding. DeAnna tried to have me write on a clipboard, but lying on my back without the ability to even sit up meant holding it up in front

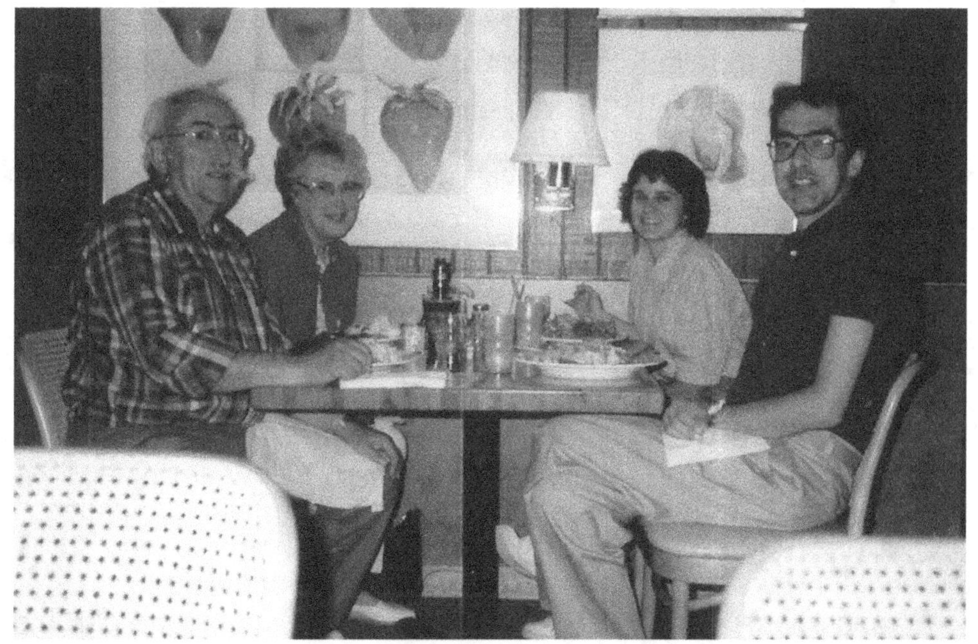

**DAVE AND CAROLYN (MY PARENTS) DEANNA AND I
ENJOYING OUR FIRST DINNER OUT - STEAK AND LOBSTER**

of my chest. And the medications I was on made my writing terribly shaky, rendering it illegible.

Intubation means no talking, no eating, and no turning of the head. I had constant phlegm collecting in my airway, and felt just plain miserable. It seemed like I was awake for the whole thirty days. The most calming and pleasant memory is the music I played on a cassette recorder. The songs of love, hope, and faith renewed my mind and sustained me.

My most remarkable memory is of the day when I was finally extubated. That nasty tube was pulled from my throat and I could turn my head, speak to my wife (though my throat was really sore) and eventually eat. I still love jello. And chicken broth. Then came the next hurdle. I was still receiving supplemental oxygen through a nasal cannula, as I had been for many years. The nurse wanted to wean me off oxygen, to which I'd become addicted. I had to train my brain to believe I could survive without it. Mentally I accepted the fact that I no longer needed it. But emotionally I was dependent upon it. So I asked the nurse to slowly turn my oxygen down, but not to tell me. The regulator was on the wall behind my head where I could not see it.

She came in later that day and announced, "You have not been receiving supplemental oxygen at all for the past hour." *Amazing!* I was incredulous. Slowly I held the plastic tube in my hand, releasing it from my nostrils, pulling it over my ears for the last time. I was free. Free indeed.

This is the air I breathe.

Even so I was only able to get thirty percent of the expected lung volume for a man my size. I was disappointed, remembering my expectation of new transplanted lungs taking giant full breaths. But doctors assured me that within a year, if I worked at it, I could hope to reach eighty percent of a normal lung volume. I would one day surprise them, reaching one hundred and three percent lung volume for a man my height, age and weight.

When released from ICU I was sent for two weeks to a cardiac care unit and placed in a private room. The risks for infection and rejection were still high. I also had to learn to stand, to walk, and to use the bathroom again on my own. There were some very humbling situations during those early days of navigating the three feet from my bed to the toilet. All those antibiotics does strange things to one's digestion. At the end of the two weeks I was discharged from the main hospital! Stepping outside was simply amazing.

Stanford had set up a special apartment nearby where patients could live after discharge. It was a block away from the main hospital building so I could walk for appointments and physical therapy sessions. They had deep cleaned it to minimize health risks for me. DeAnna learned how to change my many bandages from the chest tubes (I had seven) as they were healing. During one post visit the doctors pulled the staples from my wounds on my chest and on both sides of my back. My kids were allowed to see me for the first time in six weeks. Their prayers had been answered.

Healing takes time. That was the primary lesson during those months following the miracle of the surgery. Healing also takes

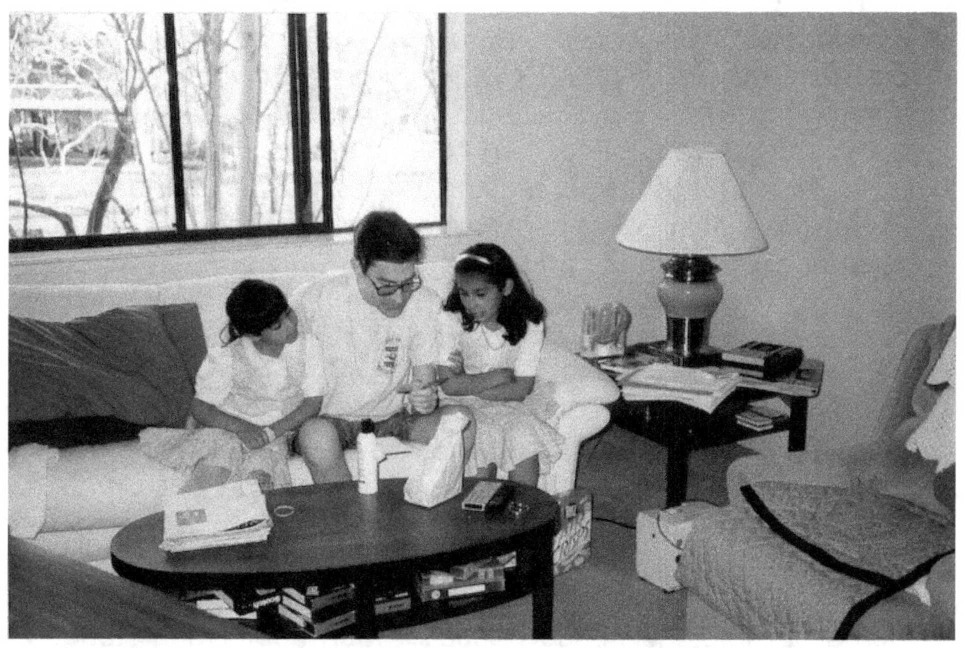

JESSICA, ME AND SHIRENA IN THE "HOMETEL" AT STANFORD

work, dedication, a belief in survival, love and comfort from others who care, and continual vigilance from professionals who understand the process.

I was comforted by many promises from Scripture, such as this one from Jeremiah 30:17, "I will give you back your health and heal your wounds," says the Lord."

That narration is just my perspective. Other lives were also caught up in the drama. My wife, my parents, and our daughters each experienced it in a unique way. My younger brother Doug, who also has CF, has a memorable story to tell. Here is the experience as he reflects back upon it:

"It was early Monday morning, January 27, 1997 - before the commuters had even begun to besiege Hong Kong Island. I made my way from our apartment up near China, down into town, past my office, across the harbor, and into a sports bar in Causeway Bay. About a hundred (mostly) Americans crowded the place, including a dozen from my men's Bible study group. It was very festive atmosphere, considering it was only six a.m. on a Monday. Ours was probably the only Super Bowl Party on earth that featured scrambled eggs, bacon, and toast. And the only "brew" being served was coffee.

It wasn't all that spectacular of a game, as I remember it. But the real shocker came when the bar-tender shouted my name, telling me I had a phone call.

"Huh?" They handed me the phone. I could barely hear my wife shouting through the phone over the noise of the game and the crowd;.

"Dan is having his transplant right now!" I began to weep tears of joy. My buddies asked what was wrong. My announcement led the bar-keep to turn down the game, while several of my buddies lifted up my brother, his surgeons, and our family in prayer.

Shortly thereafter, I abandoned the game, and wandered out into the hustle bustle of rush hour Hong Kong. The "reverse commute" back up to the countryside was easy, as I headed home to spend these critical hours with my wife and kids. We prayed. We wept. We rejoiced. We wondered. We prayed some more.

Phone calls were few and far between. Dan's family were all at the hospital- and who carries enough coins to make international calls from a pay-phone? Finally we heard that it had been an epic battle, but that he survived, barely. There would be lots more recovery before he'd be out of the woods. Unfortunately, due to the high cost of international travel, we had to just wait it out; periodically receiving email updates in the ensuing days, until he was finally released to go home many weeks later.

We didn't actually get to see Dan-the-new-man until the summer of the following year (1998). By that time, my own lungs were in terrible shape, and I was told to move back near Stanford for appropriate CF lung care, or die within a short period in Hong Kong. So as I came home, huffing and puffing. My formerly feeble brother grabbed my luggage, and helped move furniture into our home for me.

Then he and my dad painted the house we were renting. Amazing!

From that point forward - to this day - he became my survival coach. He helped me hang in through the final stages of my diseased lungs. And then he helped me pull through my own transplant odyssey seventeen years after his. When people ask me about survival rates for a lung transplant, I point to my brother and say, 'Well he's lasted twenty-three years so far, and I can't let him beat me!"

Chapter 25

"You Should Put a Zipper in."

D r. Sista turned to his colleague, "Check out the sound of this murmur." It was during a routine visit at Stanford. He sounded like he was impressed about something. Part of each follow-up after a transplant is to check the health of the lungs (pulmonary function test and chest X-rays), assess my overall system (blood work), and listen to the workings of my heart (stethoscope.) I had been told that in the case of a heart/double lung transplant it was more likely my heart that would reject than my new lungs. So my doctor paid close attention to the health of my heart. He called in a couple colleagues to also listen to the murmur.

I had no idea what a murmur was. I thought it was something like complaining. Webster says it is a, "low muttered complaint." I didn't know what my heart was complaining about; it was doing just fine as far as I was concerned. I suppose there is a spiritual lesson there. (We think our soul is fine when it actually has a fatal flaw.)

"What's a murmur?" I asked.

"It's an unusual sound that your heart is making. We are trained to recognize a normal heartbeat, and also to distinguish an abnormal one." I didn't like his implication.

I asked in an upbeat voice, "So what does it mean?" That's usually what one wants to know, particularly when the doctor has a concerned look on his face and when he calls in his colleagues for their opinions.

He continued, "It may indicate any of several things. I don't think it is anything to be too concerned about. Many people live their whole lives with such a murmur and it never amounts to anything." I listened carefully to what I call, "physician speech." Two words in the answer bothered me. The first was the word, "too." It would have been better to hear, "It is *nothing* to be concerned about," period. I thought for a moment. *"So I should be somewhat concerned,"* I thought. Personally I would rather not be concerned at all. I like carefree.

The other word was, "many." He didn't say, *"Everybody* lives their whole lives…" or even, *"Most people…."* He had said, *"Many people live…"* Naturally I figured I was not a part of the "many." I never have been. I had always been a part of the very rare, or the nearly never.

I hear doctors say things like, "I have never seen this before in my life." For example 1963 when the pediatrician said, "Nobody ever has three children that *all* have cystic fibrosis." That was one of my first recollections of a doctor talking with my parents. I didn't like being special, not in this department. But sometimes God calls us out to be a lesson for others. Most of us would rather just slip under the radar. Has God called you out to be special? Just go along with it; it's a lot easier in the end.

The natural man is prone to worry. It is an innate response and if I let my mind take control I will worry, unless I devote myself to being, "In the Master's hand." It is a lot easier to worry and question the will of God. I remember a missionary relating about facing armed jungle natives in Papua New Guinea. He had wondered at that moment if he was truly in the center of God's will. Then he simply said, "God's perfect will for you is to be in the hand of the Master." That can be difficult to experience when you are lying on a short exam table in the doctor's office and your doctor says, "Hmmm. Sounds like a murmur."

At that point he turned to his partner and said, "Dr. Patel, you should listen to this." At times like this one doesn't like to be the center of attention, especially from trained physicians. But God wanted to remind me that it wasn't about me and my heart; it was about declaring his glory. Even to a bunch of top-educated Stanford MD's.

Over the next couple months the murmur became louder. This wasn't a good sign. I was sent for an echocardiogram, which I thought was pretty neat because I just lay on a table and watched my heart beat on a computer monitor. The technician just rolled something that looked like a roll-on deodorant sick with a cable attached to it all over my chest. It was the most pain-free exam I had ever had. *"I could do this all day,"* I thought. In fact I fell asleep. When I awoke I pulled on my shirt and awaited the results. Radiologists can never tell you what they see, which always makes me feel cheated. "You have to wait for the doctor to tell you," is their mantra. I drove home not knowing the results.

A few nights later DeAnna woke up in the night. She has much better hearing than I and often wakes up and asks me if I have heard such and such.

"Hmph?" I asked while I rubbed my eyes. The noise is generally the automatic sprinkler system kicking in or the dog kicking the side of his dog house or some other unimportant event. This time she asked me if I had installed a sump pump.

"What?"

"A sump pump."

"Maybe it's the neighbor's." Our home is about ten feet from our neighbor's house and it seemed like a reasonable guess. "I didn't install one," I said, and tried to fall back asleep.

We have a king size bed which means that DeAnna has lots of room to move around during the night without disturbing me. She likes to change positions about every thirty seconds. I usually sleep on my back like a soldier at attention (which she denies) but my point is I don't take up much of the bed. She is sometimes so far away that I have to crawl across the bed to find her.

"Shush," she said, as I lay on my back. *"That's easy,"* I thought. I had been shushing for about five hours without any problem.

Then she crawled over beside me and put her head on my chest.

I was about to get the wrong idea when she said in an alarming voice, "It's your heart!" My heart was beating so loud she could hear it clear across the bed; and it had woken her up.

Needless to say my doctor told me I'd need surgery to fix my bad heart. I thought my heart was pretty good up to that point; it had been working perfectly fine. I played racket ball three times a week. I went hiking in the hills near our home. But the professionals knew better. God is like that. He can see and hear things in our hearts that we are oblivious to. We have to ask him about the state of our heart and follow his guidance. Otherwise the results will be pretty bad.

Later when I was in the admitting room for open heart surgery the doctors asked me to step into a large room near the admitting desk. A group of doctors were gathered there. I didn't know any of them; they looked like students. Stanford Hospital is a teaching hospital, which has its plusses and minuses. The plus side is that students learn to be better doctors. One also gets to meet residents from all over the world as the very best come to learn the newest and best in medicine technology. The downside is that one can easily feel like a specimen. At some appointments several students will examine me and ask the same diagnostic questions "real" physicians ask. It can get tiring. I have to repeat the same thing three times. I try and cooperate with a good spirit. I can detect from their accent and their name tag from whence they come and so I can say, "*Namaste*, (Hindi)" or "*Guten Tag*, (German)" or "*Magandang Umaga*, (Tagalog)" or "*Salam alaykum* (Arabic)." That usually breaks the ice. But sometimes if I have a fever of 104 I don't feel like saying anything except, "Please leave me alone."

On this occasion right prior to going in for surgery Dr. Sista asked the physicians gathered to be quiet.

"Do you hear anything?" he asked with a touch of excitement in his voice. There was an audible whish, ba-boom, whish ba-boom. It was my heart. They could hear it beating from clear across the room. It's not often a heart beats so loud you can hear it from fifteen feet away. The doc was very excited that he could teach a whole room full of students what a murmur sounded like. It was definitely not a small murmur. It was a full blown aneurism making a lot of racket. Well, it hadn't actually "blown," or I wouldn't have been standing any longer. But it was clearly on the way.

They signed me in for surgery. The surgeon who performed the repair/replacement was again Dr. Bobby Robbins. He'd been into my chest before so he was familiar with what to expect. He later told me the aneurism was about the size of a baseball. That sounded like I was not part of the "many" once again.

Prepping for surgery had become a rather routine thing for me, and since it's not something people like to read about I'll skip it. I will point out that the anesthesiologist is as important as the surgeon, because he or she is the one that keeps you alive during your procedure. He is like the Holy Spirit, whose role is spiritual breathing and spiritual health - which is as important as the salvation we have through Christ. It is quite possible for a surgeon to fix one's heart and do an excellent job of it, but if the patient doesn't have adequate oxygen and pain control (i.e. stay nicely asleep - but not too asleep) then everything can go bad very quickly.

When I met the anesthesiologist who remembered my transplant I told him, "It's so nice to be remembered. And incidentally, you are an excellent anesthesiologist!"

Dr. Robbins had performed my heart/double lung transplant in 1997. It had of course been a challenging experience for him, even thought I had survived. I cannot begin to imagine what it is like to have a human's very life in your hands under such dramatic conditions. Nevertheless when he met with us in 1997 following my transplant he said something I won't forget.

He smiled and said, "I never want to see the inside of you again!" But now it was time to open my chest again. I felt kind of bad for him.

I was glad he was still willing to open me up again. As the physician who *had* seen my insides he was the most competent man to return and repair the aneurism. He knew what had been done the last time and what my insides looked like. I suppose it is somewhat like taking one's car back to the same mechanic for a car's life. He knows what has been done to the car and the condition of the engine, etc. Dr. Bobby Robbins knew my guts. I readily signed the consent form for the surgery.

I am so glad that when I take life's problems to my Savior that He knows my entire life history. He knows my every weakness and he knows my specific needs. He can address them with absolute perfection. And he is willing to "go back in" as many times as is needed.

The aneurism was in a section of the aortic valve that had ballooned outwards. This had the effect of stretching the valve out of proportion. The valve is supposed to open and shut as the heart pumps, so that blood flows in one direction. When the valve doesn't shut correctly blood flows backwards and forwards. This is what makes the murmur sound. The blood is flowing back into the previous chamber. Poor circulation of blood leads to all sorts of problems. So it had to be fixed.

I had several options with the aortic valve replacement. I could have chosen a pig valve. The heart of a pig is very similar to a human heart in size. Or I could choose a Dacron valve which being artificial is prone to its own issues. If you opt for synthetic material like Dacron you have to be on a blood thinner, and that creates issues if you have any future surgeries. I chose a human tissue valve, which comes from a tissue bank. There is no blood supply to such tissue; it can be frozen and used whenever needed. Such tissue is obtained from donors just like the organs I'd received. (Be a donor!)

My defective heart valve with the aneurism was part of the transplanted heart/lungs I had received five years earlier. I had donated my own (perfectly good) heart during my transplant. I was told that a father of two had received it. So I was a living heart donor; not many can say that.

During this procedure my overall health was dramatically better than it was prior to my transplant. In 1997 I was oxygen deprived, extremely weak, had low weight, virtually no muscle mass, and was fighting multiple infections. Prior to this surgery I had been working as a mission pastor, traveling to Asia, Europe and Africa. I had gained a healthy amount of weight, had been working out at a gym with my dad three times a week, and was full of energy. But now my heart was making a lot of excess noise. It was my personal sump pump. We knew that it was just a matter of time before the aneurism burst, which would change all of the above.

Dr. Bobby Robbins opened my chest up at the same incision that he had so carefully stapled closed some five years prior. He sawed through the sternum. He cut away all the old scar. He replaced not only the enlarged portion of my heart and valve, but something called the aortic root, which is the section of artery that leads out from the aortic valve. I went home after four days. Within a week I was back at my desk answering emails and handling mission business at church.

Sometimes we are surprised by God's grace and goodness. Life can deal us a bad hand at times.

But as my card playing friends say, "You play 'em like you get 'em." That's not really bad advice. It's reality. Sometimes we have hardships that seem insurmountable and we're surprised how easy it all works out. At other times we have simple little issues that take forever to solve or maybe never get solved. Our task is not to sort it all out and attempt to control our future; it is to place ourselves in the physician's hands, sign the release, submit to the anesthesiologist, and trust in the result. We may heal quickly from our wounds, and for that be grateful, or it may take weeks, months, years, or maybe never. In every case it is critical to keep our eyes focused on the Healer and not on the wounds. I now had a new set of wires that held my rib cage together. I also got a new set of staples to give my skin a chance to merge together - and a new scar right where the old one was.

My brother Doug remarked in typical Lagasse fashion, "They should just put in a zipper." Perhaps he was right. For the day would come when I'd need to unzip it again.

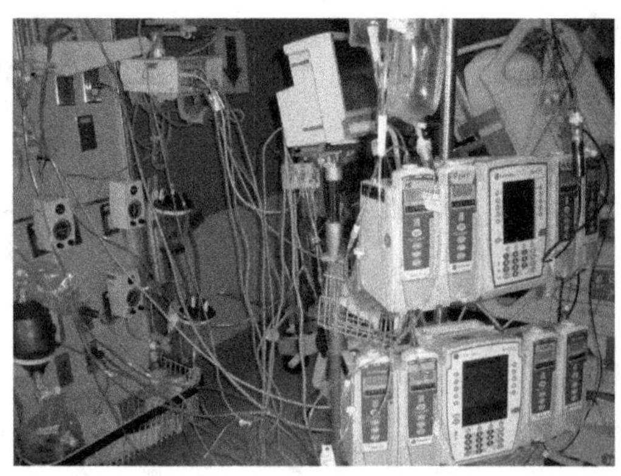

Chapter 26

Agra, India

When you are immune suppressed you are not supposed to expose yourself to dangerous situations, or to potential infections. If I'm in a crowded place, like on an airplane, I wear an N95 mask. Sure, I get funny looks from everyone on the plane. But I have only been sick from one flight out of hundreds, and I have been to forty countries. That's not to say I haven't been sick, but it wasn't from the flights.

I asked my father, Dave, and my friend, Jerry Lee, to join me on a journey to India. One of my responsibilities as the Missions Pastor at Venture Christian Church was to visit missionaries that the church supported. These dear people worked as nurses, church planters, camp directors, aid workers in refugee camps, as trainers of leaders, as professors in a seminary, and many other jobs. The founder of the seminary we were going to visit was in Bangalore, India. First stop.

The three of us landed in Mumbai and took a flight over to Bangalore to visit SAIACS (South Asia Institute of Advanced Christian Studies). We wanted to bring Graham and Carol Houghton greetings from our church, a small gift, and get a feel for their work. I would gather a report to bring to the people at home, and give Graham and his wife Carol a special night out doing something they normally couldn't afford. I was careful on my journey to only eat where the food was very safe, like in the home of this New Zealand couple. Airplane food also qualified as safe.

After our visit to Bangalore we flew north to Varanasi [bar ah NAH see]. We were visiting a single gal from San Jose who had gone to work there. The city is not noted for its cleanliness. My father, who always enjoyed a good play on words, intentionally mispronounced the city's name: "Very nasty," which though in-sensitive, was still funny. I saw more dead bodies in three days in Varanasi than in all of my life. In Hinduism it is a holy act to be cremated along the bank of the Ganges River and so bodies ar-rived continually to be carried down to the water's edge. We were told it took over a cord of wood to burn a cadaver. I saw one de-ceased man pass us, carefully wrapped in fabric and strapped to the top of a Volvo - on his way to the river. During religious festivi-ties over seventy million people also bathe in the Ganges. No, I did not bathe in it. It is one of the most polluted rivers in the world.

Our next stop was in Lucknow, where we were to change planes. The flight was delayed and, as it was lunchtime, the airline directed us inside the terminal where we were provided with a box lunch. The sandwiches were not wrapped, but they were de-licious. The soda bottles had been pre-opened and a plastic straw inserted into each bottle. I should have been more attentive to this, but it was very hot and we were thirsty. It quenched our thirst. Although it was February, which is the "cool" time of year, we were still breaking a sweat. The next leg of the flight was to New Delhi and then we had an overnight train that delivered us to Agra at one a.m. We had hoped to see India's most famous tourist site, the Taj Mahal, since we had to travel through that area anyway. We checked into a one step-above-dingy hotel around two a.m. and quickly fell asleep in a room with three beds.

I woke at five a.m. feeling really feverish. That could mean just one thing: I had an infection. I took a couple Ciprofloxacin. The pills were just a stop-gap; without serious IV antibiotics within a couple hours I knew that whatever infection was in my body it could easily become systemic. I woke my dad up. We'd had three hours of sleep. He sat up on the edge of his bed and rubbed his eyes. On the all night train trip we had been seated on wooden benches squeezed up against a mass of humanity. So we were dead tired. Come to think of it, a simple definition of India could be, "A mass of humanity." 1.3 billion and increasing.

As my wife said to me after her own trip to India some years later, "Dan, we traveled thousands of miles across countryside, and everywhere we looked as we drove along we could see people."

It was a country unlike any I have ever visited, and I have visited rural Cambodia, Thailand, Indonesia, Iraq, Turkey, Ethiopia, Morocco, and the Philippines - just to name a few. Most of the missionaries I've visited lived in hard-to-reach and out-of-the-way places, not in modern cities.

"Dad, I have to get to a hospital," I said in a shaky voice. I could feel the onset of rigors as my body began to tremble. I fought to control it. I was having trouble holding my cup of water as it vibrated beyond my control. I swallowed two Tylenol.

My dad looked at me with concern.

"What should we do?" he asked. We were in a foreign city and we knew nobody. We did not know much about Indian society, and certainly not details like how to chose a hospital. It was in that moment, however, that I realized a major shift had taken place in my relationship with my father. My dad was looking to me to decide what to do. But I was the sick one; I had the fever, felt awful, needed help. I wanted him to take the lead. But he was expecting me to work out a solution.

"Call the front desk and see if we can get through to Stanford Hospital," was my only thought. I always carried a recent medical report, and even a thumb drive that contained my medical history. I also knew Stanford would give advice and speak to a local doctor - on the fly. They could fax records, suggest treatments, tell a physician what my last antibiotic had been, provide my list of allergies, etc. All we had to do was call. Dad called the front desk from the bedroom phone. He asked to place a call to California.

"I'm sorry sir. You cannot make a long distance phone call from inside the hotel, sir. So sorry," the man said in a sing-song sounding voice. "You have to go to a kiosk sir."

Dave then asked, "Where is the nearest kiosk?"

"Oh you just walk up the road a bit. Not far. You will see one around the corner on the left. No problem." At times like that, with a raging fever in the middle of the night, in a foreign place, you just hang on to God. *"No problem,"* I thought. *"Ha!"* We pulled clothes on and the three of us set off to find a taxi. We were not about to start walking in the darkness when we had no idea what we were really looking for.

"Please take us to a phone kiosk, please," I said, with my best Indian accent. I repeated the word "please" intentionally to sound like I'd heard Indians speak . Off we went.

He pulled over beside what appeared to be a squatter's hut set back from a ditch. There was a dirt lot next to the hut where the taxi could park.

I was incredulous as I asked the driver, "Is this a phone kiosk?" I looked at the shack in the darkness. He no doubt thought I'd lost it. So I said to him, "Please wait while we call." We all piled out and went inside where a single bulb hung from a sheet metal roof. The floor was dirt. I asked about making a long distance call.

"No problem, sir." Fortunately we had cash to pay. From under a crudely built desk a traditional black phone appeared, somewhat the worse for grime and wear. I gave him the Stanford Hospital number, which he dialed. I put the phone to my head, trying not to let it touch my ear. Dave and Jerry were standing off to the side and the Indian was listening closely with interest.

"I'd like to speak to the transplant physician on call, please." I waited. I felt cold. I didn't know if I was indeed cold or if it was just my fever.

The operator came back on, "I will page him; would you like to hold?"

"Yes, please." Several minutes passed.

"Yes, this is the transplant physician. How can I help?"

I launched right in, "Hi. My name is Dan Lagasse. I am a heart double lung transplant and a patient of Dr. David Weill. My underlying illness is cystic fibrosis. I am running a fever of 102.5 degrees."

He chimed in, "You should come into emergency."

"Well," I paused. "I can't."

"Why not?" he sounded surprised.

"Because I am in India."

At that he nearly shouted, "In India?"

"Yes," I said. "In Agra, India."

"What are you doing in India!?" It was more of an exclamation than a question. I tried somewhat pathetically to give him a brief explanation. He didn't sound pleased, which is more or less what I expected. "How did you get sick?" was his next question. I thought of the last few days of activity, trying to piece together what might have led to the fever.

"Well, yesterday I was volunteering in Mother Teresa's Home for the Diseased, the Destitute and the Dying," I said, realizing how crazy it must have sounded. "We were in Varanasi." I didn't expect him to know where it was, and he didn't bother to ask. Mother Teresa's facility was not so much a hospital as a place to die with dignity. The missionary we had just visited volunteered there regularly. She washed the women's hair, cut their nails, painted their toe nails. It was a true demonstration of charity, self-less acts of love that can never be repaid. During our visit I had been assigned to wash the concrete floors beneath the beds of the men - while they lay in bed - in the tuberculosis ward. Then we set about washing their laundry in a galvanized tub. It was exhausting work and I hadn't thought to bring a mask to wear.

It is always a conflict anyway when faced with the mask question, *"Do I wear one or not?"* I often wonder how other people are going to feel when I wear a mask. *"Are they thinking that I think they are somehow contaminated?"* Or, *"Are they thinking that I am somehow contagious?"* This is often true on airplanes. I have had people change seats on Southwest Airlines when I sit down. I take care to mention to people sitting near me that I have had a transplant and am immune suppressed. Then they nod with understanding. But I couldn't converse with these men who were dying in Mother Teresa's Home. I did not want to humiliate them by wearing a mask when nobody else was. I could not talk to them because I don't know Hindi. I wanted to uphold their dignity by serving them. Anyway, I didn't have a mask to wear, so there was nothing to debate. I did realize at the time that I was putting my life at risk. But as I set about working on the floor I thought of Mother Teresa and her example. I got on my hands and knees and got busy .

I didn't have much more to share with the physician-on-call on the phone. My mind did a quick inventory of the past few days. I remembered lying on the plywood on the crowded train the previous night, of the hundreds of hands that had pulled at my clothing begging for a few pennies, and of sleeping in several scuzzy hotels. I remembered the dead cow that floated past me as I took a boat ride on the Ganges River, it's butt sticking above the surface of the water and the bird who was perched on it- like a little island, and of a dozen other things. It was, after all, India. I said no more.

"Go to a hospital and have the doctor call me when you've checked in," he finally said. I thanked him, hung up, and paid the owner of the kiosk for the call. We drove back to the hotel to get my stuff. I asked the hotel clerk for a recommendation of a hospital. He gave me immediate advice.

"Do not go to a government hospital!" he said emphatically. "That is where people go when they are going to die." I wasn't sure this was really the case but I got his message. "Go to a private hospital." he continued. "Here... I will tell you where to go," and he drew a map.

The sun was rising as we pulled up to a modest unpainted concrete building. The whole hospital was smaller than some large homes I've seen. But what was significant was the physician. He is one of the unsung heroes in our world. This physician had studied in Atlanta, Georgia and obtained his degree and his physician's license. While many Indian doctors prefer to stay in America once they have their education completed, this man chose to return to India where his knowledge and experience would save the lives of people who would never have a chance for good medical care. I happened to have been one of the lucky recipients of his sacrifice. I began to give him my medical history as he examined me.

"Listen," he said to me as I sat on the dusty bedsheet on my bed. "The president of France is here in Agra today." I had heard this fact on the news. The Taj Mahal had been shut down entirely so he could visit it. "But if Jacques Chirac were to walk into my clinic today I would tell him, 'You go sit over there," and he pointed across the room. "This here is *my* VIP," and pointed to me. I could see that for him as a physician he enjoyed the challenges of every patient's health, perhaps even more so considering my colorful history. Saving a life was more important than glory or fame. After hearing my history and talking with Stanford he prescribed me one gram of Fortum, three times a day. The IV he started was in a vein in the palm of my left hand. I assured him it was OK. My dad went across the street to the pharmacy to buy my meds; the hospital did not stock IV antibiotics.

The infusion was begun and by five p.m. my fever was abating a bit. About that time my dad started feeling poorly. He left my bedside and returned to our hotel. We were scheduled to fly on to Jaipur that same day. We were supposed to visit a Bible Training Center begun by a well known radio teacher named Anand Chaudhari. But it was clear we would miss that flight. All afternoon there were guys with jack hammers tearing up the patio outside my window. (That explained the dust on the bed sheets.) When they finally quit I fell asleep.

The following day we rented a car and a driver to take us on the six hour journey to Jaipur. It proved to be fascinating. The roadway was an obstacle course of children, camels, donkeys, buses, bicycles, pedestrians, oncoming cars and push-carts. We even saw a dancing bear chained to a tree and a guy hoping to make some money off of the poor creature.

Along the way I was able to administer my antibiotics via a gravity-fed drip. I taped the bag to the car window as we drove. (Another time I hung if from a cyclone fence while waiting for a bus.)[43]

On the night before we took our road trip my Dad called me from his hotel and said that he and Jerry were throwing up and having diarrhea. Food poisoning? Perhaps all three of us had contracted food poisoning or something similar. The antibiotics had saved me from most of the symptoms, but I had reacted to the illness a full twelve hours earlier than the others because I was immune suppressed and more sensitive. This wasn't a surprise. I was actually happy the others were sick; it meant I didn't have a blood infection or worse.

---

[43] On the overseas flight home I wired the IV bag to the handle of the overhead bin. When the flight attendant passed me in the darkness she sort of freaked out.

The entire bill for the care, including the doctor's fee, the long distance calls to Stanford that the doctor made, the over-night charge for the room, the chest x-ray, the blood and lab work, the IV antibiotics and tubing sets for the trips duration - came to just $473. (I still had to fight Kaiser to convince them it deserved re-imbursement.)

At that point we pretty much agreed that we should not have eaten the lunch in Lucknow in the airport terminal. It hadn't been prepared by the airline but rather sub-contracted to a local restaurant, and they had hand-made everything. The straws weren't even wrapped. After all we'd been through it was likely the little unnoticed thing that had mattered. That's like life; it's the little things that can cause us to stumble, that can ruin all we've worked for.

The next morning as I thanked my Indian doctor, (my VIP doctor!), I prayed a prayer of thanks. I never did see the Taj Mahal, but I saw something greater, the kindness and wisdom of a man who cared more about people than fame or fortune.

Chapter 27

Broken Bones, Broken Dreams

It was a sunny Sunday afternoon and we were having a picnic. Some kids were showing off their new stomp rocket and firing a six-inch plastic tube hundreds of feet across the grassy park. I was impressed and watched closely, after consuming my hamburger and chips. I showed such interest in their toy they asked me if I wanted to give it a try. Carefully I laid the large plastic bubble on the grass and aimed the tube (that held the mini-rocket) with its base toward the baseball diamond in the distance. I stood by the bubble and prepared to leap into the air and come down hard with my right heal - on the bubble.

I made my leap and landed hard, but missed the bubble entirely. My right heal smacked the hard packed earth. I instantly felt something stab at my heal and shoot an incredible pain up my leg. I fell to the ground and lay on my side on the grass. I looked at my tennis shoe like it was a foreign object and tried to fathom what could be causing the intense pain. It hurt too much to try and remove the shoe. I could not stand. I could not walk.

"DeAnna," I moaned, "I think we need to go to the hospital." This was not going to be a normal Sunday afternoon at the park. An X-ray at urgent care showed a fractured heal. It meant I was destined to spend a few weeks on crutches and then another few weeks in a special boot that looked like I was getting ready to ski. I eventually learned to hang my right leg over the car's console and drive with my left foot, although I don't think that was at the doctor's suggestion.

Even small plans, like a picnic, can be interrupted by a health crisis. In my case it was a stupid fractured heal. It proved to be a major interruption to just about everything I did. Most all my daily activities require the use of hands. My hands, however, were always occupied holding the crutches under my sore armpits. I couldn't even carry a glass of water to the dinner table. This was more than just a hassle. It was annoying, frustrating, and disruptive to normal life. I couldn't wait to get my walking boot as it allowed considerable mobility.

A couple years later... We were on the big island of Hawaii. Just writing that now conjures up all sorts of visions of paradise. Ahh... everybody's vacation dream. Surfing, jet skiing, kayaking, belly boarding, visiting resorts, golfing, extreme eating... and the list goes on. It is like a Disneyland for adults. Just the activity center at the airport is enough to overwhelm you. I think I collected a stack of forty brochures while we waited for the luggage carousel to spit out our bags.

It was January of 2006 and my dad had saved his frequent flyer miles from all his travels and he was feeling very generous. He was able to fly my brother's family of four, my family of four, and himself to the Big Island of Hawaii, and rent a couple two-bedroom condos with his timeshare points. This was a really big deal. Our whole family was going to enjoy ten days of excitement together. Luaus, tours, the ocean. This was going to be great. We planned to soak up the sun while our friends at home in San Jose were soaking in January rains.

One should always be careful with vacation expectations. That is one reason psychologists will tell you that a vacation can be a very stressful time. We did not need a psychologist to confirm this. It turned into what we lovingly today refer to as our, "Vacation from hell."

We should have had a clue when our teenage daughter's cell phone coverage quit in the airport and she could not converse with her boyfriend. She became very unhappy, to put it politely, and we were all immersed in her misery. The flight over was not so bad, since everyone had their own private seats and it is always too loud to converse. I also won a bottle of wine for guessing the half-way point of our plane's course, which was good for my dad, since alcohol and my list of meds don't mix. Things were still looking good as we got our rental van and economy car.

We started to get concerned when we realized that it was Saturday at 5 p.m. and all the stores were already closed. Sunday is a real day-off for Hawaiians, and Monday happened to be a holiday. We were staying in a timeshare and needed groceries. Nine hungry people can cause some discontent. Then there was some complaining about the sleeping arrangements as we hauled our bags into the gorgeous condo. I could not understand why anyone could be unhappy; the place was beautiful, and after all, *"This was Hawaii"*. But when you factor in seven hours of travel, the cramped car, no cell phone coverage, no "decent" food, and four teen-agers, I should not have been too surprised.

Things went from bad to worse in the complaining department, and our attempts at discipline and getting some cooperation were a complete disaster. We tried everything and everything failed; in fact it only seemed to make matters worse. Nobody was happy; most everyone was angry; and suddenly it didn't seem like paradise after all.

My dad was doing his best to stay out of all the issues his sons were facing with their families. Nobody wanted to do any dishes; everyone just wanted to watch the big screen TV, and there was complaining coming from all four teens. He thoughtfully invited us all to the big luau put on by the Youth With A Mission team at the Kona Resort.

I imagined the *Kalua* pig, the *Lomi Lomi* Salmon, the singers, dancers and drummers. This was an awesome experience and I knew it would be a blast even for teenagers. We were really looking forward to it as we hustled everyone in the cars and headed for the Kona Coast. Parking was a bit tight, and we had to settle for a lot up on a hill. It had old wooden steps that led down to the asphalt roadway on the steep hillside. I navigated my way down in my flip flops, wearing my totally tourist Hawaiian shirt.

The wooden step beneath me suddenly gave way and as I tipped forward I felt and heard a snap in the front of my right foot. It was just a sort of quick crunching sound. Then there was pain. Quite a bit of pain. I realized that this was not going to be an ordinary thing that just went away. I pretty much hopped the rest of the way to the luau, aided by my patient and loving wife. I stood on one foot during the entrance show, hopped along till we were seated, then allowed DeAnna to go through the food line and heap my plate with island delicacies. The show was excellent and DeAnna fetched the car so I could get back to the condo.

It goes without saying that I was not going to be doing any wonderful Hawaiian activities for the next week. Instead I hopped about on crutches, loaned to me by the local Kaiser. I was told that when one breaks the metatarsal in the foot, it is not put in a cast; it heals on its own. You just have to stay off of it. Keeping off of it was not an issue for me because it hurt like crazy when I just bumped it or put it under the blanket at night.

My Hawaiian dream vacation had just gone south. No horseback riding in Waimea. No hiking through the volcano craters, no jet skis or surfboarding. I did manage a half mile hike through a lava tube, but it stretched everyone's patience as they waited for me to navigate each step on crutches. Our daughter Jessica went horseback riding and we all did a float in kayaks down the hundred year old irrigation ditches that snaked through the old sugar cane fields. I discovered that there are ways for the disabled to enjoy the island; I just had to change my expectations. Many times dealing with illness is all about changing our expectations. When I chose to be thankful for the things I can do, rather than focus on the things I can't life is a lot more enjoyable.

But the alteration in plans is not why that vacation is our so-called "vacation from hell." The reason for that is the unbelievable stress we were under from the disobedient teens and family conflicts. I am sure the crutches did not help any, but emotional turmoil is far worse than physical disability. This is important for me to realize, especially since as a pastor I often talk to people who are in crisis. The pain of a dysfunctional relationship can be far worse emotionally than a physical injury to the body.

My next bone mishap occurred on August 6, 2006, about a week before my forty-eighth birthday. But I wasn't thinking about birthdays when the sun rose and I pulled on my work jeans. I was thinking about cleaning the leaves from the gutters at our rental home in Evergreen Valley, San Jose. (It's a guy thing.) I took my standard morning dose of 25 pills, ate some breakfast, kissed my wife, loaded my tools into our Corolla and drove ten miles across town. I always kiss my wife goodbye, because I never know when the day at hand will be my last one, and it would be a very sad remembrance for her on that day when I died if she had to think, *"He didn't kiss me goodbye."* And then there's the fact that I love her…

After parking my truck I hauled my tools around to the back of the house. I set my four legged ladder in place, which was actually an old wooden ten foot step ladder that had been abandoned by an old painter. It wobbled quite a bit, *"but if I was careful and placed it firmly on the packed dirt I should be fine,"* I thought. Later I learned from a nurse that falling off ladders is the second most common accident for men. (Cutting oneself in a power saw is the first.) But I am ruining the story.

It is important to get all of the Eucalyptus leaves off the roof at this house and empty the gutters of their clutter before the winter rains, or the gutters will fill up with water and become a waterfall dumping on everyone who passes beneath. It is one of my least favorite jobs (I actually have a lot of "least favorite jobs" as I get older) but it must be done every year, and I am loath to pay someone to do it. So I pulled my electric blower and its extension cord up onto the peak of the roof and began the noisy process of blowing everything down and away. Fortunately, the tenants were not home, so the racket did not disturb anyone.

I meticulously cleaned the gutters by hand of all the accumulated seed pods and dirt and chucked it all onto the ground, where it could be swept up later. Then I lowered the blower down using the electric cord as a rope and then tossed the rest of the cord down too. It was now time to make my descent via the wooden ladder. The gutter was twelve feet from the hard earth below. The flat top of the ladder was just under ten feet above the dirt. I sat on the edge of the roof with my feet just barely reaching the flat surface of the top of the ladder. It wobbled a bit uneasily. I felt uneasy, too. I contemplated the best way to navigate the next few critical steps.

I decided my best hope would be to turn over and lay flat on the roof on my belly, adjacent to the ladder itself and then slowly lower myself down to the point where my right foot could reach the top of the ladder. *"For some reason this was a lot simpler when I was going up,"* I thought. I could never quite muster up the same confidence coming down a ladder as going up one. *"I am sure there is a spiritual lesson in there somewhere, but I can't think of what it is right now,"* I thought as my foot searched the open air. (Getting into trouble is always easier than getting out of it!)

My right foot felt the top of the ladder. It was covered with paint and dirt from sixty years of use and storage outdoors. *"I really should get a decent ladder,"* I thought. *"This thing wobbles terribly."* My wife thought the same thing later, as we cut it up for fire wood.

The ladder at last seemed pretty stable and I lowered myself down so I could get my left foot on the ladder too. I had reached the point of commitment. There was no turning back; I had to let the weight of my body off the stable roof and put it on the shaky wood. (Now there *is* an obvious spiritual lesson in *that!*)[44]

The ladder abruptly flew to the right and I went straight down, extremely fast. I shouted something that I shouldn't print in this book. The next thing I was aware of (it could have been moments, minutes, or even a half hour) was a very intense pain in my back. I was lying on my stomach in the dirt There were leaves and garbage from the roof all around me. I was in agony unequal to anything I had experienced in life, which is no little thing.

I could not shout for help, first because it hurt too bad to even talk, and second because there was a sound wall ten feet to my left and a major expressway on the other side of the sound wall, with constant traffic. Nobody would have heard me even if someone were walking by. I just lay there in pain.

Now I wished the tenants had been home. What was I to do? I couldn't just lie there until enough time went by that DeAnna got

---

[44] The lesson is that when we decide to put our trust in Jesus instead of ourselves, we have to give complete control of our life to Him. He is either God of all or He is not God at all.

worried and came across town to find me. Fortunately I had purchased a cell phone. Unfortunately I did not have it with me. I would have to somehow make it out of the back yard by myself.

I decided, as I lay there face down in the dirt, that I would have to suck up the pain and slowly climb up from my prone position. I extended my hands to my sides and ever-so-slowly pulled my knees up so I was in a crawling posture. It hurt like crazy. I moved like a snail and bit by bit got more and more vertical. Gradually it got to where I could actually stand. I took a few tentative steps like a hundred year old man. I looked at the cursed ladder, which had a cross-support dangling free; its rusted bolt snapped in two. I realized I was going to have to get around to my car and drive home. I shuffled super-slowly along the walkway to the back patio. I did know the neighbor John quite well, as I was always borrowing tools from him when I was working on various fix-it projects there, but I didn't want to disturb him. (OK it was a stupid decision, but please remember I was in a lot of pain and perhaps wasn't thinking clearly.)

I climbed carefully into the car, keeping my back as straight as possible. I slowly backed out and pulled out into the street. I did not move my sitting position in the car seat at all as I drove the twenty minutes to our home. I parked in the driveway and shuffled slowly up to the front door. As I walked into the hallway DeAnna met me.

"I fell off the roof," I managed to groan the words to her. She didn't realize the extent of my situation.

"You are a mess," she said. I was indeed covered in dirt and leaves, but somehow I was not aware of it. "You need to take a shower," she said and led me slowly up the stairs. I was in terrible pain but did not resist.

Now the reader needs to be aware that the telling of this story is from my perspective, and no doubt my wife will seriously disagree with the narration of this part, but nevertheless, that is how I remember it.

Once I was washed, dried off, had clean underwear on and was nicely dressed, DeAnna drove me to Kaiser emergency. (It amuses me that my mom always insisted I wear nice underwear – "in case I was ever in an emergency and the hospital staff saw me." I am not sure what difference it would make if a complete stranger might observe a hole in my shorts during a crisis. But that was the mandate.) So I sat in the emergency waiting area for a few hours, nicely dressed, with clean underwear on, and waiting to be seen.

After an X-ray of my head and back I received the not so surprising news that I had four broken vertebrae. They gave me a shot in my backside, which I didn't feel at all. I was given a bottle with a few codeine pills and an appointment to see the orthopedist. The shot and the pills had no affect at all. When we got home my wife retrieved my crutches from the garage.

"See," I said, "It is good to save old things like crutches."

The orthopedist told me I had a compression fracture, which made sense to me since I fell twelve feet and landed on my tailbone. Everything in my entire spine had been compressed. Fortunately the fractures did not intrude upon the spinal cord and in time, he felt, they would heal. The breaks occurred in vertebrae T-8, T9, T10, and T11, and the cracks went straight across each bone. My orthopedist gave me a cloth device with vertical ribs built into it that wrapped around my chest tightly, and it was supposed to take some of the pressure off my spine. I am not sure if it helped, but I know it kept me from breathing deeply, which is not a good thing for somebody with a lung transplant. I wore it sporadically for the next week, then removed it, as I did not want to get pneumonia.

The worst part was trying to change position from vertical to lying on the bed, or vice-versa. I had to do it in tiny increments, so as to let the pain subside from each movement before initiating another painful move.

Two weeks later I was actually able to walk into the doctor's office without crutches. It still hurt a lot, but I have always had a high tolerance to pain, and I wanted to get a good grade on the doctor's exam. The doc was very impressed and said he had never imagined I would make so much progress that quickly. I felt I had gotten an "A."

Another (bone) break with reality came on our second trip to Hawaii. This time it was just my wife and me. We'd been married twenty-four years. It was the fall of 2008 and we were determined to have a great ten-day respite without the pressures of children, family, and a broken foot. Our expectations again were sky high. I had a long list of fun things we were going to do: hike along the *Napali* coastline in Kauai, bicycle down Waimea Canyon, kayak down the river to Hanalei Bay, surf the world famous waves, and zip line in the jungles in the vast interior. It was going to be awesome. DeAnna had a stack of seven books she wanted to read. We have somewhat different vacation expectations.

On the third day we rented bicycles from a great little shop in Kapaa on the eastern shore, Coconut Coasters Bike Rentals. The people were friendly, which was going to be very important. The seat on my bike was a little too high but I didn't want to bother the rental guy by asking him to adjust it. The bikes were the one-speed retro style, which suited us just fine. There was a wide concrete path that ran along the flat coast for five miles. We figured a ten mile trip on a beautiful day in Hawaii was right up there next to paradise.

We stopped several times to just soak in the beauty of the crashing waves, the talented surfers, the warm sunshine, and the majestic shoreline. There was one place where the bike trail jutted out a bit from the coast. I thought it would make a great photo. We could look along the expansive sea as it wrapped itself around the garden island. As we pulled up at the perfect spot for the picture I stepped down off the pedal onto the concrete pathway. I felt a familiar crack in my foot. It didn't hurt my foot so much this time but the implications were clear.

"DeAnna," I said in an even voice, "I just broke my foot." She thought I was joking. "Yes," I continued. "It is the fifth metatarsal." I felt pretty confident that I could diagnose the situation in an instant. But that's just because I had personal experience, and I assure you, some things are better learned from textbooks.

At this point I felt like there was some kind of curse on me for visiting Hawaii. I explained the sensation of the foot, the audible sound I felt; (it is a horrible thing to hear one's bones snapping) and the confidence I had that it was broken. I could not put any weight at all on the foot without excruciating pain.

Nevertheless, I was determined that we should not let this interrupt our otherwise wonderful day. So I asked DeAnna to move her bike ahead of mine and then asked a Japanese tourist to take our picture. To look at the picture today you would never know I was in pain. Pictures can speak a thousand words but they might still be deceiving.

I said I wanted to finish the ride, and with just one foot managed to pedal the rest of the ten miles. I could put just enough weight on the right foot to just move the pedal around and then place a lot of weight on the left foot to complete most of the rotation. I could not, however, get off the bike and walk anywhere. The folks at the Coconut Cycle Center happened to have a pair of crutches which they generously loaned me for the remainder of my stay. So for the next seven days DeAnna was able to read her books.

We did take one excursion in a kayak, since that involves just the upper body. Getting in and out was a bit of a trick, with some hopping and careful climbing into the boat, but it was actually a very pleasant day.

So what did I learn?

Be prepared for the unexpected and roll with it.

Plan to allow for disruptions in life and accept them gladly.

Listen to your wife's desires and be patient.

Be thankful for the kindness of strangers and willingly accept it, for it brings them joy. Don't let a discouraging incident ruin an otherwise wonderful time.

Be flexible and creative enough to look for new activities. (This is especially important as we age and find we cannot do what we used to do.)

And I also learned to adjust the bike seat so it is a good fit. A moment's prevention can save a vacation from disaster.

And finally, a broken foot (or other bones) is not the end of one's life. Such experiences can be full of lessons. One can still have dreams and pursue them in spite of the inevitable breaks in life.

Chapter 28

Thyroid Cancer & Lyme Disease

Dr. Swedenborg at Kaiser looked me in the eye and said, "If I do it right, you won't be able to see the scar at all." It was the spring of 2006.

I replied, "I am not really concerned about the scar, doctor. I have lots of scars - all over my body - and they just remind me that I am still alive!" He smiled.

He had a great smile and a great sense of humor. I thought of that each time I went in to his office to have nasal polyps removed.

"Oh, here's a biggie," he'd say, like he was playing some sort of game. He'd push his needle nose pliers in a bit deeper, grab some floppy tissue way up inside my head and give a sharp pull. I felt an audible crunch as my head jerked forward.

"Hey, you just ruined a good shirt," I said, as blood splattered down the front of my blue and white dress shirt. "Next time I'm wearing my paint clothes." He pushed his chair back from where I was and put his pliers on the side table.

"I think that's good enough for today. I'll see you again in six weeks," he said.

I egged him on, "Don't you want to get a few more? You only pulled six today." I wanted to make my visit at least worth my time and co-pay.

"Here, hold this against your nose; it should stop the bleeding." I took the hand-full of tissues.

Dr. Jon Swedenborg is one of those rare doctors who can make a bleeding and painful experience into a pleasant visit. I am not writing a Yelp review here, but I am being truthful. He has a great sense of humor and was a "Top Doc" for Silicon Valley during one of the years of my visits to him. He performed three sinus surgeries on me over three years.

I also had a primary doctor in 2006 at Kaiser, an Afghan woman who had received her medical degree from Kabul Medical University. That was indeed remarkable and I considered it an honor to get to know Jackline Saber, M.D. I asked her during a visit about an abnormal lump I had on my neck. I told her that my mother had a lump on her neck when she was young. I always wondered about it. Later in life she developed melanoma cancer on her neck, and passed away at age sixty-six. So Dr. Saber agreed to send me to the Kaiser endocrinologist to check on the lump.

The endocrinologist took several needle biopsies of my thyroid, during which time I was sure the needle was going to come out the back of my head. She withdrew about forty cc's of fluid. It was eventually determined that I had thyroid cancer. A CT scan showed a mass that was about a centimeter in diameter. Dr. Swedenborg, as the head and neck surgeon at Kaiser was the one who would perform the surgery.

"Do you suppose I could get a two for one deal?" I asked him. He smiled.

"Maybe you could put me under for the thyroidectomy and at the same time do a sinus surgery?" The sinus surgeries I likened to a rotor rooter job. I imagined some sort of whirling bladed device was thrust up inside the sinus cavity and all the polyps and tissue that shouldn't be there were cut away. Maybe it wasn't as bad as that, but that was my mental image.[45] Dr. Swedenborg agreed to the two for one deal. "Super," I said.

That was March of 2006. After the surgeries I took a look at the nice incision. Then I noted that the original bump for which I'd gone to the endocrinologist. It was still on my neck; it was a cou-

---

[45] Actually a debriding tool is exactly that. It's a set of whirling cutting blades at the end of an endoscopic cable.

ple inches away from the horizontal scar of the thyroid surgery. I asked about the bump.

"Oh; that is just an enlarged vein; it will go away with time," He said. I realized that the reason I'd gone in to see the doctor was for something that turned out to be harmless. But the visit had saved my life. I cannot stress enough how important it is for transplant patients to be vigilant about their health. Faithfully making appointments with my doctors has saved me numerous times.

After the thyroid was removed I was put on an iodine free diet for three weeks. The Kaiser endocrinologist insisted I had to be very diligent about having no iodine whatsoever. I had no idea how many of the foods I ate had iodine in them. We began to really study labels. Of course I could have no table salt. Iodine was added to salt years ago to prevent people from getting goiters. I had seen a goiter the size of large grapefruit on a woman's neck when I was in the Philippines, so I was glad for iodized salt. But besides no salt I couldn't have any sauces, no ketchup or mayonnaise, no canned foods or boxed foods, no meat, no dairy, ... and the list went on and on. I wondered how much of my meager weight I would lose on this three week diet. Perhaps I should just fast altogether. DeAnna went to work diligently making everything from scratch so I wouldn't starve. It took her hours and hours to prepare meals. She even made mayonnaise from scratch.

After the three week diet I visited the same endocrinologist again to take a radioactive pill. This pill would hopefully eliminate any residual cancer in the neck that may have snuck outside the nasty lump that had been removed. I told her how difficult it had been to make everything from scratch and to eat those meager meals for three weeks.

"Oh," she said flippantly, "You could have just done it for ten days. That would have been enough. "And you didn't have to be that picky about it." I was furious but I kept my mouth shut. I won't state her name here for obvious reasons. It is important to get as many details from a doctor as possible. What for them is routine is often a brand new experience for the patient.

When I went to the lab to take the radioactive pill the technician asked, "Have you had any iodine during the last five days?" *Five days?* I looked at the technician and tried hard not to react.

"No. I have not," I said abruptly. I didn't bother telling her I'd been on an iodine free diet for three weeks. She then gave me explicit instructions about how to get and take the radio-active pill.

"Go through that heavy metal door. Then go across the room. There won't be anyone in the room. You will see a button to push on a machine across the room. Push the button and your pill will drop down into a small container. Take the pill with the water that is next to the machine. Then go out the door on the far side of the room, get into your car and drive home. You should stay at your home for several days. Avoid close contact with your family. When you use the toilet flush two times." I was getting the gist of things. This pill was pretty special.

I followed the instructions, but about that time I was losing some of my confidence in doctor's instructions, at least some doctors. But nobody is perfect. And sometimes imperfections cause damage. However, a simple inconvenience is the kind of damage I can live with.

The surgery did in fact leave an imperceptible several-inch scar across my neck, right at the location of a natural wrinkle. It's hard to tell there was ever an incision made. Not that I cared. I was just happy to send the papillary cancer packing. For the remainder of my life I take a tiny little thyroid replacement pill, which is no big deal. I just added it to the other twenty-five medications on my list. Some scars in our lives are imperceptible to others who see us. But their story remains in our memories. And they can remind us that we are alive and have survived. That's another reason I cherish them.

In the late spring of 2006 we planned a weekend camping trip. We were headed to San Mateo County Park. I followed in my parent's footsteps in that regard, also in the tradition of the Boy Scouts, and took my family on regular trips into the out of doors. I loved it. DeAnna tolerated it. My girls liked it… sometimes. I had found a tent trailer and fixed it up, so at least the cables holding the roof up wouldn't break again. This gave the females in the family some modicum of privacy and comfort. There was a gas range so we could cook inside. There were two double beds. And a heater. Even a table. It felt like luxury to me. There was no bathroom or shower, but hey, the public shower was just up the road. You understand why the females were less than enthusiastic.

DeAnna and I love to hike. The girls like to sing, dance, compose music, act, and play the keyboard - none of which are a normal part of camping. So on this trip up into the mountains near the Pacific Ocean it would just be my wife and I. We joined another couple and had great talks by the fire and hikes around the park. DeAnna and I decided to take a six mile loop trail on our final afternoon. It began with a downhill grade on what seemed like a service road. After several miles the service road narrowed up and we found ourselves amid grass, madrone trees and manzanita bushes. *"Now we are hiking,"* I said to myself. After another mile we reached the top of a ridge and walked along a narrow path with views down into valleys on both sides. It was beautiful. Then the trail, which had been well maintained up to that point, pretty much fizzled out. We checked our map again, and yes, it was indeed a loop trail.

"Somewhere the path must continue," I said.

"Is that it?" DeAnna asked as she gazed through the undergrowth. We forged ahead, not wanting to retrace our steps for four miles and climb up the service road.

"We should just have about two miles before we reach the campground." I tried to sound convincing.

The last two miles were at least as hard as the first four, as we pushed brush this way and that and could only distinguish a trail every now and then. Finally the path widened out. With confidence we strode back to the trailhead, happy to not be lost, and to have finished the hike. It's a funny thing about hiking, I say I love it because I know it's good for me. I say I enjoy it because I do see some wonderful sights along the way. But for the most part, especially the uphill stretches, I wish I had my border collie leashed to my belt so he could pull me along.

Back at our campsite I noticed a tick on my arm. I flicked it off onto the ground, and thought no more about it. But I should have. I didn't realize they sometimes carry a disease.

One evening a week or so after the camping trip I saw a red spot on my leg. I had no idea what it was. A few days later the red spot had a white, skin-colored spot in the middle of the red spot. It looked like a bull's eye. The following day the whole thing had grown larger by half an inch, and the next day another half an inch. Everybody in the family had a look at it.

"Hey," said Jessica, "I know what that is." I smiled and waited. She was seven. "That's Lyme disease." I had no idea what Lyme disease was.

"How do you know that?" I asked her.

"We studied it in science in school today," she said in all seriousness.

DeAnna looked Lyme disease up on WebMD. The symptoms showed a characteristic bull's eye, according to the website. A few pictures looked remarkably similar to my leg. I remembered the tick I'd flicked off my arm. Perhaps he had a cousin that found my leg irresistible. I was beginning to put two and two together. I called my primary care physician at Kaiser and was later referred to an infectious disease specialist. When I saw the doc I showed him the red circle and I said I thought it was Lyme disease. He told me there were no cases of Lyme disease in Santa Clara County.

"But I was in San Mateo County," I said. "Doesn't it look like Lyme disease?" I asked. I told him about the tick I'd had on my arm. I mentioned the bushes we'd whacked our way through on our hike.

"There isn't any Lyme disease reported in San Mateo either," he said.

"Then what is it?" I asked. He looked momentarily confused.

"It's just a rash. Or some kind of infection," he guessed.

The following day I was sitting at my desk at work in my office at church. Suddenly I felt a sharp jab like a needle had been shoved into my big toe. But I was sitting immobile and wearing tennis shoes. Tammy, my admin, ran into my office when she heard me shout.

"What's wrong?" she asked.

"I don't know. It felt like a needle was forced into my foot." I pulled my shoe and sock off. Everything looked fine.

That night we read more about Lyme disease. It seems that the bacteria, which is carried by the tick and is inserted into the flesh when a person is bitten, travels to the person's central nervous system or brain. In some cases the bacteria attacks random nerves which can cause pain, such as in joints. I figured that might have been what I felt in my foot. One medication to treat Lyme's is an antibiotic, Doxycycline. I happened to have some left-over pills in my drawer at home so I prescribed myself a two week course.

Lyme's disease often goes undiagnosed. Some people never have the telltale bull's eye on their body. The damage can be debilitating: brain damage, permanent nerve damage, arthritis, fatigue. I was grateful I had a clever daughter and a drawer full of medications. I have had no lasting symptoms from the tick bite. I realized it could have been much worse.

Some years in our lives, or seasons of our lives, are full of difficulties. Like when we were raising teenagers. Or as in the case of my year 2006. But much of the time if we just persevere we will find that kids do grow up, sicknesses do get better (but not always) and bones do heal.

There is a spiritual illustration from that year. I hope I learned it. This world is full of lawlessness, of evil, of bad stuff. But those who persevere and remain faithful to their walk with God will endure and be rewarded with life. Matthew 24:13 says, "But the one who endures to the end, he will be saved."

Chapter 29

Stranded in Reno with a UTI

It was going to be a nice get away with my wife, a romantic three day trip to Reno, Nevada. Well, it was also a car show, but that was secondary (at least for my wife.) Hot August Nights is pretty well known as one of the premier hot rod and custom car shows in America. It had become so popular that it was limited to six thousand cars. People drove their rides (or had them trailered) from up and down California and the western states.

I had been working on a 1936 Ford coupe in my garage for some time, and my hot rod mentor, Gilbert Crum, was going to be there with his brother Russ and their 1957 deep blue Chevy. Gil had done most of the build on that car and he was the inspiration for my getting involved with my own old Ford. Gil and Russ planned to stay at their timeshare in nearby Sparks, Nevada. My car wasn't drivable yet so DeAnna and I drove our reliable Toyota Corolla from San Jose up to Reno, a five hour drive.

We checked into the Atlantis Hotel and then wandered around the parking lot looking at street rods. She did her best to have fun as she watched her husband chat with complete strangers about headers, manifolds, transmissions, paint jobs, etcetera.

"Oh, that one is nice," she'd say. "I like the color." I realized that like anything, appreciation comes with developing knowledge. Some of the guys I met seemed like they practically worshipped their hot rod. They sat for hours, even days, in their folding chairs beside their blown Willys or their chopped Merc just for the opportunity to tell some other guy about their pride and joy.

For me, my car was just a rod, not my god. The truly crazy ones were the guys who pulled up with a massive box trailer, with their car inside. They never drove the car; they just showed it. For them it was a piece of art; it had nothing at all to do with transportation.

I woke on our first morning in Reno with lower abdominal pain.

"I don't want to be sick," I groaned to DeAnna. I knew that being immune suppressed as a post transplant patient put me at a much greater risk for infections. There was a fine line between the two. The immune system had to be suppressed so the body wouldn't see the lungs and heart as foreign and reject them. But the immune system had to also do the normal function of attacking foreign germs. Well it looked like my immune system had missed a few bacteria and I was getting sick.

As I went to the bathroom I felt a terrible burning.

"DeAnna," I sadly said. "We are going to have to find a hospital." We both knew that getting IV antibiotics was the only way to combat an infection; tablets were not of sufficient strength to be effective. That meant I had to get to an emergency room quickly. It does not take long for an infection to spread throughout the body of an immune suppressed person. This was also going to ruin the car show for me.

"I'm sick of being sick," I said to nobody in particular. Every time I got sick it was a total disruption of my life. I had to accept that healthy or sick, my life is still my life. The apostle Paul put it this way, "I have been crucified with Christ and I no longer live, but Christ lives in me. The life I now live in the body, I live by faith in the Son of God, who loved me and gave himself for me."[46] When I was sick, I still belonged to Jesus, and His grace allowed me to live a life of faith, not despair.

But it is very hard not to feel despair when first confronted with a fever of 103 degrees. Daily life stopped. The car show was over before it even began. Our vacation was done. Hospitalization was beginning once again. I did not know if I'd ever live to come to Reno again for this annual one week show. I guess one could say going to that show was on my bucket list. And it was going to remain there.

---

[46] Galatians 2:20

We drove our Corolla north on Virginia street to the Saint Mary's Regional Medical Center[47] and checked into their emergency room. In a record amount of time a doctor inserted a PICC line (peripherally inserted central catheter) into my upper arm and started me on Erythromycin.

At the time I was on Kaiser insurance and it took a couple days before their team decided to transfer me (by ambulance) from Reno, Nevada, to a the Kaiser facility in south San Jose. I could not believe that an insurance company could make such a ludicrous decision, but I was just the patient, so I had no voice. The ambulance would have to cover a five hundred mile round trip drive to deliver me to San Jose. Unbelievable. DeAnna and I discussed it and decided it made best sense for her to check out of the Atlantis Hotel and drive our car back home alone. I would be following later in the ambulance. So much for our vacation.

Hospitals have strict policies about personal possessions. Basically they don't want you to have any valuables, less somebody steal them and they get blamed. Since I am (or was) so compliant I gave all my cash and credit cards to DeAnna, as well as my luggage. We kissed goodbye, knowing that the next day an ambulance would bring me to the San Jose Kaiser and we'd be together again. She left the hospital, drove to the hotel and checked out. Then she began the long drive home.

The following morning a nurse came into my hospital room and mentioned that my St. Mary's doctor had reported my improving progress to Kaiser. I had been recovering very well. The prompt administration of the strong antibiotic had attacked the UTI (urinary tract infection) and my fever was gone. She said I was well enough to be discharged that afternoon. It took a moment for her news to sink in.

"You mean I won't be transferred by ambulance?"

"No," she said. "Kaiser has decided you are well enough to be driven home by your wife. The discharge nurse will be in shortly." I was dumbfounded.

Quite honestly I thought it was pretty funny. I knew that nothing is a surprise for God. He knew that DeAnna and I had made

---

[47] https://www.saintmarysreno.com

the best decision we could with the information we had. He knows all things. "As the heavens are higher than the earth, so are my ways higher than your ways and my thoughts than your thoughts."[48] So this was no surprise to God. I gathered my few belongings, all which fit into a small bag. I only had my driver's license for identification. I did not have a single penny and no credit card.

As I put my coat on and walked down the hall to leave the hospital, knowing there was no one to meet me at the exit, and nobody to pick me up in a car - not to speak of somebody to drive me five hours back to San Jose, my mind was racing. What should I do? To whom could I turn to?

Suddenly it occurred to me that my friends Gilbert and Russ, who had driven their '57 Chevy to the show, might be at the Atlantis hotel showing their car. They were the only people I knew who would be in Reno. *"Perhaps I could walk to the Atlantis,"* I thought. It was a bit over six miles, pretty much straight down South Virginia street. *"There must be a bus. If I could get a bus ride there at least I might find Gil and Russ,"* I hoped.

"Can I have a dollar fifty for the bus?" I asked the nurse who walked beside me towards the exit. I explained how Kaiser had told me I'd be taken by ambulance to San Jose, so my wife had left the previous day in our car. I explained how I had given her all my money and belongings.

She looked at me gently and said, "I'm sorry," our hospital policy is to never give any money to patients." My eyes widened.

I began, "But I have no money at all. I just need a bit to get the bus." I realized I must have sounded like a thousand other desperate people she'd met in life. Now I was one of them.

"I'm sorry, but no."

I walked outside into the fresh air and thought, *"Hmm. Looks like a nice day for a walk, even a long walk. At least I don't have anything to carry."* I always delight in those first few moments when I am discharged from a hospital and walk unencumbered into the out of doors. It is amazing to me how God's presence becomes more real in times of need. When a person has walked

---

[48] Isaiah 55:9

with God and learned to trust Him in the little things, then big things don't crush him or her. God is bigger than our circumstances. Certainly being homeless in Reno (with a PICC line in my arm that would need an infusion that night) is not that big of a deal, not to God. I suppose the worse case scenario would be to either ask DeAnna to drive five hours back to Reno to pick me up, or if I got sick again just check back into the hospital. I continued to walk the three blocks from the hospital towards South Virginia Street. My heart was surprisingly light.

"My peace I give unto you," Jesus said in John 14:7. "Not as the world gives... let not your heart be troubled." In spite of being in another state and so far from home, and without even money for food or lodging, I had no sense of fear or worry. I just continued walking. I looked up the street ahead and saw that there were a lot of street rods parked along South Virginia Street. *"Hmmm. I came here to look at cool cars. I might as well take my time and check out these cars as I walk toward the hotel. After all, I did not come to Reno to visit St. Mary's Hospital!"*

I turned right and began walking down the side walk. It looked like they had blocked off that part of the street so that show-participants could park their vehicles up and down the road. With 6000 cars to feature, the organizers had to arrange for many display venues.

I walked about half a block and I saw it, a bright blue '57 Chevy. Two-door hard top. Corvette suspension, Corvette engine. Tuck and roll custom interior. No-post window. That's the thing about custom built hot rods: they are, as expressed in hot rod lingo, "one-off." There is no other car like Gilbert's and Russ' Chevy. Nobody was seated by the car showing it, so I sat down on the curb and waited for the owners.

Thirty minutes later Russ walked up.

"Hey; I thought you were in the hospital!" he said in his jovial way.

"They sprung me," I said. "Oh, and by the way, DeAnna left for San Jose yesterday. They were going to send me home by ambulance but they changed their minds." Russ was quick to figure things out. He was also very resourceful. His own plans were to stay for a full week to participate in the show. He wasn't going to be retuning to San Jose himself for a while. But he had a friend.

"You know," he began, "I have somebody who is going back to San Jose this afternoon. Let me check with them and see if they have room for you."

So I was only really homeless and helpless for about thirty minutes. But it was enough for me to appreciate God's provision in bizarre situations, and to be reminded again of His faithfulness. My alma mater is Westmont College in Santa Barbara. The school song is the great hymn, "Great is Thy Faithfulness." The words came back to me:

Great is Thy faithfulness, O God my Father,
There is no shadow of turning with Thee;
Thou changest not, Thy compassions, they fail not.
As Thou hast been Thou forever wilt be.

Great is Thy faithfulness! Great is Thy faithfulness!
Morning by morning new mercies I see;
All I have needed Thy hand hath provided—

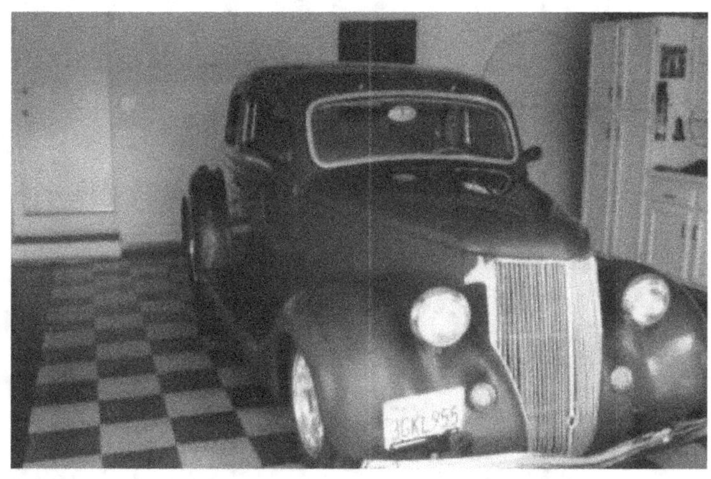

MY FINISHED '36 5 YEARS LATER IN 2011.
WE DID MAKE ANOTHER TRIP TO RENO...

Great is Thy faithfulness, Lord, unto me![49]

---

[49] penned in Franklin, Kentucky by Thomas Chisholm (born 1866). Thomas became a schoolteacher at age 16 in Franklin, Kentucky. Later he worked for a newspaper and then became a pastor.

Chapter 30

Aortic Stenosis

Turning to DeAnna I said, "Those are big banana trees. Don't you think we should take them out?" I looked at the line of giant palms that separated my father's yard from his neighbor's. "I know Mrs. Bailey would sure like it. She has hated these trees ever since dad planted them." She was an original home buyer, like my parents, back when the Los Gatos subdivision had been built up against the southernmost hills of Santa Clara Valley. That was forty eight years ago. Now all the homes had very mature trees growing. I fetched my DeWalt saws-all from my truck. This was going to be fun.

There is nothing like cutting down trees that makes a man feel, well, manly. I watched with joy as the first one fell across the lawn. I chopped up the smaller pieces with loppers. Then I hauled them down a hill and out to my truck which was parked fifty feet away at the curbside. Then it was time to make the return walk back up the the front lawn and through the narrow side gate. Wow. That was just part of one banana palm tree. I counted the trees. Thirty-three.

"This is going to take some time, dear," I said to my faithful and hard working wife. She began hauling them as I cut them. She could only manage the lighter leafy portions. I cut the trunks into chunks and loaded them into old recycle bins we'd salvaged years ago. The full bins seemed to weigh a hundred pounds. I couldn't lift them so I drug them across the lawns. The tree trunks were full of water.

I had most of the trees cut down and was in the process of hauling another bin out across the front lawn when it happened. I was suddenly overcome with a feeling of complete fatigue.

"I'm going to sit down," I announced to DeAnna, like it was some big deal. I plopped myself down on the grass. "Wow," I'm tired," I said, as I lay back on the grass and looked up at the October sky. "Those banana stalks are full of water. Man they're heavy." Then I passed out.

It was 2008. My dad had just died as a result of an accident in that home two month's previous on August 29th. We guess that he felt faint and lost his balance while carrying a plate from his living room into the kitchen. He'd lived alone for the ten years since my mom had passed. He'd hit his head on a cabinet and then wandered around the house looking for a bandage, all the while gushing blood from his forehead. He was taking a blood thinner.

DeAnna had phoned him and Dave had said he was busy cleaning up a lot of blood. She immediately drove over and took him to Kaiser where he was bandaged up and put in a room for a night of observation. Because of the blood thinner he had a huge shiner on the right side of his face. After complaining to his nurse of a headache the next afternoon he went unconscious and then passed away. His thinned blood had been seeping into his skull and pushing his brain stem off to one side. There had been a fracture that the radiologist hadn't seen in the CT scan. No coagulants had been administered.

After his memorial service we had begun cleaning up and repairing his home with the help my brother Doug, his wife, and some friends from church. Now it was just DeAnna and I working on some of the landscaping projects.

Looking at me laying there unconscious on the front lawn, DeAnna was frantic. "Dan, Dan!" she shouted. I didn't wake up. She felt for a pulse and couldn't feel one. She thought I was dying. I lay there, eyes wide open, staring up into the blue sky, unblinking. She knew she had to call 911, but she didn't have a phone. She ran to the neighbor Mrs. Bailey's home and knocked on the door. No response. In her mind all she could think of was the death of my dad that had just happened. It was horrifying. She ran down the street to another neighbor and just opened the people's front door.

"Call 911, she shouted in a panic." A man and lady responded. She ran back up to where I lay on the grass. Suddenly I blinked my eyes and responded to her. I sat up. She told me quickly what had happened.

"Well I feel fine," I said. And then characteristically, "There is no way I am taking an ambulance ride to a hospital." So she cancelled the 911 ambulance request.

Instead she drove me to Kaiser and we waited in the emergency department, not far from where my father had passed away. We waited there for six hours before a doctor saw me. While waiting I anticipated they would want to start an IV and I was thirsty so I requested water. I wanted to hydrate so my veins wouldn't collapse.

"We cannot give you anything to eat or drink without doctor's orders," I was told. Finally, the doctor examined me and made the startling pronouncement that I was dehydrated.

"Perhaps that's because I was not allowed to drink anything since I got here," I said with a bit of attitude. And then with sincerity, "Why did I pass out?"

"It's likely because you were dehydrated," he said. "You need to drink lots and lots of water." I knew it had been hot and I knew I had worked hard. But I didn't feel dehydration would cause me to pass out. I decided not to argue. I was sent home.

Two days later I was helping my friend Bruce while he tiled the floor in my dad's bathroom. My brother and I had decided to solicit our friend's help to dress up the home a bit so we could rent it out. Bruce was a retired fireman. He was down on his hands and knees laying tile. He marked the cuts he wanted with a pencil, then I would take the marked tile down the two half-flights of stairs and out to the side yard where the tile saw was set up. I made the cuts per his marks then ran back upstairs to give the cut piece to him. He then handed me the next piece that needed a cut. Bathrooms are small and have many odd shaped corners and edges so there were lots of cuts to make. I was on my fifteenth piece of tile when I felt light headed. All day long I had been consuming huge quantities of water, per the doctor's instructions. Not wanting to fall, I sat down on the concrete on the side yard by the tile saw. A breath or two later I felt really weak, so I lay flat on my back.

I passed out.

Somebody hollered for help. Bruce came down to my side. He could find no pulse. When a fireman can't find a pulse it's not a good sign. My brother had been sanding and repainting the intricate woodwork of the front door of the house. He ran down the stairs to the garage level and rushed to my side.

"Dan," he hollered. "Breathe! Breathe!" he could only see a slight rise and fall of my chest. That's the last I remember.

Perhaps ten minutes later I came back. Again I felt fine.

"Have you been drinking enough water?" everyone asked me.

"I have drunk more water today than any day of my life!" I said. "Except perhaps the week dad and I hiked across the Grand Canyon and back!" I was ready to get back to work. Doug, however, took over the running up and down the stairs to pass the rest of the tiles to Bruce.

The next day we decided to tackle the garage. Our dad grew up in the depression and ever since that time of severe austerity he'd had a tough time throwing away things with a useful value. Every plank or piece of odd plywood had been used to make shelving or cabinets. Invariably these held other things that might be useful someday. All the cabinets had been painted with left over paint of various colors. We decided all of it would not appeal to a prospective renter, so we tore it all out. I borrowed a large truck from a friend at church and we filled it with odd shaped boards to haul out to the Kirby Canyon Landfill. Two guys joined me to haul it away.

A dozen switchbacks led us to the top of the dump. We had a magnificent view of Morgan Hill and the south valley. We began throwing boards off the truck. When the truck was empty we were all tired and ready to drive home. I sat down in the bed of the truck. Then I lay down. DeAnna's father Steve was at my side. My last thought was, *"I'm going to die at the dump. What an undignified place to die! Maybe they can just bury me here; that'd be cheap!"* Like I said before; one shouldn't put too much stock in a person's dying thoughts or words. I wasn't "all there." I do remember it was a rotten thing for my father-in-law to have to see.

There was no 911 service at the dump, and the entrance was at least a mile away down the windy dirty road. Once again, after about eight or so minutes I awoke. Steve drove us home. We all agreed I needed to see a doctor, and not at Kaiser. The next day I was able to get a waiver from the cardiologist at Kaiser to be seen at Stanford because I was a "multiple organ transplant." If I'd only had my lungs transplanted and not the heart as well I would not have qualified under my insurance to switch to the more expensive facility. I booked an appointment.

I had to park rather far from the main clinic entrance which made me a bit late for my appointment - so I was walking as fast as possible. A couple of times I jogged for a short distance. I hated to be late. I went in at the south entrance and headed down the carpeted hallway. I was right beneath the sign indicating the cardiologist clinic when I felt light headed. *"Whoa!"* I sat down on a bench on my left. People were walking up and down the busy hallway. I realized I was going to pass out, so even though it was embarrassing I lay on the brown low pile carpet in the middle of the hallway, my arms at my sides. My last image was of a passing Sikh wearing his black turban. He eyed me like I was some sort of whacko who'd lost his marbles.

In my next conscious moment I was surrounded by ten or so medical personnel. A moment later a gurney appeared at my side. I said I was fine; I just had to get to see my doctor.

"His office is right down the hall," I said.

"You are not going anywhere; just lie there," someone said with authority. I felt a bit embarrassed.

"One, two, three," and a group of them lifted me up onto the gurney. Off I went down the hall.

"I guess I'm going to miss that appointment," I thought.

It was determined after an echocardiogram and other tests that I had aortic stenosis. That meant there was a kind of hardening of the flaps of the aortic valve. It is unclear why it happened to me. But whenever I exercised, and my heart was restricted to force blood to the muscles in my extremities, the stiff valve flaps would stick shut. This stopped the blood flow to my head, hence the light headedness.

Then without any blood flow at all, i.e. no pulse, the rest of my body went limp. Lying quite still on the grass, or the concrete side yard, or the bed of the truck, or the hallway at Stanford - meant my muscles no longer needed any extra blood to work hard. So my heart could relax. When the heart relaxed it expanded. This permitted the valve to open a fraction and the heart could begin to pump again. My heart had in effect stopped each time. I was told it was a serious condition. *(Really?)*

That was the precursor to opening my sternum a third time. Dr. Bruce A. Reitz performed the surgery. A zipper would have been nice.

"I had the heart on a bypass for five hours," he later told my wife. He continued, "I wondered, really wondered, if it would start again on its own when I completed the eleven hour surgery. I just prayed. It was a miracle to see that heart start pumping again. All I can do when I'm done operating is sit back and watch it. And it started! Usually a heart can only re-start after a four hour operation. Your husband has a really strong heart," he told her. He went on, "The surgery took so long because after the two previous surgeries there was very little tissue to reattach the heart to. Each time all the scar tissue has to be removed, so there is healthy fresh tissue where it can re-attach." DeAnna breathed a huge sigh of relief as I lay in ICU in recovery.

Sometimes life has tiny (or not so tiny) warnings about dangers ahead. We can heed those warnings or ignore them to our own peril. God's desire is that nobody perishes. He gives us indications of his power and majesty in creation all about us. Those are magnificent reminders of his power and presence. He tells us of his perseverance and faithfulness in the changing of the seasons, in the cycles of the stars and planets, in the recurrence of the tides. He tells us of his strength in the height of the Redwood tree, of the breadth of His love when we look at the expanse of the oceans. All of nature declares His glory. We can chose, however, to ignore it.

God gives us truth about forgiveness and healing when our bodies heal from infirmity or wounds. We need not give up hope when everything seems to fall apart and we are flat on our backs. We can see his love in the perfection and beauty of a Yosemite or a Grand Canyon. We can chose to respond to Him and give Him his due place in our lives. Or we can refuse to see the Doctor and miss out entirely on getting our hearts fixed.

Go see the Doctor. You need more than just water. You need living water.[50]

---

[50] <u>John 4:10</u> Jesus answered her, "If you knew the gift of God and who it is that asks you for a drink, you would have asked him and he would have given you living water."

Chapter 31

"Have You Been to the Track?"

I took a good look at the dinosaur. He gently swayed his head in a mechanical sort of way. In the distance was a man who looked to be walking with his wife; they were dressed in primitive clothing. They were actually stationary, made of artificial material. The sign in the foreground explained how the fossils of many dinosaurs on display were so complete and in perfect shape as to support the theory they had been destroyed in a catastrophic event, such as a flood. This would be consistent with the account of a worldwide flood such as is described in Genesis seven to eight.

I stepped outside of the Creation Museum in Petersburg, Kentucky. DeAnna and I had flown to Kentucky in May of 2009 to visit her cousin Gwynn and her family. I sat down on a bench to cool off in the southern heat. It wasn't working.

"I think I need to get my temperature taken," I said to Gwynn's husband Karl, a dentist by profession. He hunted up some Tylenol for me. I took it.

After a stop at the museum's petting zoo we climbed into their fifteen passenger van; (they had six kids) and began to drive back toward their home in Louisville, a hundred plus miles away. Karl knew the importance of getting me to a hospital fast. A huge storm was moving in and rain began to pour down on their vehicle. We were buffeted by gusty winds. I knew I was getting sick. Not nausea sick, but infection sick. I was sweating. Next to me were six kids joyfully singing, "Ninety-nine bottles of pop on the wall…"

It's a rotten deal when you are sick on vacation. For one thing you don't get to use your sick days off; you are using your vacation days - but you're sick. Plus it's that awareness that everything you'd planned has suddenly been thrown out the window and instead you have to reorganize your plans.

"I'm sick of being sick," I again mumbled to nobody in particular.

Once in Louisville DeAnna and I loaded our rental car with our bags and headed north. We had booked the only existent timeshare in southern Indiana for our vacation. We wanted to stay near DeAnna's cousin Gwynn and husband Karl. The resort was in a town called French Lick. It was the weirdest name of a town I'd ever heard. But that's probably because I've lived in cities all my life. A quick search shows hundreds of strange names for places. Like Oddville, Ordinary, and Okay, in Kentucky. The timeshare in Indiana turned out to be all three. It was an *ordinary* building. It looked like the low income housing project we'd worked in in San Jose. It was *odd* because there was absolutely nothing of interest in the vicinity to see or do, accept a casino, which held no appeal. And it was *okay* in so far as there was a jacuzzi in the unit, only it was next to the kitchen. No matter; my body felt very chilled so this was just what I needed. Or maybe not, as I was to later learn. I filled it with hot water and enjoyed a long soak.

We were booked to stay a week, but after just one night in the "resort" I knew I should really go to a hospital. I called information and found the contact information for two hospitals. I wanted a PICC line as it would make life so much easier. Generally when the fever has subsided I can be discharged with the PICC in place to finish the course of medication, even if it is for six subsequent weeks. So I asked the hospitals if they were familiar with a PICC and if they had trained people to insert one. It requires an ultrasound device to detect the deep down veins in the upper arm. Jasper Memorial Hospital had the proper equipment so we planned for me to be admitted there.

I packed a few things and DeAnna drove us in our little red rental car. I was sad I'd messed up our mini vacation with my wife. She had endured so much, it was awful to ruin another get-away. I was taken right in when we got to emergency. I met Dr. Sellers, who was the nicest doctor I had ever seen in any emergency department. His silly humor helped lighten things up. Their PICC specialist came right into emergency and they hurried to start an IV. It was imperative to get antibiotics going as soon as possible. We were literally racing against the infection. I lay on a bed and waited for a room. I was impressed with the place. They certainly weren't crowded. But then, we were way out in hicksville, or "Lick"-ville. They drew blood from several locations on my body, to rule out a blood infection. I had had such an infection before and knew they were life threatening. About forty percent of people who become septic (a blood infection) die, and that is far more than the combined number of Americans who get prostate cancer, breast cancer, and AIDS. It is also a difficult illness to diagnose, since a fever can be caused by a lot of things. How do you know where the infection started once it has spread to the blood and multiple organs?

I had been septic before and had developed endocarditis, an infection of the heart. This causes permanent damage. Dr. Sellers was especially alert to this infection developing again and perhaps getting worse. He wanted to not just do an echocardiogram, where the heart is looked at through the outside of the chest, but a similar procedure that is done with a view from inside the body. The scope is sent down the esophagus and the heart is viewed from the backside, right through the wall of the esophagus. I was all game. But the gastroenterologist was unable to thread the thick black tube down my throat, even though I had been sedated. This concerned him. Without a proper assessment of my condition he feared his regional hospital could not help me best. He wanted to transfer me.

The task of contacting and updating family and friends falls to my spouse. Everyone expresses concern and prays each time I am hospitalized. I have never been one to like visitors, except immediate family. Hospital stays are pretty routine and I prefer to just sleep whenever possible. Hospitals are terrible places to try and rest, and adding guests, who I feel need to be entertained, is an added stress. I prefer quiet. The best visit I ever got was when three men from a group I meet with monthly came. The group is called, "Hearts for Jesus." It's a pun; we all have hearts that belong to our Lord, and we all play the card game hearts. When we normally meet we have a meal at the home of the host, and then we play three games of hearts. We share whatever needs we each have, and finally we pray for one another. It has been a time when we really bonded as men. So during my gall bladder removal Don, John, and Darrell came to see me at Stanford and we played cards. That was a fun visit.

DeAnna called her parents and our daughters from the hospital in Jasper to give them an update. Our girls were now grown and living in San Jose. Our oldest, Shirena, was nineteen and preparing to get married. She was with DeAnna's sister Judy in Auburn and shopping for a wedding dress when DeAnna reached her.

"How sick is he?" Shirena wanted to know.

"Well, he is very very sick," DeAnna said, trying hard to sound strong. She has always been honest with people, not trying to cushion reality with false hopes. "He could die," she said. Shirena's eyes teared up.

"I will cancel my wedding," she said. "I can't get married if dad dies." DeAnna tried to talk reason and put some hope into her.

"Even if dad dies," DeAnna began, "You will still be alive. You will still love Josh and will want to get married. And you should. Your life will not stop when dad dies. And we don't know that he will die. You will go on living and you should keep on living. Go ahead and shop for your dress." She did find a beautiful dress and she looked beautiful when married in September 2009. (I officiated.)

A day later Doctor Sellers was able to transfer me to a larger hospital in Indianapolis. As I was rolled out of the building in Jasper he stopped the bed and handed me a toy. It was a green Shrek flash light. He was being funny - with a note of sincerity.

"Let this light your way," he said. I could see the genuine concern in his eyes. As I write this I hope he knows I am still alive. He was a super doctor. The ambulance raced off and two and a half hours later it delivered me to a transplant center, the Saint Vincent Indianapolis Hospital.[51] They had specialists for everything.

Their tests revealed that I did indeed have a blood infection. It becomes more difficult to diagnose when a patient has already begun antibiotic therapy, so the preliminary blood draws when I was first admitted were important. I would have also fared better if I'd gone in much sooner, instead of driving around in Kentucky and southern Indiana, and sitting in a hot tub. Lesson learned.

May in Indianapolis means one thing to everyone in Indiana, as well as to every car racing enthusiast in America: the Indianapolis 500. While I lay in the hospital I looked up facts about the race on the internet. I was feeling better now that the fever had abated. When the right antibiotic is administered my fever is usually contained within three days. I still had to stay for tests and assessments of organ damage, but I was feeling much better. I even ordered nice big meals from their telephone. You could get any food at any hour. Each patient was provided a restaurant style menu.

"This is excellent," I emailed my brother. "You can order a cheese burger with mushrooms and bacon in the middle of the night if you want!" The room was also equipped with a system so patients could sit in bed with a computer keyboard and write emails on the in-room TV monitor and send and receive email. Doug did some poking around from his home in Colorado and emailed me that the Indianapolis 500 has a special day before the big weekend when they let the public come in for free and view the track and see some of the timing trials. These trials are important because they determine the position of the cars at the start of the race. If you are a fast driver then you are positioned up in front and have a preferred spot. This free-entrance day happened to be the coming Thursday, just two days away. I sadly thought, *"No way. I don't feel that great to be discharged in two days. But it's a nice thought."*

Wednesday I was feeling better and Thursday morning better yet.

---

[51] https://www.stvincent.org/indianapolis/

"Say, doc," I asked the cardiologist. "Did you know that today they open the track for people to come in for free just to visit the track?"

"What do you mean?" he asked in disbelief. "You have never seen *the track*?" He said the last two words like it was the holy of holies on the temple mount in Jerusalem.

"No, I haven't," I said. He was incredulous.

"You *have* to see the track," he said. My mind went to work.

"Well do you think I might be able to get a pass to leave the hospital for just a few hours?" I knew that hospitals sometimes did this. Back when I was a fifteen year old patient at the Children's Hospital at Stanford in Palo Alto the nurses used to encourage long term patients to get out of their beds and get some exercise. They would unhook our peripheral IV's, put some heparin in the line so the veins wouldn't clot, and send us off to shop at the Stanford Shopping Center. Or we'd take a hike across the creek and go to the Allied Arts Guild in Menlo Park. So I was hoping that this cardiologist could probably swing a pass. I mean clearly he could see the necessity of sending this California boy to see *the track*. He thought for a moment.

"First you will need to get clearance from the Infectious Disease specialist," he said as he was leaving my room. "We work as a team and we all need to be on board with each decision."

A few minutes later the Infections Disease doctor came into my room. I was glad to see him. He had the same reaction.

"You *must* see the track!" He was visibly excited, like a father who sees his son pull in his first fish. I was jazzed. I was going to see the Indianapolis 500 track, just two days before the actual race! I knew I could never see the actual race. For one thing I didn't have a ticket and for another thing I knew my wife would have no interest in it. And I would not want to put her through the agony. Oh, and then there was the fact that I had a blood infection.

Before leaving my room the infectious disease doctor said, "We will have to run it by the transplant specialist first, however." My heart sank just a bit. Then I thought, *"Surely, if these two top notch specialists were all for me getting a pass to see the track, then the transplant doctor should approve too."* I emailed my brother Doug that things were looking good. I would probably get the pass.

An hour later a woman in a white lab coat came in my room. I didn't recognize her. She identified herself as the transplant doctor. I sat up on the edge of my bed and gave her my best, *"I am healthy,"* look. She was the head of the team overseeing my care. A note of caution registered in my brain. I told her about the free day at the track for people to come and see it.

"I have never seen the track," she said in a monotone. She didn't appear at all impressed. Suddenly I was concerned.

I continued, "I would really like to get a few-hour pass to go down the street to see the track." It was literally just two miles away. She looked at me like I was from Mars. I could sense it coming.

"You have a *blood infection*," she began with as much authority in her voice as she could muster. "You likely have a *heart infection*." She stressed it like I'd just had two legs amputated. "You had a *heart/double lung transplant!*" her voice was rising. Then the clincher, voiced up a few decibels, "There is no way you are leaving this hospital to go see the race track!" She said the word "no" like I was a three year old who wanted to drive a car. And the words, "race track" came out like it was a useless, meaningless, value-less, less-than-intelligent tourist attraction. I sank back down into my mattress.

Most astonishing, two days later I was released to go home. The bitter irony remains with me to this day. I never did get to see *the track*.

However, we did drive by it ever so slowly on our way out of town, holding up traffic just a bit. The Indy 500 was full underway. I decelerated to two miles per hour as we crossed an empty crosswalk adjacent to the edifice. We could hear the massive roar of the turbocharged 700 horsepower engines as they whipped around the turns. I caught a glimpse of the jumbotron as we passed a gap in the stadium. I could smell the exhaust. *"Wow,"* and, *"What a bummer,"* was all I could think of. If only more women were into racing I might have gotten that pass.

I pulled out onto the interstate 65 and headed south toward Louisville where we would catch our scheduled return flight to San Jose on United Airlines. Instead of a week in the timeshare I'd had exactly a week in the hospital.

Approaching downtown Louisville we saw billboards advertising Churchill Downs. A smile crossed my face.

"Hey, why not check that out?" I asked DeAnna. She was game; what a woman! We pulled into the gravel parking lot and it was half full of cars. Parking was free, my kind of place. We could hear the starting bell ring and the clop, clop, clop of horse hooves racing around the dirt track as we passed through the turn styles. We past through the stands and looked for a seat. A pack of horses were raising clouds of dust as they raced for the finish line. It was a quiet sort of race compared to the Indianapolis 500. One horse power still makes for an interesting race, I guess.

A horse race and an auto race both find their contestants ending up at the spot where they began, a line drawn on the ground. It's not unlike the race of life. Do we just end up where we began? Genesis 3:19 says, "By the sweat of your brow you will eat your food until you return to the ground, since from it you were taken; for dust you are and to dust you will return." So our bodies end up back in the earth. From dust to dust. Some would want to believe that that is all there is. We are but dirt. Period. End of story. Lights out? Race over.

In 2 Timothy 4:7 it says, "I have fought the good fight, I have finished the race, I have kept the faith." The faith of the apostle Paul, who wrote the book to his friend Timothy, can be expressed in the next verse. "In the future there is laid up for me the crown of righteousness, which the Lord, the righteous Judge, will award to me on that day; and not only to me, but also to all who have loved His appearing."

That is how I want to finish this race. How about you?

Chapter 32

Elk Rut

Doug's black Chevy Tahoe pulled to the side of the road and we slowly got out. It was the time of year when the elk rut in the Rockies. We were some of the privileged few who were able to watch them across the field, as the males competed for access to the female harem. The drive up to Estes Park in Colorado had been strenuous, as had the setting up of the camp for my brother's family. Doug and I decided to drive back down the mountain a few thousand feet to a hotel to spend the night. We'd left his wife Dawn and their granddaughter Rachel there to enjoy the camping experience, while we enjoyed real beds. Doug was fighting cystic fibrosis and was in the middle of a self-administered IV antibiotic regimen. He needed oxygen full time, so it was simply a better idea for us to sleep in a clean hotel.

Early the next morning we faced the brisk Colorado air and hustled into his truck again for the two hour drive back up to eight thousand feet. I was driving, and enjoying the heated seat in the Tahoe. Even with long underwear I felt the chill; being skinny is not all it's cracked up to be. I started feeling warmer and warmer as we climbed the winding road up into the National Park. I shut off the heated seat but I began to sweat.

"Doug are you hot?" I asked. He wasn't. I knew then that I was in trouble. I had a fever.

We were a long long way from any significant hospital, but I knew I had to get help fast. I took my temperature. I had learned a long time ago to travel with a thermometer. Even Doug had one - a fancy one that you run around your head and it gives an imme-diate digital reading. 103. Yikes. I had also learned to always carry

Tylenol. But sometimes I forget things I've learned. Like this time. We pulled into the campground.

We began going from campsite to campsite shamelessly begging strangers for Tylenol. The third site yielded results. I quickly swallowed two 600 milligram capsules. Then we drove to the campground entrance, explained our situation to the ranger on duty and he called an ambulance. Ten minutes later one appeared and the EMT looked at me skeptically. I said I needed to get to a hospital asap. I didn't look very sick to him. No broken bones. No big cuts, bruises or blood.

"Why, what's the problem?" I have learned to summarize my medical condition in an abbreviated way, partly out of frustration and partly to speed things up.

"I'm a cystic fibrosis patient with a heart double lung transplant. I am running a 103 degree fever. If I don't get IV antibiotics within two hours this infection will be systemic and I will likely die." I handed him my pre-printed list of my 26 oral medications to make it real. His eyes widened a bit. He took my temperature.

"Get in."

The drive back down to the Estes Park Medical Center didn't take long. We were delayed a bit by tourists who'd parked their cars in the middle of the street to look at a black bear who'd climbed a tree. During the drive two nice EMT's (they looked like kids) tried in vain to find a vein, as we bounced along in the ambulance. In spite of my protestations that I have no peripheral veins anymore, phlebotomists, nurses, med techs, and doctors are always certain they can, "find something." Of course these guys couldn't. I had grown accustomed to getting stuck with needles.

We arrived at the Regional Medical Center. The challenge was that the center dealt mostly with altitude sickness and broken bones from rock climbing and skiing accidents. They were not a fully equipped hospital. When they rolled me in I gave them my spiel. I explained that I probably had a blood infection and needed Vancomycin and Merepenem by IV immediately. That's when I got really strange looks. Most patients don't know the antibiotics they need, nor even that they have an infection. I knew what I had been given during my last hospital admission and it was likely the same bug.

I gave further history and gave the admitting doctor my Stanford physician's phone number. I told him my password to My-Health Stanford so he could go on-line and read my history and also see the list of the twenty-six oral medication I take. I think he was a bit out of his depth. He suggested I be transported to the big hospital in Denver.

"That's four hours away," I said. "By the time I get there, am admitted, and then they find a vein, it will be five or more hours. The infection will have spread, threatening my life." He said to wait and he'd see what he could do.

At last a nurse appeared and said she was going to start an intravenous line. I showed her the choices on my arms and hands that might offer vein access. She poked me a few times. I had to remind her to use alcohol wipes before she stuck me with a needle, and also to wear gloves.

"Sometimes that isn't necessary," she said.

Undeterred I responded, "With me, it is always necessary." Maybe it was the fever that gave me the attitude, but I wasn't feeling much patience for teaching a nurse IV protocol.

She succeeded in starting a tiny catheter in the knuckle of my middle finger of my left hand. It barely functioned but there was a small blood return. They could only get a small sample of blood to test for a blood infection. They were skeptical. I convinced them they could use the pediatric blood-infection-detection kit. It only required half as much blood, and still returned acceptable results. They hooked up a bag of saline and a bag of Vancomycin. I was all set. I was so very thankful for these folks way up in the Rockies. They saved my bacon. They loaded me back into an ambulance.

I had a great time chatting with the two EMTs Chris and Bill on the four-hour ambulance ride down to the University of Colorado Hospital in Denver (UCH). The IV in my knuckle held up fine and I got a dose of antibiotics. We arrived at emergency and I was eager to get admitted. The problem was the doors were locked. By now it was the middle of the day. Chris peered through the glass window and could not see anyone. He rang the bell. No answer.

He rang again. Still no answer. I was a bit unhappy, as I lay there on the gurney in the cold. It is never any fun to be an emergency patient, even with all the experiences I've had. It always seems like a real emergency to me, but never to anybody else. For them it's business as usual. *But to not even unlock the door?* Finally Chris found the UCH phone number on his cell phone. He called them and somebody opened the door. They had no explanation for the locked door and the vacant admitting desk. (Although perhaps it had something to do with the neighborhood. This hospital had a lot of gun shot victims and drug overdose patients.)

After admission I at first received IV antibiotics through my knuckle - but my fever did not drop. When that site failed an IV was begun in a vein in the top of my foot. It wasn't working very well. You can imagine my delight when a PICC tech came into my hospital room (on a Sunday afternoon when his department was closed!) and started a functioning line. I was impressed.

My biggest concern was when my fever shot up to 103 the next morning. The LVN (licensed vocational nurse) knew my temperature had risen sharply. She said she'd notified the nurse. The nurse, however, left for the day and didn't pass along the message. My request was passed around and around and finally I was given just 400 mg of Tylenol. It didn't even touch my fever. I began shaking uncontrollably, not even able to hold a cup of water to drink through the straw. I had rigors; a violent shaking of the entire body. It was not until Doctor Zamora, who heads the transplant team at UCH, came in to see me during his rounds that I received enough Tylenol (1000mg) to lower my temperature. One reason it took so long, a nurse confided in me, was the nurses were all terrified of Doctor Z. He was a large man, with a rough disposition who could be quite intimidating. It had taken four hours of misery to get my message to him so he could write a simple order for 1 gram of Tylenol. When he arrived I let him know of my displeasure.

I have learned that it is important to encourage those who work hard and who sacrifice to serve patients, but also to give suggestions - even strongly, when it can improve patient care.

At the same time, for the sake of my own spiritual health (and obedience to Christ), it is key to be thankful in every situation.

"Give thanks in all circumstances; for this is God's will for you in Christ Jesus."[52] When I paused to reflect I realized I had a lot to be thankful for! I had the strangers at Estes Park who gave me Tylenol. The rangers who fetched an ambulance. The patient doctor at the regional medical center who listened carefully to me and ordered Vancomycin. The clumsy nurse who got an IV started in my finger. The friendly drivers who got me to Denver. The fellow who worked on Sunday and miraculously got a PICC line started. And even for Doctor Z, who oversaw my care and discharged me in record time. And then there was the fact that I was still alive. I was thankful for that too.

Initially Dr. Z. thought he would have to transfer me by medical jet to Stanford in California, since I had had three heart surgeries and the current infection most probably involved my heart. He surmised that I had endocarditis as well as pseudomonas bacteria in my blood. Pseudomonas is one of the primary bacteria that is present in cystic fibrosis patients. In spite of the lung transplant I remain susceptible to it. It is found everywhere in nature, even in drinking water. It does not cause sickness in the normal population, but for people with CF it cannot be eradicated, just nocked down a few notches with strong antibiotics. Eventually it destroys the lungs.

Once the fever was gone I was discharged with the PICC still in place in my arm. I was given a box full of IV meds, a pump, and some bags of saline, so I could administer the meds myself while I continued my travels. The next day I was with Doug at his cabin at 9,100 feet where together we built a deck extension, stopping periodically to run his or my IV meds. It was so good to be out of the confines of the hospital room. It really does feel like a prison. When admitted I am put in a strange room, am rid of my clothes, give up my personal space, lose my privacy, relinquish control of my body, and cease getting any real sleep. It is not easy.

Doug was struggling with a very low lung volume. He was at perhaps 30% of normal. His own lungs were deteriorating from CF. Years earlier, he'd qualified for a transplant, then he bounced back, and regaining some lung function. In spite of his current di-

---

[52] 1 Thessalonians 5:18

minished lung function he had not yet decided if he wanted to take the huge risk of getting a transplant. He knew there would be many new challenges being immune suppressed and recovering from surgery. As it was he was still managing to work from home. Adding onto his deck at his cabin was a bit crazy. For both of us.

"Hey bro, we are out of deck screws," he said as he emptied the box. And then with a hint of suggestion, "I have some more down in my shop."

Catching my breath I replied, "Yeah, you want to go downstairs and get them?"

"Well," he said and took another breath, "They are in the garage on the shelf to the left."

"Does that mean you want *me* to get them?" We were at a much higher altitude than I was used to, so even with my new lungs each breath was a challenge. "OK, I'll get them." I took my sweet time; I figured Doug could use the rest. I paused after each few steps as I made my way back up the slope to the deck.

In the end we managed to add sixteen feet of decking and railing to expand the redwood deck. Doug was happy with his finished deck. It meant he no longer had to climb stairs to get wood for the stove. He now had a nice rack right outside the patio door.

It has always been deeply satisfying to each of us to accomplish something tangible with our hands. After our father Dave Lagasse died we went through his things. Inside his worn Bible was a scrap of paper with the words from 1 Thessalonians 4:11. "Make it your ambition to lead a quiet life: You should mind your own business and work with your hands, just as we told you." It was a verse he had put into practice, long before either of us knew it was even in the word of God.

God creates. And Genesis tells us He created us in His image. This means that He made us also to create things just like He created - and also to take joy in the things we create.

God said when he finished his creation, "Behold it is good." When we create something we can delight in the strength and ability we have been given to make something about which we too can say, "It is good!"

I flew back home on my scheduled flight with United Airlines. After my follow-up care I continued on two antibiotics every six or eight hours for the next five weeks.

Before I was even finished with the home IV treatment I was to have another brush with death. This one was serious enough that the whole church was praying for me.

Chapter 33

Coma

Back and forth I sprayed the pearl blue paint on my street rod. It was looking really nice. I made sure the air hose remained behind my back. My buddy Mark Oswald guided the long red hose so it would never touch the fresh paint. Faces were pressed against the glass on the outside doors of the paint booth as "newbies" watched to see how a car was painted. The occupational center in San Jose had a state of the art paint booth.

This was the final touch after eight years of effort. My 1936 five-window Ford coupe with a rumble seat had taken a long time to completely restore. When I'd bought it on eBay in August 2003 it was rusty, had broken windows, and was completely gutted inside. Seven years later it was nearing its transformation into a street rod. It now boasted a three-hundred-thirty horsepower Corvette engine with four-wheel disc brakes, Mustang suspension, rack and pinion steering, a beautifully designed interior, air conditioning and a complete sound system. If this were a story about cars I would go on and on. But these are stories of scars that tell stories. And this story is particularly grim. At ten p.m. on a Thursday night Mark and I finished pulling the paint tape and masking paper off the car. I had been in the paint booth for three hours. The heated booth had dried the paint. I fired the car up for the short drive home.

Friday morning I went about business as usual. I went to Denny's Restaurant at seven a.m. where I meet each week with some retired guys for breakfast. Then I took care of some paper work, ran some errands, and worked on some projects around the house. In the evening we headed to the home of friends who had twin girls. We were taking our friends Sterling and Tiana out to dinner at a Greek restaurant. At their home we chatted with their baby sitter about snacks their girls were allowed.

After some small talk I said, "Some of my...," and my mind went blank. I was searching for a word but it wouldn't surface. I couldn't think of it. From the context of the dialogue somebody figured out the word.

"You mean, 'friends?"

"Yes, that's it," I said, feeling foolish for forgetting such a basic word. *"How could that happen?"* I wondered.

I told DeAnna that the same morning, while at Denny's I had trouble remembering another common word.

I told her, "At the time I could picture the food in my mind, but I couldn't think of the name." The word I couldn't remember was "carrots." I simply couldn't think of it. It really bothered me. I was talking with the guys and had stumbled in mid sentence. They looked at me.

"Never mind," I'd said. "Senior moment." It was actually more than that. DeAnna made a mental note. Something was up.

I didn't get out of bed the next morning. DeAnna woke me and started asking me questions as I lay there. I didn't answer. (This is abnormal for me.) I had a blank stare on my face. She asked me if I knew who she was. I shrugged my shoulders. Deeply worried she got me out of bed. I stood in front of the clothes closet and looked at the clothing. I wasn't sure what to put on. She began helping me get dressed, the anxiety rising inside. As I got dressed she asked me another question. I turned and looked at her. We were just a few feet apart standing by the closets. I could not answer. I thought I knew what she wanted. I understood her, or did I? But I could not speak. It's not because I didn't want to speak; I just couldn't. I smiled at her and buttoned my shirt. She asked again. And again I could not speak.

"Do you understand me?" she asked in a serious tone. I nodded my head. I wasn't concerned for some reason. Everything seemed fine; I just couldn't talk anymore. But DeAnna *was* concerned. She asked a few more questions, and got no response.

Guiding me over to my end table she took out some medications, which I keep in colored pill boxes in the top drawer. She held up a, "morning box for Saturday" and asked me if these were the right medications I should take. I didn't answer.

"Well you'll just have to trust me," she said. I did trust her. She put the pills in my hand and I took them. Then she took me by the arm. "Let's go," she said. "We are going to Stanford." I am blessed to have a wife who though she never sought employment as a nurse is nevertheless a registered nurse. And I guess one could make the point that she has had plenty enough work caring for me.

She decided to do the driving, and I was very content with that. I watched the scenery go by in full awareness of what was going on. I just could not speak. DeAnna pulled into the small emergency lot at the back of Stanford University Medical Center. A parking attendant asked if we needed assistance.

It was a euphemism for, "This parking is reserved for emergency situations." DeAnna assured him it was an emergency. She hung the disabled placard on the rear view mirror. We walked through the double doors into the building. She was holding onto my arm to guide me. But I knew the way. I surrendered my pocket knife to the guard as we passed through emergency security. And that is the last thing I remember.

If it were not for my wife and the people who work at Stanford emergency this would be a paragraph penned by somebody else. I am told that as I entered the emergency waiting room and prepared to check-in with my insurance and personal information I had a grand mal seizure.

This guaranteed immediate attention. I lost consciousness. My muscles in my entire body contracted causing me to fall down. For maybe twenty seconds the muscles contracted. But then a second phase began of seizing began, the clonic phase. The muscles went into a rhythmic contraction, flexing and then relaxing. I know this from reading on the web. I have never watched a seizure. Unfortunately my wife and children have. It is perhaps the most terrifying experience one can imagine. Their loved one looks like he's dying. There is no controlling it, instead there is a frenzy of spasms and muscular convulsions, perhaps loss of bladder and bowel control.

At Stanford the nurses and doctors and emergency personnel jumped to assist. I thank God I was in that emergency room and not on highway 85, or even at home getting dressed in my bedroom. Or at the restaurant the night before. The seizure did not stop after the standard two or three minutes. Instead it continued non-stop … beyond thirty minutes. This is called status epilepticus. The only way to stop the constant spasms was to induce a coma. This stopped the brain activity from causing any more damage. So much time had elapsed, however, that there was a strong concern that my brain may have been permanently damaged. Seizures are caused by electrical irregularities in brain activity, and continually seizing means the normal flow of electrical activity (which we know as thinking), has become thoroughly randomized. Or something like that. It's hard to explain; I just can't put it into words…

That was Saturday morning. I was still in a coma. As word was spread among our family and our friends at church, prayers were offered up to Jesus. Jesus, as recorded in the Gospels, healed people, even some who had seizures. He raised his friend Lazarus from the dead. The Bible says to pray in Jesus name because he can heal the sick. Chip Ingram, the lead pastor at Venture Christian Church, led the congregation during the Sunday services in prayer for me. Many appeals were made to heaven as I lay in a coma in ICU at Stanford. Specialists worked me over to assess my situation and administer the right drugs. I remained in the coma all day Saturday in ICU.

Our daughters were told about their dad's illness when DeAnna called them. They were out of town. Jessica had a break from work and was visiting her sister Shirena in Roseville, California, near Sacramento. They were shopping at a mall (of course) when DeAnna reached them on the phone. Jessica was able to and wanted to come. Shirena wanted to come too, but she had a job.

"Mom, should I come?" she asked, trying to make her decision.

"You need to decide, Shirena, and just accept that decision no matter what happens. If you lived in another state and were too far away you wouldn't even have a choice." She continued, "We don't know what will happen; dad could die. But you also know that he has bounced back from some really scary situations. So we just cant know for sure." I think Jessica's prompt decision to drop everything and drive three hours and come was because she didn't want DeAnna to be alone. In 2008 Jessica had been alone in ICU at Kaiser with my father when he lay unconscious. Doctors had said it could be days or weeks before my dad passed. DeAnna and I had been with him for eight hours, had talked and prayed with him, and had said goodbye and goodnight. It wasn't clear if he had even heard us. Doctors doubted it. Jessica was with us the whole time and said she wanted to stay with her grandpa. Ten minutes after we left his side he passed away. Jessica had been alone with him. It was a terrible shock for her. So she realized the importance of being with somebody when they are really sick. You never know if you're saying goodbye.

DeAnna's parents Steve and Rena rushed up to Stanford Hospital to join Jessica and DeAnna by my side. Doctors were monitoring my brain, keeping me unconscious, trying to assess the cause of the seizures. Was it the paint fumes I'd inhaled for three hours? That can cause toxicity and lead to seizures. Or had I messed up my medications? Maybe I missed my anti-seizure medication. I had several pills that all looked alike. My blood work showed no trace of Gabapentin, which is the anti-seizure medicine I'd taken since college. Later I thought I'd perhaps loaded the pill boxes incorrectly, doubling up on my enzymes (for the pancreas) and missing the Gabapentin. Often drug manufacturers change the appearance of meds and I would have one pill that was very similar to another. With twenty-six medications they could easily get confused. Or did I have an allergic reaction to IV Immipenim? I'd been administering it to myself for five weeks already, to combat the infection I'd gotten in Colorado. This drug has a possible side effect of seizures. Three days passed.

Then I opened my eyes and saw that I was in a familiar place, the Stanford ICU. The head of the hospital bed had been raised. Both my arms were strapped to the bed rails. My head felt like it was wearing some sort of cap. I saw DeAnna at my side and a team of doctors standing at the foot of the bed.

"How are you feeling," somebody asked.

"Fine," I replied. "Can you undo this velcro from my wrists, please?" I was happy to get those loose. I wondered if in my unconscious state I'd tried to hit somebody or something. (I did that once before.)

"We want to do a few tests. Can you touch your nose?" I was familiar with the neurologist's routine. Touch your fingers together. Squeeze the toes. Look at this light in your eyes.

"Look at that spot on the wall over to your right. Now look up at the ceiling." They examined my retina and looked for abnormalities. "We are going to do another EEG." I realized the cap I was wearing was the electro encephalogram device. It records electrical activity along the scalp. Wires and caps continued to monitor my brain activity for the next several days. I passed the time with Doug who had flown out to be with me. I beat him relentlessly in cribbage.

"He was still having mini seizures during the time he was sedated," the neurologist told DeAnna. "Even though he was sedated and not moving, his brain activity showed seizure activity." I was eventually allowed to get out of bed. DeAnna was relieved. The ICU nurses seemed irritated when I got up. I think they like their patients to stay where they're put. I was soon discharged.

The whole congregation was shocked to see me join them for worship the very next Sunday. The last they had heard was that I was in a coma on the precipice of death.

At discharge a couple new medications were added to my long list and some more routine appointments added to my others. Now I got to see the neurologist on a regular basis. (Whoopee.) This was in addition to the dermatologist (skin cancers), cardiologist (heart surgeries), the arrhythmia doctor (for abnormal heart rhythm), my transplant pulmonologist (to monitor the heart and double lung transplant), the otolaryngologist (sinus surgeries), the ophthalmologist (cataract and glaucoma exams), the endocrinologist (thyroidectomy), the gastroenterologist (colonoscopies), the nephrologist (chronic kidney failure), and my primary care physician so I can get a physical. Ha ha.

But the scar of loosing my mental capacities and the crushing blow to my nervous system of the status epilepticus reminds me that Jesus still heals. I feel like Lazarus.

Chapter 34

Uncle Dan's Head

Dr. Nayak approached DeAnna who was seated in the waiting room, "Mrs. Lagasse, take a look at this!" He had just finished my sinus surgery.

DeAnna has never been squeamish about looking at pictures taken during surgeries or procedures. I am sure it's her nurse's training. I have had four heart catheterizations, and I always requested a copy of the final photo of my healthy arteries to share with her. Kind of like a five-year-old coming home from his kindergarten art class. *"Hey, look what I did today!"* I have had fourteen bronchoscopies, as it was required every year after my transplant.[53] Each time I asked to have a photo of my bronchioles to share with her. I figured it was boring and perhaps nerve wracking sitting in the waiting room all that time. It was the least I could do to show some of the reason she'd waited. Cracked ribs, broken feet, an X-ray of a broken wrist I'd gotten while jack-hammering concrete in our back yard. Fun photos.

But this was different. I was still lying sedated in the surgical unit. It was Doctor Nayak who was sharing a picture today. He held up a color photo printed on HP paper.

"Can you tell what that is?" he asked. It was like some sort of game show. She took a careful look at the picture. She knew of course I was having sinus surgery done. Dr. Nayak was doing the last (hopefully) of a series of three operations on me. This is subsequent to the six others that previous otolaryngologists had done. Dr. Nayak had developed a set of operations that opened

---

[53] I was able to stop having these around ten years after my transplant. It is done to diagnose rejection of the lungs.

up successive sinus cavities. His theory, which has proved to be true, was that my recurrent blood infections were a result of pseudomonas bacteria in the sinuses entering my blood stream. This bacteria was never completely eradicated in the sinuses. Just like the bacteria in my pre-transplanted lungs it was impossible to wipe these little buggers out entirely. And the frontal sinuses, which lay at the top of the head between and behind the eyebrows, present a particular problem.

In some people with CF, the walls of the sinuses continually get thicker and thicker. This creates tiny spaces where there should be large open areas filtering the air we breathe. Sometimes polyps grow. The problem was with the harbored pseudomonas bacteria. My frontal sinuses were very small, no bigger that the end of my little finger. They were in fact compacted shut entirely. They were full of pseudomonas. Dr. Nayak, never one to mince words, called them a, "festering pus-filled nasty germ factory." I think you get the picture. He liked to use down-to-earth vocabulary along with the technical stuff. I liked that, it demonstrated his humanity. Even if it did seem a bit silly. It went along with his wide grin and hilarious laugh.

And so while I was still sedated in another room Dr. Nayak was sharing a bit of his joyful personality with my wife in the waiting area. He held up the picture and gave her the quiz question.

"What do you think it is?" he asked again. She stared at the curious photo, trying to gain perspective. Obviously it was something in her husband's head. She could see the pink tissue and the dark hollow areas of sinus cavities. But right in the middle of the photo was a small black slender angular object that was clearly out of place. It looked to be about a half inch long. She didn't know what it was.

He smiled. "That is a drill bit," he said with obvious satisfaction. "It broke off in your husbands head! I was drilling an opening between the left frontal sinus and the right frontal sinus. There is a bone right here." He pointed in the center of the photo. "It separates the two sinuses. In your husband these spaces are so small that they don't drain; they clog up. So by removing the bone he will have a bigger space that can drain easier." We knew this from the pre-surgery consultation. But he reviewed it for her.

"That was a brand new drill bit too," he said. "I am going to write to the manufacturer and tell them it's defective." She looked at him with eyes wide open, still thinking of her husband with a broken drill bit in his skull. "Oh," he said with a grin, "Don't worry. I got it out." And with a final chuckle he said, "Your husband is doing fine. I printed the picture because I thought you'd enjoy it." In fact she did.

She went home and posted it on Facebook and asked her friends, "Who knows what this is?" She received forty replies within an hour. The closest guess came from our nephew Aaron.

"Is that something in Uncle Dan's head?" he asked.

A sense of humor is indispensable when fighting multiple illnesses, tragedies, or major trials. We had learned to laugh at life's hurdles from our parents who had handled rough patches with a smile. It's not about being careless or flippant in the face of adversity. It's about keeping the big picture in focus. Take life a little less seriously. Roll with it.

I bought a sweatshirt on a rafting trip once. It said, "It's not the destination; it's the journey." While I believe that knowing my destination is heaven is essential to inner peace, I also know that enjoying this journey of life, with all the rocks and trees that interfere with the bouncing raft - is what makes the trip a blast. The boat careens down the class three rapids, bouncing off boulders hidden beneath the white water. That's what makes the trip worthwhile. Yes, there are slow patches when we look up at the majestic trees and mountains. The guide points out the hawk and then an eagle high in the blue sky. Then he points over the edge of the raft at the trout in the Green River. Those quiet times are important too. We need an appreciation for the quiet.

But without a good laugh during out sometimes hectic moments the stress can overwhelm us. "A joyful heart is good medicine, but a crushed spirit dries up the bones."[54] It's good for the doctor to laugh, and it's good for us to laugh too. That keeps us all healthy. It also clears the sinuses.

---

54 Proverbs 17:20

Chapter 35

The Sneeze

I reached forward to grab the slice of pineapple and ham pizza on my paper plate. I had to be careful not to drop it on the fellowship hall floor. The chairs around the table were so close together I could not pull my chair up to the table. The guy seated on my right hacked and coughed a few times. The fellow on my left was blowing his nose into a paper napkin. He wadded it up and set it carefully beside the four others he'd already deposited between his paper plate and mine. Then he sneezed.

Normally I would have left the table long ago. But this time I felt it would be offensive to the men around the table. It was an evening Bible study of ten men. We'd become good friends. Three of the guys were in a classic car club together and another a motorcycle club. We laughed together, prayed together, studied God's word together, and ended our time by eating junk food together. It was usually a really good time. But this was February and it was cold and flu season. Then there was that sneeze. I tried not to think about it. I excused myself and drove home.

It was an unusually dry winter for San Jose that year. I had undertaken a project in my back yard reminiscent of my brother's and father's plans. Maybe it was a Lagasse thing. Each of us had built a waterfall in our back yards. My dad and brother had put koi fish in theirs. I decided I would recirculate my waterfall into the swimming pool. That would mean no pond slime to clean up and no fish to take care of. I poured a concrete base and was mortaring in staggered slabs of green quartz over which the water would spill. A self-priming pump was buried underground. It drew water up from a hidden pipe in the pool. I had a stone-cutting circular saw blade in my angle grinder and I was happily cutting slate slabs to fit together like a puzzle.

My nose dripped. I wiped it off on the sleeve of my work shirt. *Maybe it's the cool morning air,* I thought. A few moments later it dripped again. Now I began to wonder what was going on. I have a condition called dry mouth, which essentially means that my mouth is dry all the time, as are my eyes and nose. It is a side effect from taking so many medications for so long. It's a small price to pay, but it does mean waking up with a very dry mouth, having to flush my sinuses, and using eye drops in the middle of the night. It also means, however, my nose never runs. Or drips.

On this morning I had work to do and so, like a typical male, I put off going to the doctor. After all, it was just a few drips. A few days later I was in for my scheduled check-up at Stanford with my pulmonologist, David Weill, M.D. During these check-ups my litany of meds are reviewed, a pulmonary function test (pft) is done to check lung volume, and routine chest x-ray and blood work are completed. It ends with a consultation with Dr. Weill. As almost an afterthought I mentioned my dripping nose. He then performed a nasal swab. Within fifteen minutes the result came back. It was positive. I had the flu.

I only remember one other time in my life when I had the flu. I had awoken with so many aches and pains, and a raging fever, that I told my wife I thought I was going to die.

She laughed and then said, "Now you know what it's like! I'm actually glad to hear you feel that way. After all you've been through you certainly know what it feels like to die. Now I don't feel like such a wimp, because the flu does make you feel like you're dying!" I sensed that I'd been somewhat less than sympathetic during the times she'd had the flu. Oops.

This flu, called RSV, however, was different because I was immune suppressed. It was a whole different ballgame. It really was life threatening. The reason lies in the immune response. My body was detecting the virus and my immune system was working overtime to fight it off. The heightened response would not just mean attacking the virus, it would also attack my transplanted heart and lungs. The maintenance dose of immune-suppressants that I took were woefully inadequate for such a situation. Instead of oral prednisone I would now be given IV methylprednisolone. I was admitted to a private hospital room. This room was special in that it had a negative air flow ventilation system. No air could leave the room and be re-circulated throughout the rest of the hospital. The reason was not just the flu virus, it was the medication I would be given. It was a mist delivered through a special pump.

My hospital bed had been rolled away from the headboard by about a foot. A machine that looked like a big-block car radiator was set in place. It was in fact a deluxe HEPA filter. A mist tent was then fitted over the hospital bed where I lay on my back. My face and chest were covered by the tent. A large plastic hose was fitted to the wall and the medication was placed in a nebulizer. I wore a mask which was strapped to my face. *"This was going to be a blast,"* I sarcastically told myself.

Compliance is essential to survival as a transplant patient. I had learned to be compliant as a cystic fibrosis patient all my life. I followed doctors instructions. Simple as that. "Compliance" is really just the medical term for, "doing what you're told." It is simply obedience. Only I think if hospitals told their patients, "You are disobedient," it would somehow be politically incorrect. So it's called "non-compliant." Maybe it looks better in the patient's chart.

"The patient is non-compliant," she types into the computer. What the nurse is really trying to say is, "This patient is a pain in the ass and he won't do what he's told." That would be the truth.

But I did as I was told.

"Go to the bathroom before we hook this up," my nurse said. I went to the bathroom as told and when I was back I hung two urinals on my bed rails so I wouldn't have to crawl out of the tent in the night. Once under the tent I was supposed to stay in place. I climbed onto the bed and squeezed beneath the plastic tent.

"If you need a nurse during the night, push the button on your control, but only if it's *really* important. It will take some time for them to come," he said. I had seen that everyone who came into this isolation room had to gown-up with a yellow gown, put on latex gloves, and put on a blue head cap. Every person went through this routine. During the night when I was getting the mist it would be even more severe. Each person who entered had to put on the normal personal protection get-up, and also wear a canister strapped to their back. It completely filtered the room air. They wore an airtight mask with hoses running to the canister, and over their head another shield that looked like the one in my garage that I wore when grinding steel.

No young female nurses worked in the room while I was receiving the medication; because the drug was known to cause sterility. It was serious stuff. It was also pricey, thirty thousand dollars a dose, I was told. The plan was to give it five consecutive nights, unless I tested negative for the virus. Each morning after the dosage was finished, people came in (all suited up), and they then sent all my bedding and my gown to some hazmat service, (or maybe they threw them away). Then they washed down all the walls. I was sent to the shower to clean off any of the medication that clung to my skin. It was all quite interesting.

The antiviral was only administered for four hours each night. That is the time when there is the least need for patient interaction. No blood pressure, temperature, or oxygen checks. No food delivered or removed. No doctor visits. No nurse or CNA shift changes. No visitors. No nurse charting 26 oral medications. You get the idea. Hospitals are non-stop activity. From one a.m. to five a.m., when it was relatively quiet, I would be receiving the brand new mist-delivered anti-viral medicine. Most people think of antibiotics when they think of infections. But those are only good for bacterial infections. Until recently we have not had any anti-viral drugs. Viruses were left to run their course, leaving people sick and miserable for extended periods of time. As may as fifty thousand people died from the flu each year in the US (up until 2020). Some years it had been much fewer. This particular year I did not want to be part of the statistic.

In addition to the mist I was given the methylprednisolone to combat my body's natural effort to attack the virus, as it would have caused my lungs and heart to go into rejection. One side effect of that drug, besides bizarre dreams if one can sleep, is being acutely awake. All night and all day long. I did not sleep for forty-eight hours straight. I lay in the mist tent listening to the rise and fall of the machine's motor, watched the mist flow out of the holes in the mask and fill the mist tent. I jammed my glasses over the plastic mask to try and see the TV through the plastic tent, but they misted up. In spite of being a big blur I watched every movie in the hospital system. Even the ones for kiddies.

I thought back to how I'd gotten sick. I do not blame the guy next to me for coughing, or the guy for wiping his nose and sneezing. It would have been nice if they had covered their mouths, however. Ultimately it is my responsibility to avoid infection, even if it means vacating my table and being thought impolite for leaving the situation. Shaking hands is one of the worst things for passing germs. I learned a trick to avoid it in public. I carry something in my right hand and smile warmly and voice a greeting. My close friends know to give an arm bump or something else non-contagious. My wife also caries hand sanitizer, which she squirts into my hand after close contact. The responsibility lies with me, however. And it is up to me to seek immediate medical attention when I have a fever or a nose-drip.

Each of us is personally responsible with the physical life we've been given. It is also true with eternal life. "For we will all stand before the judgment seat of God. For it is written, as I live,' says the Lord, 'Every knee shall bow to me, and every tongue shall give praise to God.' So then each one of us will give an account of himself to God."[55]

There is a virus called sin. And we all have it. There is but one way to cure that virus. It's not a new problem. Two thousand years ago there was a follower of Jesus named Thomas. He is remembered for having doubted if Jesus really rose from the dead. Many people relate well to him. They call him doubting Thomas.

Thomas said to Jesus just before Christ was going to his crucifixion, "Lord, we don't know where you are going, so how can we know the way?"

Jesus answered, "I am the way and the truth and the life. No one comes to the Father except through me. If you really know me, you will know my Father as well. From now on, you do know him and have seen him." Jesus said, "I am the way, the truth, and

---

[55] Romans 14:11-12

the life. No man comes to the Father but through me."[56] He made an exclusive claim like no other man has ever made.

Thomas was fortunate to be present in the upper room after Jesus was raised from the dead. "Then He [Jesus] said to Thomas, "Reach your finger here, and look at My hands; and reach your hand here, and put it into my side. Do not be unbelieving, but believing."[57] It was the scars of Jesus that testified of the reality of his death. It was those scars that proved he had gone to the cross, died, was buried and rose again. And those wounds had already become scars in his hands and side.

One of these days doctors will be one drug short in the treatment of Dan Lagasse. I will perish, just like the rest of the people of this world will one day perish. I have no fear, however. That is because I know the way and the truth and have eternal life. I am confident that I too shall see heaven, and will walk alongside my father, my mother, my brother and most importantly, Jesus.

You've read these stories of these illnesses, injuries and scars. I write them for you, the reader, to think of the meaning of life, of its brevity, and of its fragility. They are my stories, different from yours. But as fellow humans we share a common brokenness. Illness afflicts us all. And we all have that virus called sin. One day you too will face death. It could be *you* laying in ICU, as an aneurism bursts and your heart fails. It might be *your* life that hangs in the balance as organs begin to shut down and go septic. Perhaps it will be a fever that rages out of control from an untreatable infection. Or maybe you will get cancer and have your pain and senses dulled by infusions of morphine. You might be the one laying in a hospital bed, or in a wreck at the edge of a freeway, and you will be wondering,*"Was being a good person enough to merit heaven? Has my life counted for anything of eternal significance? Have I chosen the right path? Has being tolerant of everything and anything given me an assurance of eternity, or do I have a nagging fear of my own mortality?"*

---

[56] John 14:5-7

[57] John 20:27 from the New King James Version

I have stood at bedsides and seen the final groan of the mortal body as a soul departs the earthly shell and travels off towards a life of eternity. I know with confidence that those who've called out to Jesus in this life will meet Him in the next. I have seen their hope, their serenity, their peace - even in their final moments of earthly existence. If these stories have said anything to you I hope they have communicated that a life without God is just a life. A life with God is everything.

You can begin a new life right now by calling out to the one who can begin it. Say His name out loud. "Jesus." It's not a magical mantra; make it a genuine calling to the living eternal being whose name is Jesus. God knows your thoughts. It does not take a lot of faith to just speak to Him out loud. And eternal life has nothing to do with living a perfect life or doing more good deeds than bad. That's religion, and that is a man-made thing. It's a hopeless spiral that ends in death. Jesus was the only one who lived perfection. If you read the Bible from cover to cover you will not find one person, not one, who lived a life of perfection, except Christ alone. So stop for a moment and call out to Him.

"Everyone who calls on the name of the Lord will be saved."[58] Call out to him, "Jesus." He will take the rest from there. Say His name like you mean it and when you meet Him you will find life. With all your scars, your wounds, or your broken life - you will find purpose and hope. Often it is *because* of our scars that we turn to Him. He heals the broken hearted. And our scars serve as reminders that we have survived. We have learned lessons during life, and we continue to live.

---

[58] Romans 10:13

Chapter 36

Back to Iraq

Sometimes I have heard a still small voice telling me to do something. It's not audible, rather it is something in my heart or in the Bible that assures me to take a specific path. The Holy Spirit talks to us through the Word, through our conscience and in our hearts. "To obey is better than sacrifice," the Bible says.[59] When I have such a conviction that I know is from God I want to obey it.

So in the summer of 2014 when IS (Islamic State, also called ISIS) took control of the city of Mosul, and thousands of historic Christians and Kurds fled their homes, taking absolutely nothing with them but the clothes on their backs, both my wife DeAnna and I were deeply moved. We had lived in Iraq. We had been guests in the home of an Assyrian family when we adopted two Kurdish abandoned children in 1991. We had spent years learning Kurdish. Our hearts were struck in a deeply moving way.

So during this upheaval I asked my wife, "DeAnna, what is God saying to you about this crisis?" She replied that her heart was deeply moved. We bowed our heads in our kitchen and prayed together for the incredible suffering these people were enduring. We talked about it. We were experiencing the kind of grief one feels when a loved one has died. You cannot speak. Feeling overwhelms you. There are no words to describe the agony in the soul. People whom you love are hurting, so you hurt too.

In the following days an idea began to take form in my head - and in my heart.

---

[59] 1 Sammuel 15:22b

"Why not take a team of experienced men to Iraq and bring some relief to these suffering people?" I asked myself. *"God, would you want me to take some initiative in this?"* I prayed. The answer seemed clear; we had done this before. We had been to Iraq and we spoke their language. We knew their hearts. I remembered well the words of a young woman as we sat in a crude tent in 1991, after Saddam Hussein had driven 1.5 million Kurds up into the mountains of Turkey and Iran.

"Why has God done this to us?" she cried out. "What have we done to deserve this?" I knew that bringing answers to their emotional and spiritual suffering was as important as bringing them food, security and shelter.

The idea began to take shape. Because of the imminent risk associated with IS and their horrific acts of terror, I would invite only mature men who had cross-cultural experience. It had only been a few days since the journalist James Foley had been beheaded by IS. His crime: he was an American. Therefore by their definition he was an "infidel". Christians are also "infidels" according to a strict observance of parts of the Koran. For this reason I did not want to recruit young men, or men who had children at home. They had to be men who were completely sold out for Christ, men who were willing to die serving Him, if He called them to go. And they should have skills, cross-cultural experience and knowledge of foreign languages that would make their contribution meaningful.

In November 2014 I began to call, email and visit men who I have known through the years of my ministry. One had served in Iraq in the US military; he had lived in Mosul, the city that ISIS had overrun. Another one had lived in Egypt and spoke Arabic. One had sent short term teams all over the world. Another had lived thirty years in Pakistan and Afghanistan. I invited my brother who had just received his double lung transplant. He had experience living in a restricted country - one that was hostile to Christianity. He was accustomed to high risk and was willing to die for Christ. In all I invited twelve men. I was encouraged. Most of the men replied by saying, "I will pray about it."

I waited eagerly for commitments. One by one they said they could not come. My disappointment was great. From the initial twelve whom I had invited, I decided that eight would be a good number. Then it was down to four. Eventually it was just two, a longtime friend and myself. I decided that the timing just wasn't right.

"I need to give these men more lead time," I told myself.

Winter in Iraq is cold and miserable. I waited until the worst of the snow was passed. I knew that March marked a turn to the beginning of spring. March 21-23 is the Kurdish New Year festival called *Newroz*[60]. It is significant to them as the beginning of the new season, and new life. I did not want to wait too long for the journey. I knew the weather in summer in Iraq is unbearable. 125 degree heat is not uncommon. I had been there in 120 degree heat in 1991 and nearly died from dehydration and pancreatitis. I did not want to repeat that experience. So I set March as a possible date.

The next step was to contact people in Iraq with whom we could work. I have developed many contacts all over the world as a missionary and also as a missions pastor. I have visited forty-three countries and in each I spent time with resident missionaries. As the missions pastor at Los Gatos Christian Church I interfaced with the leaders of many mission agencies. So I began to contact them and ask who they had that was at work in Kurdistan, Iraq. In all I contacted twelve agencies. I received positive responses and invitations from ten.

The trip began to take shape. Of all the men I invited, however, only the one said he could go. His name will remain unmentioned, as it would jeopardize his security in future endeavors. I will call him Joe. Joe had served with an NGO in Pakistan and Afghanistan during the times of war and upheaval. He was accustomed to high risk. He also spoke local languages and had a real heart for the needs and sufferings of the poor and oppressed. He said he would join me.

The purpose of the trip was to assess the work of agencies who were meeting humanitarian needs. Our focus would be on long term work to address felt needs and to strengthen the church. We would gather as much information as possible so that

---

[60] *"roz"* means "year" in Kermanji. *Newroz* is "New Year"

my home church (now called Venture Christian Church) could become involved in sharing the love of Jesus with those in Kurdistan. What kind of short term volunteers could add value to the work being done? Where is humanitarian aid having the most impact? What kind of long term workers were needed and what kind of skills should they have? These were our questions as we planned the trip.

As I booked my flight to the Middle East I reviewed my itinerary. I had arranged to meet with the local leaders of the ten agencies. The journey would last eighteen days, six of those would be spent traveling there and back and the rest between the two cities we would visit, Erbil and Dohuk, Kurdistan. I planned for Joe and I to meet with each of the ten leaders on ten separate days. Five days in the capital of Kurdistan, Erbil, and five days in the northern city of Dohuk.

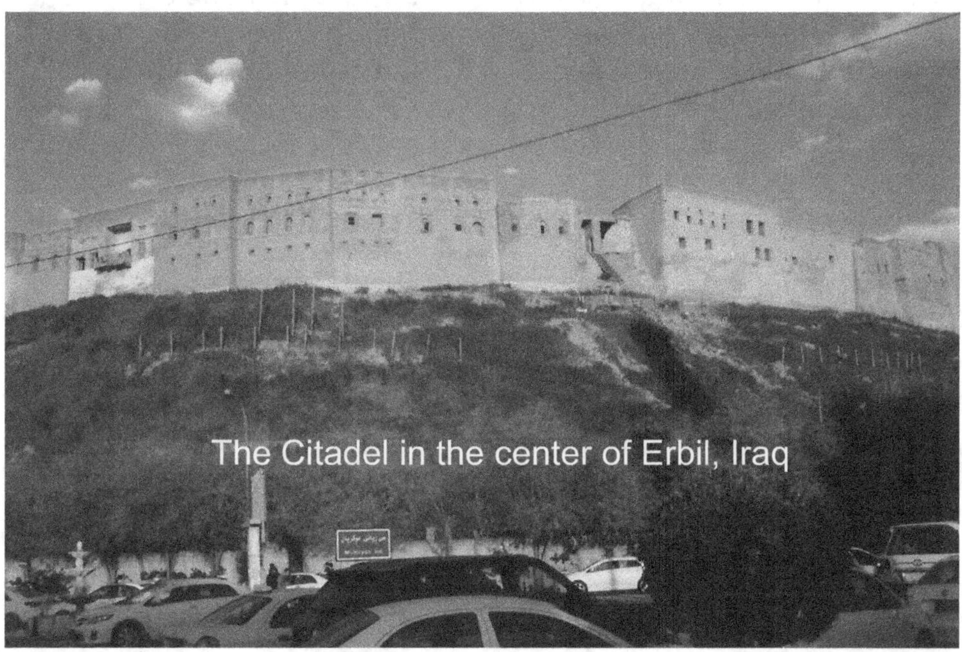

The Citadel in the center of Erbil, Iraq

There were many obstacles during the month of February as I established our itinerary. First were the flights. Joe was in Dubai and so I planned to fly via Dubai to Erbil. I found a great bargain on United Arab Emirates that took me round trip from SFO to Erbil, $1,260. I was delighted. Then quite unexpectedly Emirates cancelled it's flights into Erbil for no given reason, but they rebooked me on their associate airline FlyDubai for the leg from Dubai into Erbil. I was fine with that. Then the next day FlyDubai cancelled their flights into Iraq. Again no reason was given. I began to scramble to find an airline for Joe and I to get from Dubai into Erbil. Qatar Air had an expensive flight, and after checking with Joe I booked two seats. I breathed a sigh of relief, but not for long. One of my contacts in Erbil emailed me saying all the Qatar flights had been removed from the arrival board at the Erbil International airport. Qatar never contacted me that their flights were cancelled, but they too had stopped flying into Iraq. It was back to the drawing board.

In the end we were able to fly on Royal Jordanian, but that meant flying from Dubai clear across Iraq to the Jordanian capitol of Amman which was their hub. Then after a couple hours lay over we had to fly back across ISIS controlled Iraq to our destination of Erbil. Fortunately it was in the middle of the night when we flew and we were at 30,000 feet.

Another hurdle was travel insurance. All the companies I contacted had excluded Iraq from their insured countries. I found one company, Roam Right, that offered insurance. I purchased their "Elite" coverage, which agreed to fly me back to the "hospital of my choice." If you have read this far in this book then you know why that was important to me. With my medical history it was unlikely any hospital except Stanford Hospital could navigate my complicated medical history.

Finally it was recommended I purchase K&R insurance. That stands for Kidnap and Ransom. I was surprised such a thing existed. It turns out there are a lot of factors that make negotiating with terrorists very expensive. Getting a quote from companies took over four weeks; it seemed they were either not very motivated or just didn't want to sell the insurance. In the end they quoted me $1,600 for two weeks of coverage. It goes without saying that I already felt captive by the company and I declined the coverage.

The real time consuming work was setting up appointments. There are confidentiality issues to deal with when working with people whose lives are in danger daily, and whose very presence in the country could be jeopardized if certain communications were made public. And for that reason I won't mention any of their names nor their organizations here.

I departed San Francisco for a fifteen hour flight to Dubai on March 12th, 2015. There were two empty seats in my row so I was able to sleep most the journey. I arrived in Dubai in the middle of the night and passed through immigration and customs rather quickly. I had just two small carry-on bags (one of them was full of just my medical supplies) and Joe met me shortly after I exited the terminal. Everything in Dubai is over-the-top. It is of course home to the tallest building in the world, and boasts such things as man-made islands in the shapes of palm trees, and an indoor ski slope in the middle of their dessert. Dubai wants to be the best of the best in the entire world. They are doing a good job of it.

Their construction boom is financed by their huge oil revenues. All the labor is performed by foreigners. There are Filipinos at work in the airports because their English is good. Pushtuns from Afghanistan do the cleaning and hauling of trash. Taxi drivers were from Bangladesh. Electricians and Plumbers are from India. Expatriates from seventy-five different countries outnumber Emirati locals by a ratio of nine to one. I spent my day and a half in Dubai in a guest house with Joe, recuperating from the long journey.

In the middle of the night Joe and I boarded the Royal Jordanian aircraft and flew to Amman and then to Erbil. At the brand new Erbil International Airport we took a shuttle to their domestic terminal and then were picked up by our first host. It was four a.m., but I still found it strange as I bedded down on a pad on the floor and the room started getting light. The sun was coming up.

At nine we woke, had showers, then headed downtown to a guest house that would be our base for the next week. Joe and I absolutely loved interacting with people on the street, with taxi drivers, fruit vendors, family run restaurants, barbers, etc. The Kurdish language spoken in Erbil is Sorani, which has many similarities to Kermanji (the language I had learned) and also to Farsi (which Joe could speak.) We wrote new words and phrases in small notebooks so we could practice them throughout our days. Learning language is a way to build friendships with people. It demonstrates we care about them and their culture.

The center of Erbil has an underground market, surrounded by modern shops with all kinds of goods. Adjacent to the market is a plaza with fountains and seating areas, where thousands of locals gather to meet one another. Above the plaza is an ancient citadel. Erbil claims to be the oldest continuously inhabited city in the world, with evidence that people have lived there since 5000 BC. Thanks to the no-fly zone established after Saddam in the 1990's, Erbil and all of Iraqi Kurdistan have been able to build their economy in relative security. There has been astounding progress in transforming the region (and the capitol of Erbil in particular) into splendid cities. There were tall buildings everywhere. Construction cranes dotted the horizon. Office buildings and glass towers filled the horizon. In addition there were satellite cities that had sprung up around the capitol.

In some of these areas, and in some of the unfinished buildings downtown, refugees from Mosul (which ISIS had taken over) had found shelter. In one unfinished mall every floor of the concrete structure was host to dozens of families living behind plastic and hastily constructed enclosures. A public school in town had been transformed to house families. Shipping containers were moved onto the property for some families, tents erected for others. At the school there was clothing strung up to dry between posts in the outdoor hallways. People gathered around their tea pots in what once were student hallways between classrooms. The playground was crowded with children eager for attention. The need was incomprehensible. A four year old boy hung onto my leg the entire duration of our visit at the converted school. I invented a game of *herre herre* (run, run) and *werre werre* (come, come) to keep the children occupied.

Much of our personal visits with the leaders focussed on what they were doing, what their goals were, what needs they had in personnel and resources, and an evaluation of ways our home church could come alongside to partner with them. It was helpful to both parties. Each day Joe wrote an assessment and emailed it to our church. We took photos and videos to help communicate the needs and opportunities.

On March 19th I woke at two a.m. with a stuffy head. For most people this would be no big deal. But for me it was a signal of things to come. Bad things. I was dead tired and didn't even feel like getting out of bed to flush my sinuses. I had brought with me two bottles of .9% saline with which I could flush my sinuses. Even after nine sinus surgeries I am still prone to polyps, narrowing of the sinuses, and chronic infection. So when my head is stuffed up it means there is an infection that has gotten out of control.

Joe and I were sharing a simple room and I tried not to wake him as I rose to go down to the community bathroom. I slipped on my house slippers and quietly shut our bedroom door. Nice bathrooms in Iraq, as in much of the Middle East, are completely tiled. The floor and all the walls were all tiled right up to the ceiling, which also was tiled. There was no shower stall, but there was a shower head and a drain in the floor. This too is typical. We were grateful we had warm water and even a western toilet. Most of the Middle East feature "squatty potties" which are basically a ceramic fixture placed in the floor, with two sculpted places to put your feet. We were even blessed with toilet paper. Not to be taken for granted!

I blew my nose, but my head did not clear. I felt rather warm. I took my thermometer and found my temperature to be elevated. Another bad sign. My throat had that feeling one gets from post nasal drip, a creeping soreness. Yikes. I was getting sick.

I remembered well the last times I had gotten a fever. Each time I ended up in the hospital with sepsis. Any infection in my body can get into the blood stream and attack critical organs like the heart, kidneys, or brain. Once multiple organs come under attack death is imminent. I knew I had to make a choice. The only reason I had survived previous infections was because I had gotten to sophisticated hospitals within two hours of getting a fever. Each time I was given multiple IV antibiotics that ran three to four times a day, for six consecutive weeks. What were the chances of getting that kind of advanced treatment in Erbil? I think you know the answer.

That next day Joe and I were scheduled to travel four hours to the north and east to the city of Dohuk. Most of the huge refugee population was centered in the region around Dohuk, since it is located closest to Mosul. Mosul was the de-facto capitol of IS, since their invasion and conquest of the city in August 2014. Of the 2.7 million refugees in Iraq the majority of the settlements are around Dohuk. It was important that Joe and I get there to assess the work of NGO's in that part of Iraqi Kurdistan. To travel to Dohuk we would drive towards Mosul and then skirt to the right of the city and drive through the mountains to Dohuk. At least that was the plan.

Being sick changed everything for me. I swallowed two 500 mg tablets of Ciprofloxacillin, an antibiotic I like to carry with me when I travel, for just such instances as this. Then a thousand milligrams of Tylenol. But I knew that an oral antibiotic would not eliminate the infection. I had not successfully eliminated an infection with an oral antibiotic since I was fourteen years old. I always require IV's. But I figured it would help.

I sat there on the edge of the bed, with its purple fitted sheet, red blanket and orange bed spread (it was an inexpensive guest house) and realized I had two choices. Either I continued my trip with Joe or I turn my back on Kurdistan, most likely forever, and head home. It was an agonizing decision to make. I talked to God about it. I knew that Joe could continue the itinerary and finish the plans I had laid. He was highly competent and experienced. He knew how to travel by himself in risky regions of the world. He knew the questions to ask and the sensitivity required. He could send home a detailed assessment. But I wanted to go with him so bad it hurt.

Two a.m. became three a.m. I tried to sleep. Four a.m. came and finally I fell asleep. Joe told me later he knew I had gotten a stuffy head because my annoying snore had become a freight train. Even with his ear plugs he heard the racket. He typically rose at six, ate a simple breakfast and did his exercises. I slept through all of it. Finally I woke at nine a.m.. He had left me a note saying he'd gone to the bazaar to talk to people. The note lay on the carpet beside my bed where I would see it first thing. I was jealous. I would much rather be at the bazaar than facing a trip back to the US.

I did not feel any better after washing up. I knew I would only start feeling worse each hour through the day. I thought about the four hour ride up to Dohuk. I have traveled many times when sick. It is agonizing. Particularly when running a fever, with a hacking cough, a sore throat and a runny nose. And then, when I reached Dohuk what would I do? I'd be a liability, not an asset. To go would be selfish. It would also put me much further from getting any medical help.

And throughout my deliberations I thought of my dear wife. I remembered clearly her looking me in the eye just before I left our home. We were standing in our living room surrounded by my leather coat on the sofa and my two small black bags on the floor. She stood just two feet from me and looked up into my eyes.

"Dan," she said in a grave voice, "You come home to me." They were brief words that carried the gravity of all our years of travel together. They conveyed the weight of all her concerns and prayers. Included in that sentence were all those hospital cots she had slept on at my side. She knew, as I did, that I could die in Iraq. Yes, God had called me to go, but she did not want to lose me. She knew in her heart that I was determined to make a difference in the lives of the Kurds. But she did not want to bury me at age fifty-six.

Now I was sitting on the orange bedspread in Erbil, and looked at my stuff scattered about on the desk, the end table, the rickety wardrobe, and my drying laundry on the back of the door. There was just one question in my mind, *"Do I pack my bags and call the travel insurance company, or do I call Joe on his cell phone and go downtown to join him in the bazaar?"* I wanted so bad to go onward to Dohuk, but I felt the same small voice of the Holy Spirit giving me direction. And on top of that I could hear DeAnna's voice calling me from almost twelve thousand miles away. What should I do?

Chapter 37

"You Come Home to Me"

I looked at my belongings and decided I would begin to get them organized. *"Pocket knife and scissors must go in the check-in baggage,"* I reminded myself. *"All medicines must go in the carry-on bag."* I had decided to go home. The compelling message and the expressions of my wife were overwhelming. I felt her love. I imagined the grief she'd experience if I died in Dohuk or was struck down somewhere on a long journey home. I knew what I should do. It is important to serve the Lord and heed his call. However, he also calls men to love their wives. I knew that for me this call to love DeAnna was more important in this moment than my life calling to love the Kurds. So I packed my bags.

Then I called Roam Right, the travel insurance company from whom I'd purchased the "Elite" package of coverage. This was a wise thing to purchase anytime I traveled, regardless if it is to Denver or Dohuk. I had never had to use the travel insurance, however. The travel assistance office on the US east coast was seven hours ahead of Erbil time. I reached them on my cell phone and explained my situation to them, including the fact that past sinus infections had caused me to become septic. They said I needed to first go to a local hospital, be examined in an emergency room, and then have the ER doctor contact them. I said goodbye.

Next I called the man with whom we had an appointment that day and cancelled. Then I called a Jordanian believer who was the chief financial officer for a large NGO in Erbil. We had met with him the previous day. He said he would be happy to come around noon to pick me up. He had his own car. Most people in Erbil take taxis, very few have their own cars. I finished packing and ate some breakfast in the community kitchen. The electricity was off in the building so there was no hot tea. It is not uncommon for the power to go off. Kurdistan is still part of Iraq, but the central government in Baghdad had not been distributing the agreed upon proceeds from the sale of government oil. So there had been power shortages and all government employees were not being paid. It was a reminder that I was still in a third world country. I wondered what the hospital would be like.

Our Jordanian friend arrived and drove me across town to the PAR hospital[61]. I was very impressed. It was one of the many new buildings and featured an all glass five story front and had marble tile inside. The emergency room was orderly and clean, had eight beds, and only one was occupied. A Kurdish doctor, Dr. Kew, met me and immediately devoted all his attention to my case. His English was excellent; learning English is highly valued in Kurdistan. It is a preferred language (for the Kurds) to even Arabic, which is spoken throughout Iraq. Dr. Kew listened carefully and most importantly, believed me and took my personal assessment of my health seriously. I have found that many medical personnel don't truly listen to me, and ignore my personal diagnosis. *"They are professionals and they know better,"* is their attitude. They simply don't realize that I know my own health and medical history. I know my own body. How many times have I watched an IV nurse stick me over and over, then finally agree with me that, "I am a hard stick." Then they ask me where my good veins are located. Ha!

"Here, try this vein in the palm of my hand." Their eyes get real big.

"I have never put an IV in anybody's palm before," they say.

"Well, I have had IV's three times in that vein," I tell them. In the end they put the IV where I show them. It's a painful lesson. Pun intended.

Dr. Kew agreed that I should be flown to Stanford Hospital where my complicated medical history could be properly addressed.

---

61 http://www.parhospital.org

"We simply don't have the specialists and equipment here to help you," he honestly said. He called Roam Right to tell them I should be transported to the US. He said I was healthy enough to travel. They told him they would fax a form to be filled out and faxed back. We both anticipated a swift emergency evacuation. After looking at my veins he decided to give me an intramuscular injection of an antibiotic, Ceftriaxone, rather than attempt to put an IV in. I unbuckled my belt and bent over. Ceftriaxone is a broad spectrum antibiotic and should address whatever bug was present. Joe had arrived at the hospital and together with our Jordanian friend we discussed going to the restaurant next door to the hospital. We knew it would take some time to work out the evacuation. We headed for the entrance. My cell phone rang.[62]

It was Roam Right on the phone and they told me, "It will only take a short time."

"What is a 'short time?" I asked.

"Quickly," she said.

"How much time is quickly?" I persisted.

The lady thought for a moment and replied, "Oh, a couple of hours." When you are standing outside a hospital running a fever and waiting to be transported home, "two hours" does not seem like, "quickly." I said I would await their call and hung up. We decided to go get a bite to eat.

The restaurant next door was called *Paradise*. This seemed funny to us since the hospital was called PAR. Many people who go to hospitals don't make it.

"First you go to PAR," Joe said, "Then you get the rest of the word…. and end up in Paradise." We all hoped true paradise was not too imminent for me.

Joe had decided to stick with our itinerary and travel to Dohuk in a car with friends of mine, Christine and Greg Callison, that lived in Dohuk. I phoned them. They just "happened" to be in Erbil that day on an errand. They explained that it is much safer to drive with a hired driver to Dohuk even though it is six times more

---

[62] This was a $20 cell phone that I purchased in Erbil. It contained a SIM card for a specific number of minutes. The phone I'd brought from the states did not work in their network.

expensive than a taxi. Chris said there is a greater risk of dying in a traffic accident on the highways than being taken hostage or killed by a car bomb. Taxi drivers are paid by the trip and they take great risks to arrive quickly. The hired driver known to Greg was a safe driver. Since the Callisons were in Erbil and not far away they drove to the restaurant Paradise to see me. It was wonderful to have dear friends join me during my final hours in Kurdistan.

There was such a mix of emotions passing through me. I felt a deep appreciation for my friends and their willingness to help me in this crisis. I felt the love of my wife that motivated me to return home. Then there was the passion I felt for the Kurds and for the refugees who were in such dire need, and finally my yearnings to stay in Kurdistan. I also felt a bit of guilt that I had the resources to fly twelve thousand miles to a safe country and stay in a top notch hospital while 2.7 million souls struggled to just survive after losing all they held dear. Many had lost family members, women had been raped and sold to ISIS as slaves, Christians had been beheaded or shot, Shia Muslims had been executed... the list goes on. But here I sat in an air conditioned restaurant with four precious friends, awaiting an emergency jet to fly me around the world. Why am I so blessed?

Word came from Dr. Kew that he had gotten through to Roam Right and they had given permission to evacuate me. I was relieved. But the relief was short lived. Roam Right had decided (against Dr. Kew's advice) to fly me to either Amman, Jordan or to Istanbul, Turkey. I was shocked. I dialed the number for Roam Right on the cheap cell phone I'd purchased in Erbil. There was too much noise in the restaurant to hear even the ringing so I stepped outside onto the sidewalk. Roam Right answered. Above the sound of the traffic I tried to hear the voice of the insurance agent and also make my point for flying back to the US. I explained that I had purchased the "elite" package that assured me of being flown to the "hospital of my choice." The agent countered with a clause that allowed Roam Right to fly a person to a third country until they became stable. I told them I was stable already. They said I needed to be evaluated more. Above the roar of the traffic we argued. I explained that I was a heart double lung transplant patient. I told them I was immune suppressed, and that I had been septic four times.

"I have no IV accessible veins," I said. "I have to have a PICC line inserted in order to get IV antibiotics." The agent said she was not a medical professional and did not understand what I was saying. I asked to speak to a doctor.

"That isn't possible," she said. Finally she said I could speak to a nurse. When the nurse came on the phone my line went dead. My SIM card minutes had run out. I could feel my heart rate go up. I sat down on the front steps of the restaurant to try and relax. The sun was going down. Joe handed me his phone and I dialed the long distance number again. After waiting on hold forever and wondering if Joe's minutes would also run out, I was reconnected with the nurse.

I explained my complicated history again (which was also included in the faxed document they had received from Dr. Kew.) The nurse was clearly exasperated with me, as I was with her.

"Please," I said. "I have a first world problem. But you want to fly me to a third world country. They cannot help me. They won't be able to start a PICC line unless they have intervention radiology. I have two stents in my heart. I am immune suppressed and require special treatments to treat the flu. Neither Istanbul nor Amman does double organ transplants," I thought of every rational argument I could think of. "Why would you send me to Istanbul?"

"We are wasting time here," she said and then shut me down with, "You need medical care. Do you want to go to Istanbul or not?" I was clearly stuck. Either I accepted their decision or I stayed in Iraq. It was no decision at all. It was an ultimatum.

"I will go to Istanbul," I conceded. I tried to quickly reorient myself to this new reality.

"When will the jet come?" I asked.

"We have to find out which company can provide us with a jet the soonest. Then we will know whether you will be flown to Amman or to Istanbul. We will let Dr. Kew know." Unbelievable.

After another interminable wait we learned that I would be flown to Istanbul. Dr. Kew from the Iraqi hospital was puzzled since he had said I should be sent to Stanford, but we realized I had no choice. *"There is a time to fight and a time to accept reality and rest,"* I thought to myself. I tried to wind down and relax.

I had to be admitted to the PAR hospital for the night as the emergency flight would not come until the next morning. I did not look forward to another new hospital and all that admission entailed. The hospital's emergency room was now completely empty and the hallways were dark. It had taken an entire day just to get this far. My supportive friends soon departed after some emotional goodbyes.

Joe whispered in my ear as he gave me a hug, "Don't worry Dan. This trip has been a success." He knew what I was thinking and feeling. I was feeling it had been a failure. I had come all that way and had only met with five NGO leaders. Joe, however, said he would be going on to Dohuk and would meet with the others on my list. It was agonizing to accept the fact that I was not going to see more of Kurdistan. I loved its people and its culture. I prayed that God would use my small part of the journey and this small effort in his greater plan.

I walked down the long darkened corridor in the hospital toward a big sign that said, "Admitting." I wasn't sure whether they were saving electricity or there had been another brown out. I felt alone and far away. *"I can do this,"* I said to myself. *"God is with me."* I approached a young man sitting all alone behind an imposing desk. I told him I was supposed to be admitted for the night. He began the requisite paperwork.

"There is a required deposit of $1,000 sir," the clerk said with a straight face. That was a shocker! No worries though, I put my credit card on the counter. "No credit cards, sir," he said. "Only US dollars or Iraqi dinars." My eyes opened wide. He wanted cash!

All my friends had left the building over ten minutes ago. I realized if I didn't have $1000 US, I wouldn't be admitted for the night. Immediately I was thankful for Joe's advice to me in San Jose to put ten $100 US bills in a money belt, "for an emergency." Neither of us had any idea that a deposit of this sum would be required in this instance.

But my relief quickly evaporated when I remembered I had cashed one of the bills in Erbil to purchase Iraqi Dinars to buy food, lodging and pay for taxis. Joe insisted on several occasions that he pay for all our other expenses since I had purchased his air travel from Dubai. If he hadn't done that I would have had even less money in my money belt! I prayed a prayer of thanks. Then I wondered how much other US currency I had randomly placed in the money belt as I was packing in California.

I opened my shirt and unclipped the belt. I unzipped its pocket and began laying the cash on the counter. "One hundred, two hundred, …. nine hundred," and I paused. Then I began counting some twenties I'd slipped in. There were exactly five.

"There you go," I said. "One thousand US dollars." I looked at my remaining money. I had four one dollar bills. I held them up for the clerk to see.

"This is all I have left," I said. His eyes grew wide. I was reminded of God's promise "For my God will meet all your needs according to his glorious riches in Christ Jesus."[63]

As I entered the spartan bedroom I immediately noticed the unmade bare plastic mattress. The admitting nurse (male) quickly set about putting a fitted sheet on it. Then he handed me a blanket. I realized then that they didn't use top sheets. *"When in Rome…"* I mused. I wondered how many people used the same blanket.

The room was clean and spacious. There was just an oxygen outlet above the headboard. Other than that it could have been a simple hotel room. As I closed my door I could see many people seated in the hallway on the floor near to the doorways of various rooms. It is normal for an entire family or at least many loved ones to be near to a hospitalized person. At the very least they bring food, but more significantly they are a comfort and provide companionship. The admitting nurse was shocked that I was alone.

"Have you no one with you?" he asked with surprise.

"God is my companion," I replied. It probably sounded trite to a Muslim, but I meant it sincerely.

A while later four men came in to work on my IV. After several attempts and much searching they were able to start a small line

---

[63] Philippians 4:19

in a vein below the ball of my ankle on my right leg. It made walking an impossibility, but at least it was IV access.

I was wakened at four a.m. to prepare for the flight. It took no time to get ready, since I had slept in my clothes. A Turkish man in a tight leather black jacket and black pants was to be my escort. He spoke good English, but did not want to talk to me. He acted aloof, as if this whole experience was a major inconvenience for him. Maybe he wasn't an early riser. He helped me get into a wheel chair and brought me down the elevator and out to an ambulance.

The ambulance drove me to Erbil's domestic airport terminal. There I was transferred out of the hospital's ambulance and into the airport's own ambulance. It was a security measure. A male nurse stepped up to the side door and asked me several questions. Then he completed a form that verified I was healthy enough to travel. The ride across the tarmac was brief.

They opened the double doors of the ambulance and the cold morning air swept in. I looked through the doors and could see a small jet waiting for me.

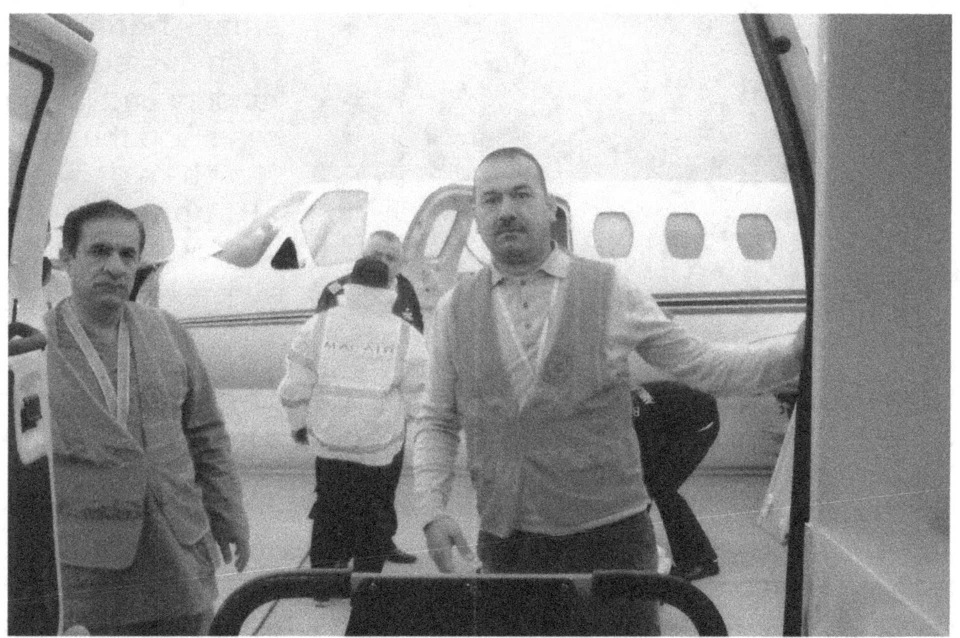

"Can you walk," somebody asked?

"I can hop on one foot," I said. I didn't want to remove the IV, since it seemed to have worked during the night. *"Perhaps I can use the same IV when I get to Istanbul,"* I hoped.

There was a gurney in the small cabin, beside three other large well worn leather passenger seats. A lady nurse climbed in. She spoke no English but I could see she wanted to do an O2 saturation so I obliged her by providing a finger for the clip. She seemed satisfied that I was in a safe O2 range. The jet began to taxi. The nurse set the large monitor box on the seat opposite me. I motioned that I would like to use the seat belts to keep me in place on the gurney. The buckles were jammed between the wall of the cabin and the metal rails of the gurney.

"No, problem," the nurse said, as the jet began to taxi out to the runway. She left the buckles unfastened.

I noted there were oxygen tanks laying in the isle on the floor.

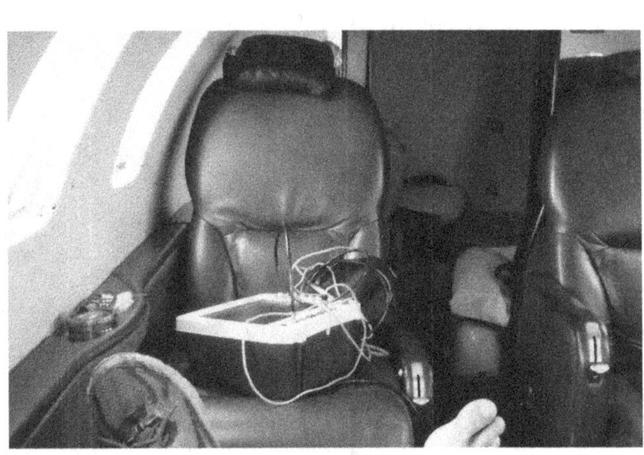

They were rolling back and forth as the jet increased its speed. My small bags had been tossed in at random and lay on seats and the floor. Nothing was strapped down. The jet began to shake as we rolled for take-off. The nose came up. I began sliding down off the gurney. My left hand grabbed what it could of the window frame; my right reached across the isle and held on to the leather seat. We lifted off.

The flight plan carried us over northern Kurdistan toward the Turkish border. This avoided ISIS held territories in Syria. Or at least it allowed us to gain sufficient altitude (I guess) to minimize being shot at. At the heart of it was the assurance that God was in control. *"He does watch over even the sparrow, a plane should be no problem,"* I was reminded by a still small voice.

The landing and transfer to an ambulance in Istanbul went smoothly. A customs agent came out to the ambulance to process my passport. The flight had been over two hours and there was no bathroom on the small jet so I began to think about my need to use one. None of the three men in the ambulance spoke English and I knew it could be an hour ride or more to the hospital. (I had been to Istanbul several times before.) From my reclined position on the gurney I used hand signals to indicate my need.

"Ah," they smiled. They understood. Good. I anticipated they would hand me some sort of urinal but instead they handed me a plastic bag. They pulled the van to the side of the freeway and stopped. I eyed the plastic bag with skepticism, but they assured me (again with hand signals) that all would be fine.

Indeed there was some sort of valve in the top of the bag, so when I had finished the contents were securely contained. I started to place the sealed bag on the floor beside the gurney. But they insisted I give the full bag to them, for whatever reason I couldn't fathom. To my horror they opened the side door of the ambulance and chucked the entire bag out onto the side of the road.

"No problem," they said. *"Welcome to Istanbul,"* I thought.

The Acibadem [ah gee Bah dem] Hospital[64] was a beautiful ten story glass and marble building in the heart of downtown Istanbul. Its emergency room was well equipped and quite crowded. The attending physician took my medical history and became more and more alarmed as he heard of all my past ailments. He ordered a full consultation with a cardiologist, a pulmonologist, an ENT, the infectious disease specialist, and an internal medicine physician. I forgot to tell him I'd had brain surgery as a youth, and was thankful I'd forgotten to mention it. I am sure he would have sent me to see a neurologist. And if I'd mentioned the cancers I'd had there would have been an oncologist visit. And my thyroid removal would have caused me to visit an endocrinologist. As it

---

64 https://www.acibadem.com.tr/hastane/international-hastanesi/

was it took an entire day just to see the five specialists and oblige them with their litany of tests.

Finally I was admitted to a room on the ninth floor. Acibadem would not accept the IV in my foot ("It wasn't from *their* hospital," so could not be trusted,) and four attempts by four nurses in ER to start their own IV had failed. A female anesthesiologist came in to my patient room to start my IV. She seemed very annoyed that she had been called to start a simple IV. We did not exchange any pleasantries since she could not speak English. I just smiled. In the end she was able to get an IV started in the knuckle of my right thumb. The floor nurse arrived and hung a bag of liquid from a pole. I could not read what was written on the bag as I don't know Turkish.

Later my nurse entered with a pill and a cup of water. I looked at the foil package and did not recognize the medicine. I asked what it was. She did not speak English. I already take twenty-six medications (for lots of different things) and I am leery about any new meds.

"Why should I take it," I asked? She smile and shrugged. I left it on the bedside table and she walked out.

The view from the window was certainly five star. I could see the strait that separated European Istanbul from this side, which was in Asia. I recognized a mall way beneath my window. Some five years earlier my wife and I had dropped our daughter Jessica off at that very mall to hang out with the daughter of a friend we were visiting. We had been in Istanbul on a trip to encourage some missionaries. The two girls had gone to a movie there while DeAnna and I took the missionary couple out to dinner.

But this visit was a lot different. I thought of DeAnna. She was so far away. Would I live through this to see her again? We had been unable to talk by phone, although she had gotten word of my illness and transport to Turkey. I looked at some of the Acibadem information material on the desk in the room and noted the hospital had internet. I was thankful I had brought our iPad and even more so when I was able to log on. Before long DeAnna and I were emailing and then Skyping with one another.

DeAnna worked on trying to get me medical help and advice by contacting my physicians at Stanford. They were reluctant,

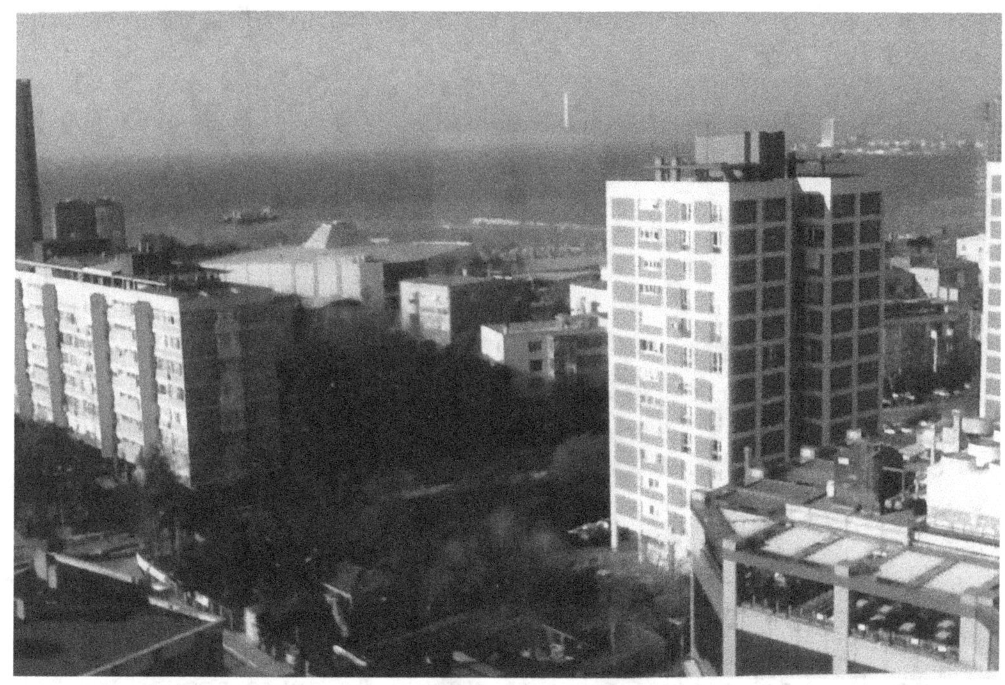

however, to interfere with any medical treatment I was receiving at another hospital. So they did nothing. She prayed and asked others to pray. "Cast your cares on the Lord."[65] This has been our way of life since we were young. Jesus cares and listens. Yet it was very frustrating and fearful for DeAnna when her husband was so far away and she felt helpless to assist.

She searched the internet to see what the pill was that the nurse brought me. I had given her the Turkish name written on it. It was the equivalent of Thera-flu. This is an over the counter flu medicine. It would have been laughable if the situation were not so serious. I most likely did have some kind of flu, but there is no way this pea-shooter drug was going to take down my illness. The last time I had had the flu I had been treated at Stanford University Hospital and been given a newly developed anti-viral medicine.

Because my immune system is compromised a virus is potentially fatal. The wonderful people at the Acibadem hospital didn't

---

[65] Psalms 55:2

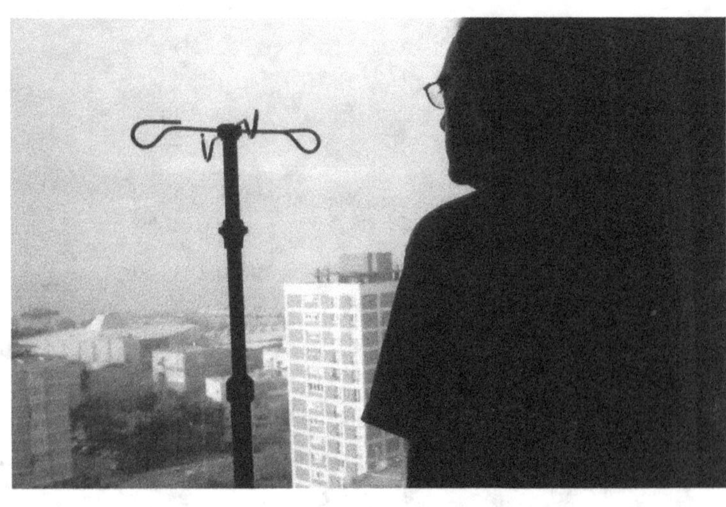

have the means to help me. The new drug Stanford had administered was given to me for five consecutive nights. How well I remembered that horrible mist tent and the sweaty mask that misted medicine into my airways.

I didn't think Thera-flu was going to do the trick. It treats a common type A or B flu virus. (I later learned I was afflicted with the RNA virus.) Both DeAnna and I knew that time was of the essence in attacking any infection quickly. As hours passed the risk was increasing of me developing a secondary infection which could enter my blood stream and destroy vital organs like my heart, kidneys, or brain. I needed to get home fast. I remembered what it felt like to be septic.

I also knew a virus would stimulate my natural immune response. *"I should be getting a massive dose of immune-suppressant medicine,"* I thought.

It was not a situation the Acibadem hospital could handle, even after all the great consults I'd had with their five specialists. They apparently did not understand organ transplantation, at least in my situation. I tried to communicate this to the travel insurance company but was given multiple layers of bureaucracy. They would not fly me home from Turkey until I first completed some more forms. First I had to get a signed (and translated) doctor's "clear to fly" approval form. Acibadem had provided me with a wonderful interpreter, and she managed to get this form completed in record time. She faxed it to the company, gave me her personal phone number for emergencies, and then left for the evening and took the bus to her home.

Several hours later I received another email from Roam Right. They now wanted a three page medical summary completed. This was very frustrating. What could I do? Why hadn't they asked for this the first time? There was nobody at the hospital with whom I could speak English. In desperation I telephoned the interpreter. Although she had barely settled into her home for the night, she took a one hour bus ride back to the hospital, found the appropriate nurses and my medical records, completed the form, located a doctor to sign it, translated it into English, and then faxed it to the insurance company. She again said a sweet goodbye (may the Lord bless her) and left to take the bus back home.

Several hours later I received another email from Roam Right. This time they wanted copies of the reports from each of the five specialists I had seen. These would also have to be translated into English and faxed to them. Only then would Roam Right decide whether to transport me home.

I was livid. As DeAnna and I skyped we discussed the situation. It seemed ludicrous for the company to make such demands. Clearly they did not understand (or perhaps care about) the gravity of my situation. I wondered if it might be cheaper for them to fly me home in a wooden box rather than a seat on a plane. Sometimes such thoughts are better left unspoken, but I blurted it out to DeAnna. I immediately regretted having said it. She was sitting in California, without any real sense of my degree of illness, and was no doubt wondering if I was going to die in Turkey.

The reality, however, was that I no longer had a fever. I was mobile, though confined to my room, was eating fine and sleeping fine, and simply needed to go home as fast as possible to address what I figured was either the flu or a sinus infection. I composed a final email to Roam Right. I asked them quite directly if their doctors knew more about my medical condition than the doctors in Istanbul who had treated me and granted me clearance to fly home. Then I asked for the names and addresses of the doctors with whom Roam Right worked. I wanted to know the names of the people who were making these life-and-death decisions.

Perhaps they finally realized I was serious and would hold them accountable. I received an email within minutes that said I was free to purchase a ticket and fly home. It was close to eleven p.m. on Saturday night. I quickly went on line and checked flight schedules. There was a nine a.m. flight each day to San Francisco from Istanbul (via Los Angeles.) But I didn't have time to be discharged and catch the Sunday morning flight. Discharge from a hospital takes several hours and certainly doesn't happen at 6 in the morning. So I booked a seat for Monday morning. Thankfully Turkish Airlines accepts credit cards, because all I had was the four dollars. And fortuitously the hospital covered the ride to the airport terminal. Wow!

I did not run a fever during my flight home, nor even need to take the Tylenol I carried. I was so relieved just to be in the air and on my way to get reliable medical care. When I arrived in San Francisco the emotional relief was indescribable. I knew I was not out of the woods yet. But at least I was in a place where I could be treated with some hope for recovery. I gathered my bags and called DeAnna on the phone. She met me curbside. Neither of us could speak for several moments as we hugged one another.

"I'm so glad you made it," she said.

"I love you so much," I replied. "You know," I continued, "When I left home you looked me in the eye, put your hands on both of my upper arms and said with clear conviction, "You come home to me." They were just five words. But I knew you meant them from the depth of your heart. It was those words that helped me make the decision to leave Erbil and not continue on to Dohuk. Dohuk would have been five hours from the hospital in Erbil. I knew I shouldn't take the risk. It was so hard to say goodbye to Kurdistan and return to the US. But I know how much you wanted me to make it back to you. I know how much you sacrificed to let me go. And I knew it was the right thing to do, to come home to you."

"Really," she asked? "I don't remember saying it."

I had spent one night in the hospital in Iraq and three nights in the hospital in Turkey. Then after five more miserable nights in the mist tent at Stanford I made a full recovery.

It took multiple letters, a complaint filed with the California Department of Insurance, and four months of waiting before Roam Right finally agreed to pay the benefits agreed upon in the insurance policy.

Chapter 38

One More Time

Even though I walk through the valley of the shadow of death, I will fear no evil, for you are with me; your rod and your staff, they comfort me.
Psalm 23:4

The doctor looked me in the eyes and asked, "Do you know where you are?" I lay on a hospital bed in a daze. "Do you know what day today is?" he continued. My eyes rolled shut.

Back in the fall of 2013, I went to my cardiologist Dr. Kiran Khush at Stanford Health Care. She listened to my chest and told me I once again had a murmur. An echocardiogram later confirmed Dr. Khush's diagnosis. The valve was not shutting properly. I knew of the murmur, but this was my first visit to this cardiologist.

"How severe is my faulty heart valve?" I asked.

"Well, it is serious," she replied.

"So," I continued, "If I walked in here off the street, and I had never had any other health issues, what would your recommendation be to me?"

Without hesitation Dr. Khush answered, "I would recommend you have it surgically repaired."

"Well then," I asked, "Why don't we repair my valve?"

"Because," she replied, "Doing this surgery on you, would most likely result in a fatal event."

"That's 'hospital-speak' for death," I responded. "You mean I'd die." I was never one to beat about the bush.

"Yes," she replied. "There is a 95 percent chance it would be fatal. You have already had your chest opened three times. First for your heart/lung transplant, second for the aneurism and valve repair, and the third time for aortic stenosis. Your aortic valve is once again the faulty valve. Each time your chest was opened they cut through the sternum. This bone is about a half inch thick before it is sawed through the first time. Then, after it heals, it reaches about half that thickness - roughly one quarter of an inch thick. After the second surgery, the bone again grows back to a thinner thickness. One problem with opening up your chest for a fourth time is that the bone would not heal to sufficient thickness."

She continued, "Your last surgeon, Dr. Bruce Reitz, stated in his notes that your chest should never be opened again." My wife and I both remember him telling us this sober news during my recuperation. Apparently there had been very little healthy tissue for Dr. Reitz to complete the repair of the aortic valve. Old scars had to be cut away, since only healthy normal tissue will heal together. That surgery (October 2008) had taken five hours to complete, and had left Dr. Reitz praying I would survive. He said it was amazing that the heart began pumping again after he'd completed the repair.

Since fixing the murmur was no longer an option, my wife and I accepted the fact that the murmur might slowly get worse. The aneurism might get larger, like a balloon slowly being inflated. We knew that at any moment the balloon could burst, causing the heart to pump blood into the chest cavity whereby death would quickly follow. Doctors might try to rescue me, but it would be of little point. The best thing to do was to live life to the fullest, obey and trust the Lord each day, and rejoice in the unbelievably long and wonderful life God had given me.

A couple years had now gone by. I visited Dr. Khush annually and had my echocardiogram done. Each time the report showed insignificant change. I did what all of us do, I grew complacent with my health.

Then DeAnna was injured. My wife and I own a rental property and had decided to redo the yard ourselves to make it conserve water. 3000 square feet of grass was taken out and replaced with drip irrigation to 75 new plants. Part of the work was to put in a french drain. DeAnna accompanied me to the rockery to buy a yard of rock for the drain. Our truck had a sturdy flat cover over its bed, and the rockery wanted the cover removed. It was far too heavy for DeAnna and I to do alone, in fact DeAnna had weak wrists and had told me she didn't want to help. But we needed the rock. One of the employees agreed to help us remove the lid, provided we verbally agree not to hold them accountable if there was an accident. I'd taken it off many times so I quickly agreed. I tilted the huge cover upwards on its shocks. Then put the tailgate down.

DeAnna stood on the open tailgate as the employee and I disengaged the hinged end of the cover. As we lowered the now-unhinged lid downwards DeAnna tried hold up her end. It was still over her head when her right elbow gave out. The cover came down and smacked her on the head, sending her down to the bed of the truck. It was just a millisecond moment in time but it changed the rest of her life. She had seriously injured her neck. It was a full year before she got a correct diagnosis and another four months before she could have surgery.

During the same year I began having recurring blood infections. Six times I was admitted to Stanford Hospital and put on IV antibiotics. Each time I seemed to recover, only to again run a fever. The source of the infection remained somewhat of a mystery until August 2016. Dr. James Mooney, my pulmonologist told me that perhaps the aortic valve was harboring the bacteria and continually infecting my blood. He gave me an immediate referral to the cardiologist. The cardiologist first ordered an echocardiogram. When the echo tech looked at my echocardiogram he was visibly disturbed. Afterwards the technician asked me to remain in the waiting room while he got the doctor. The doctor came to me in the waiting room expecting me to be weak and immobile. But I said I felt fine.

Meanwhile DeAnna had been searching to get the diagnosis for the incredible neck and back pain she was experiencing. Doctors could not see the damage on X-rays and MRI's to her spine. Finally she learned that she had multiple injured discs and a pinched spinal nerve. She would have to have the injured discs replaced and the vertebrae C4-C7 fused together. She was finally scheduled for spinal surgery at UCSF in October 2016. She waited expectantly.

In September I went to see a cardiovascular surgeon, Dr. David Woo, about my damaged heart valve. After some discussion he agreed to take on my case. The chances of survival were very slim, and he was the only surgeon at Stanford willing to attempt it.

How well I remembered Dr. Khush's words, "It would most likely be a fatal event." However, Dr. David Woo did about four hundred valve replacement surgeries each year. We sat in his office and looked together at the color display of my heart beating on the computer. He pointed to the valve flapping about aimlessly.

"That is going to kill you," he said emphatically.

"Is it something you think you could fix?" I asked.

"It is very risky," he began and he laid out the grim scenario.

"Well, I know where I will go when I die," I told him. I belong to Jesus and have perfect peace."

"Hmm...," he paused, "You should have all your affairs in order."

"They are," I replied. He then explained the surgery and made a surgical date for one week away.

I went home and wrote out my memorial service, asking my brother and Bob Blincoe to lead it. Bob had been instrumental in our lives when we lived in Iraq. Then I (finally) donated a bunch of clothes so my wife wouldn't have to deal with them. There is nothing like imminent death to make one realize the futility of one's belongings.

Monday morning came and I checked in for surgery. The routine was familiar, but the outcome was anything but certain. DeAnna was in too much pain to even be a passenger in a car so she couldn't drive me to the hospital. Our daughter Jessica packed up her life in Southern California and immediately moved home to take care of her critically ill parents. God bless her.

Once I had been intubated, had my chest and arms shaved and cleaned, had venous and arterial access lines placed, was catheterized, connected to oxygen and temperature sensors, hooked up to blood pressure monitors, had EKG wires attached, and who knows what else… Dr. Woo began by sawing open my sternum. He found that before he could replace the aortic valve he would have to chip away significant calcification.

"I used chisels just like those in your garage," he later told me with a smile.

But he couldn't perform this while my blood circulated. With blood flowing through the heart the loose chips of calcification would be transported through the blood stream and could block arteries or end up in the brain, which could cause a stroke. So Dr. Woo had to stop my heart during that part of the operation. He also had to drain my body of blood. He told me he lowered my body temperature way down in what was basically a controlled hypothermia. He wanted to minimize the damage to the brain from oxygen deprivation, but it was very risky.

Once he completed the aortic valve replacement he saw he needed to work on a second valve, the mitral. Then he repaired the tricuspid valve, stitching an annuloplasty ring in place. The entire operation took twelve hours. Dr. Woo was not anticipating the extra valve work, nor the length of the surgery.

Afterwards I lay unconscious in ICU, fully intubated and surrounded by machines for two full days. I had not awakened as they had planned. My brother Doug flew in and was present with me for the entire time, as was Jessica. DeAnna had to content herself with telephone updates. She remained at home, laying prone on her back most of the time. When I did not come out of the anesthesia, Dr. Woo explained to Doug and Jessica that it was possible I had had a stroke during the surgery, or that possibly I had had a brain seizure. It was also possible that I was brain dead, he said. He did not want them to get their hopes up; my body had been through a huge ordeal.

At one point Jessica decided to sing to me, though I was unconscious. She is an accomplished soloist and she knew I had asked her many times to record her singing the song "My Redeemer Lives."[66] It was a beautiful piece she'd sung at our church and she knew I loved the message. This time she was singing for a much smaller audience. It was just me, Doug, a couple nurses,

---

66 listen to this song at https://www.youtube.com/watch?v=XRW-jr_PnbQ

the doctor, and the Lord. She climbed up beside me onto the hospital bed in ICU and sang it a cappella. We never will know for sure this side of eternity what spiritual impact her faith and singing had. But I did finally stir.

When I awoke and was extubated my mouth was dry, my throat hurt, and I was indescribably tired. Everything around me was a blur. I was aware of Doug's and Jessica's presence. That's when a nurse asked me if I knew where I was.

"Stanford," I said with a touch of disappointment and familiarity, and promptly went back to sleep.

My periods of wakefulness lengthened during the next two days and nights. I frequently asked for ice chips to soothe my throat. The ICU nurse was concerned that my swallowing reflex was not really functioning yet, so I had to really beg for the ice chips. Jessica and Doug took turns spoon feeding me ice. At last I was given permission to swallow something substantial. Jello. Gotta love that Jello.

While still in ICU the doctors decided to remove one of the lines that ran from my neck inside a vein down into my heart. I think it had been used to monitor my heart during the surgery. I said I'd prefer to be conscious when they did the procedure. I have a high pain tolerance. Maybe it's practice. The nurse removed the dressing and tape. She gave the line a tug but was unable to pull it out. The doctor came and tried. Then the surgeon gave it a go. They brought in an Xray machine to take some pictures. Then they tried again.

"Does this hurt?" I was asked as they tugged with force.

"Not really," I replied. But they were unable to budge it.

They then rolled me down to intervention radiology where they could get a live Xray picture of my lungs, heart, and neck to see what the hang-up was. As I was moved onto the operating table I again asked that I not be sedated. As I watched them work I was amused at how cavalier the technicians and doctors were about surgery. I realized that most of the time the patient isn't aware of the jazz music playing, of the jokes being told, and of the discussion about various options to solve real-time problems.

They had quite a dialogue about this particular line and why it wouldn't come out. It turned out to be an actual snag. I have two stents in my superior vena cava (SVC) that date from the time of my heart/double lung transplant. They were placed there due to complications that arose at the time of the transplant. They are metal coils that hold the vein open. This SVC is a large vein that runs from the heart up into the brain. The troublesome line they were trying to remove was not a flexible catheter like one a person gets for medications. It was a coated electrical wire that was intended to monitor my heart's rhythm and pace during and immediately after surgery. This wire had gotten snagged inside my superior vena cava on one of the stents.

As I lay there discussing the problem with them we talked about various options. I rolled to one side and they gave a tug. Then I rolled back to the other side. Another tug. I bore down with my abdomen and they tugged. Still no progress. Then they decided to insert another wire down a vein into the stent itself from the right side of my neck. The troublesome wire was positioned on my left side. Picture an equilateral triangle with my head at the top and two wires running down the sides.

"Should we use the five or the seven?" asked one of the guys wearing green. I assumed this referred to the diameter, or maybe the length of the new line they would use.

"I'd like to try with the five," the surgeon said. The tech perused all his gear that lay out on a long table.

"Mmm… I don't see a five. Here's a seven, try that." Such was the banter. I realized that a lot of surgery is literally flying-by-the-seat-of-the-pants medicine.

After at least thirty minutes the surgeon was able to push and twist the end of the entangled wire from the coil of the stent and free it. He then gave a very slight pull and it slipped right out. Phew. I gave him a sincere heart-felt thanks.

The next obstacle was breathing. I had retained a lot of fluid in my lungs, heart, and surrounding tissue during the extended surgery. It made it very difficult to breathe. My lung doctor stopped by and said my lungs were full of fluid. He said it might take months for that to dissipate.

Since by now it was evident I had not had a seizure, a stroke or worse, I was moved to a standard room. I was able to call DeAnna on my cell phone. I was eager for her to know I was fine.

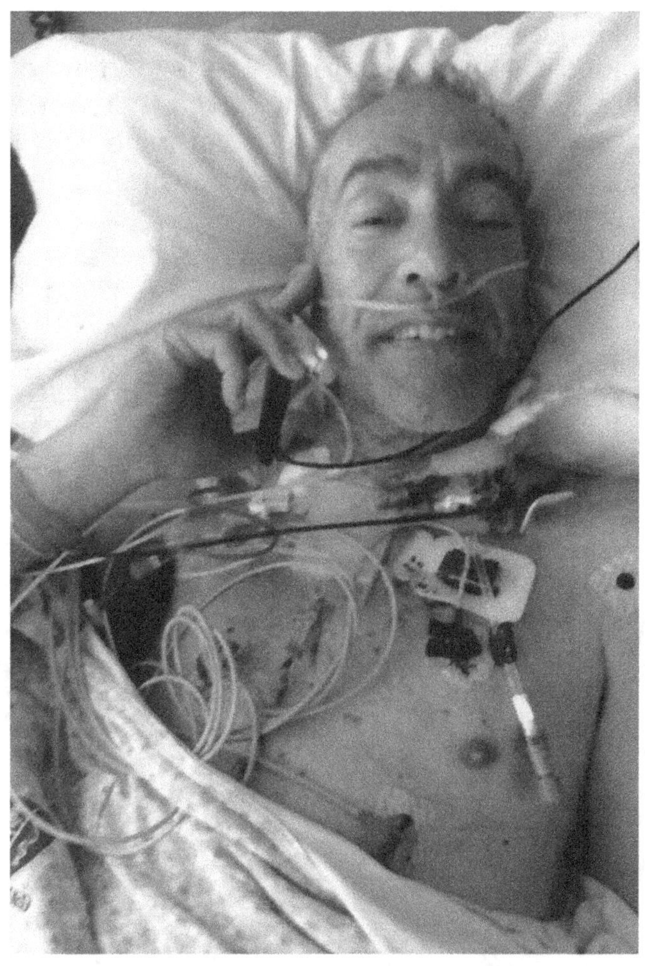

In spite of the chest tubes, the EKG lines, the wires running to the heart, the IV line, the O2 sat, and the blood pressure cuff, I was happy as a clam. I had been given pain medication in ICU - which at the time was putting me right to sleep. So I quickly weaned off of it and just took some acetaminophen each day.

Doug and Jessica stayed by my side until I was discharged. It had been nine days.

The whole experience was another reminder that my life and my future is in the hand of God. Nothing can take me out of his will if I remain submitted to Him. When I pray, "Your will be done on earth as it is in heaven,"[67] I also mean I want God's will to be done in my life. I desire for His will to be done in my family, nation and across our world, but it is only by individually submitting to Him that we can be assured of remaining in His will.

We present ourselves as a living sacrifice. Scripture says to us, "Do not conform to the pattern of this world, but be transformed by the renewing of your mind. Then you will be able to

---

[67] Matthew 6:10

test and approve what God's will is--his good, pleasing and perfect will."[68] So I consciously seek to conform to the pattern of Scripture - not to the world. And I renew my mind with that Word. So when faced with a 5% chance of survival I can have confidence. To the believer in Jesus, there is no "fatal event." Living with Christ each day is an everlasting event.

It is His Word, hidden in my heart, that guides me. It is assurance that even when I "walk through the darkest valley"[69] God is with me. He will never leave me nor forsake me. Not in the simplest times, not in the most difficult times, and not even the last time.

---

[68] Romans 12:2

[69] Psalm 23:4

Chapter 39

Final Thoughts

God's word has taught me about humility, trusting Him alone, about knowing Him personally, serving Him, and loving others. If I hadn't been reading and memorizing His word from the time I was fourteen until the present, I would have just endured these events without any realization that God was working in me through it all. Without the regular input of His word I might be aware of God's existence, but I would be missing life's principles and guidance that come from actually reading His scriptures. There is no meaning or purpose for somebody who is experiencing hardship apart from God; it is just plain misery. But when one is grounded in Jesus life has an entirely new purpose. We are born to give Him glory. We can do that in health or in sickness, in life or in death.

Jesus himself has multiple scars that don' just tell a story, they have brought us salvation. Some are familiar with the biblical phrase, "With his stripes we are healed."[70] One thinks first of the deep gashes created by the lashing Jesus received prior to his death. Those cuts must have looked like stripes across his back. We are healed because we have eternal life that is a result of Him paying our debt with his death. The scars that are in His hands and feet tell of the price He paid on the cross. They are the most significant scars in the history of mankind. They are the wounds that rocked the eternity of mankind. They paid the enormous debt of man. Our debt is that we are condemned to eternal death and separation from Him because of our load of sin.

---

[70] Isaiah 53:5 from the King James Bible

Many people have a problem with saying, *"I am a sinner."* I was watching a video recently where a fellow went around in a modern shopping mall and asked teen-agers and young adults some questions about right and wrong.

"Is it wrong to steal?" he asked.

"Of course it is," was the prompt answer.

"Have you ever stolen anything?"

The kid thought for a few seconds and then replied, "Well, yeah. I have." So the cameraman continued with another question.

"Is it wrong to lie?"

Each person he interviewed agreed it was wrong to break these simple laws of life. Then he changed the wording and asked if they had "sinned." To a person they slowly each admitted on camera that they had sinned. They had lusted, lied, stolen, etc. and that they were by their own admission sinners. Most people are just never confronted with their own behavior. They think that because society is "tolerant" that they somehow get a free pass. Well, there are no free passes. Someone has to pay.

"All have sinned."[71] Jesus paid the obligation (our debt) for our sins so that we can receive complete forgiveness. It's like when my daughter gave my wife and I passes to a movie theater recently. She of course had to pay for the passes. But we got to enter the theater without paying anything. We couldn't get in without the passes. My daughter had to pay the "debt" for them. What did I have to do? I had to accept the pass and present it at the door to the kid who collects tickets.

He recited his line, "Welcome to our theatre; I hope you enjoy the show." At least in heaven we won't have to pay ten dollars for popcorn.

Since Jesus paid for our entrance into heaven he then teaches us in His word how to live here on earth, how to follow Him. He doesn't just give us a pass to heaven. He teaches us to love others, and to love Him with all our hearts. Sometimes we won't learn those lessons easily. But we can learn them if we are in His word and see His purposes in life's challenges.

---

[71] Romans 3:23

Some might read these stories and think, "Well that worked for you, Dan. You were healed." But I want to tell you that as I suffered with cystic fibrosis I wasn't healed. I did, in fact, pray several times to be healed. The apostle Paul asked three times to have his thorn-in-the-flesh removed (which most commentators feel was some type of illness), and God told him basically, "No." He had to just contend with it and press on. I also prayed and asked Jesus three times to take away cystic fibrosis. But God clearly said, *"No."*

I realized that if God said, *"No,"* then He had a good reason for it. So I suffered. I sucked every breath in for twenty years with increasing difficulty. I endured the humiliation of caring around a sputum cup with me everywhere and spitting into it.

So God chose *not* to heal me of CF. He did of course heal me when I was dying on the operating table after the transplant and was doomed to die. And as you've seen He healed me many other times as well. But life is not about getting healed and being released from all our suffering. It is about knowing God and experiencing Him intimately. It's about bringing Him glory in our life and death.

You can begin to experience this by asking Him to take control of your life. Open His word and read how others did this. They believed Him by faith, like Abraham. They were told to be born again, like Nicodemus. They declared Him to be their King, like Nathanael. They left their profession of fishing and became His disciples, like Simon, Peter and Andrew. They simply followed Him. One thing is sure, when you leave your past life and turn to Jesus and make Him Lord of your whole life it will radically change you. You will still experience this fallen world and your decaying body will still annoy you. But you will have the Holy Spirit alive inside you; the Lord of Lord's will come to live in the temple that is your heart. And you will be continually changed.

And will I continue in this body to suffer? Probably. However, it is not in vain. For, "We also glory in our sufferings, because we know that suffering produces perseverance; perseverance, character; and character, hope. And hope does not put us to shame, because God's love has been poured out into our hearts through the Holy Spirit, who has been given to us."[72]

I will surely die one day, as every person on earth has done. But I remain joyful. For whether I live or die, it is for His glory. "For to me to live is Christ, and to die is gain."[73] Simply put, I am alive in Christ. That concept is communicated well in this verse, "I am crucified with Christ: nevertheless I live; yet not I, but Christ liveth in me: and the life which I now live in the flesh I live by the faith of the Son of God, who loved me, and gave himself for me."[74]

And remember the promise the Lord gave to DeAnna when I was so critically ill in 1995? The Lord said, "Dan is going to make it. He is going to live. You will one day see him holding his grandchild." A tremendous peace overwhelmed her.

That day came in 2016.

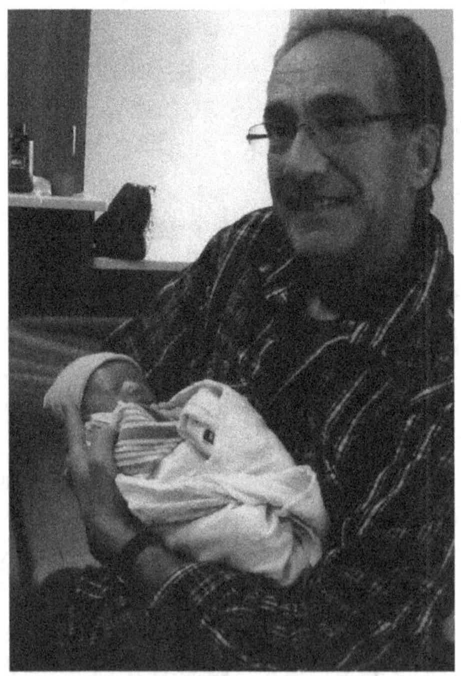

---

[72] Romans 5:3-5

[73] Philippians 1:21

[74] Galatians 2:20

DeAnna took this picture just a few hours after our grandchild was born!

Chapter 40

Doug Lagasse

On November 22, 2013 my awesome brother Doug, after waiting (on and off) for several years for a double lung transplant, received a pair of lungs at the University of Colorado Hospital (UCH) in Denver. After his transplant he went back to work as a culture and security trainer for an international Christian humanitarian non-profit. He continues to travel to difficult places to serve others in need. He is married with two adult children and a granddaughter. He received lots of attention when he was in the recovery room recuperating from his transplant. Although both our parents are deceased, DeAnna, I and our daughter Jessica were able to come. Of course Doug's wife Dawn, their

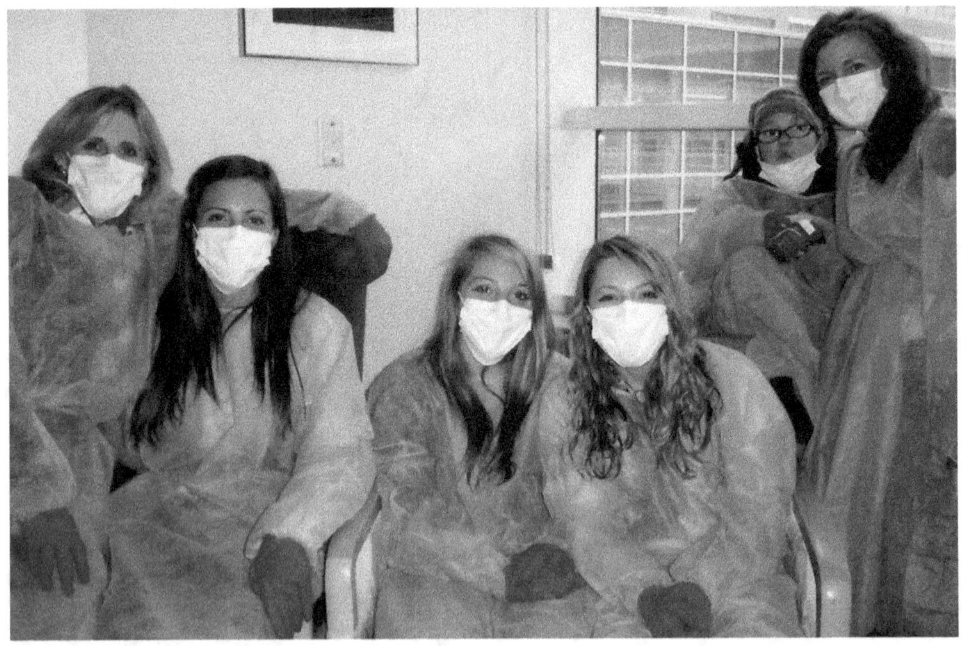

children and their granddaughter were able to be at his side. Pictured here (left to right) is a gaggle of females: his sister-in-law Laura, three of Doug's nieces, his granddaughter and Dawn. Doug writes about his experience:

"Despite my chronic lung disfunction, I had been inspired by my older brothers to pursue a full and purposeful life. I became critically afflicted with cystic fibrosis in my thirties. As the infections took hold, my lung function dropped over the years, but I was still able to carry out my international work.

When my lungs got down to 20% function I qualified for listing in September of 2011. I was fifty-one. But in that qualification they discovered an aortic stenosis which needed to be addressed before transplant. It was a catch 22 situation. My heart would not survive the lung transplant, but my lungs would not survive a traditional heart surgery. Cardiac surgeons lobbied for my case, and I was able to receive the newly developed Trans Aortic Valve Replacement (TAVR) in March of 2012. It did not require opening my chest. After that operation I had to be on blood thinners for six months. That further delayed getting re-listed for my transplant.

I was put back on the active list In September 2012. I got a call in November, went in, gowned and scrubbed up, and got the IV started. Advanced directives were signed and sealed. Then a friend of the deceased donor came forward and revealed a critical detail about the donor. Apparently he had been huffing all kinds of strange intoxicants (without parental knowledge). Doctors realized the lungs were too brittle for transplant. So I was sent home, disappointed, but grateful to have avoided those defective lungs.

I waited a full year after that; including four continuous months spent as in-patient at UCH. I was placed on ever-changing combinations of antibiotics to attempt to keep the infections at bay. I did as many daily lung treatments as I could tolerate, and required ten liters of oxygen at rest. I was down to just a 15% FEV1 (Forced Expiration Volume for 1 second) for a person my age and weight. By pushing a wheel chair that held my oxygen tanks and my IV pole, I still managed to walk up to five miles every day around the hospital. Eventually I was deemed too fit to be in the hospital and I was sent back home - with all the machines and tubes - to continue my wait.

My lungs were shot. I tried to remain upbeat during the long ordeal but it was difficult. I needed a transplant, but new lungs were not forthcoming.

I am O positive, which seemed to be a disadvantage. Any lungs of this blood type could go to any needy recipient. Other patients were accepted ahead of me because they were deemed to be sicker. With a low population density, Colorado did not have many organs available. I was offered the opportunity to be listed at other transplant centers on the east or west coast, but we chose to stay at our home in Colorado where we had a fuller support system for the recovery process.

Whenever I was hospitalized over the years I made an effort to continue my job by internet, and tried to be an encourager to staff and visitors. But toward the end of my old lungs, I was intertwined with life-supportive and pain-relieving mechanisms, tethered on all sides by tubes and cables, not able to move, unable to speak, and not really hearing much over the noise of the machines. I spent days staring at the acoustic tiles on the ceiling of my hospital room. I felt pretty useless. What could possibly be the purpose of such an existence?

I considered the possibility that all I would have to do is to stop trying to survive, and I could quickly be in heaven. But my beloved wife expressed her opposition to that option, and she asked me to keep on fighting. I decided that living would be the loving thing to do for her.

Then, in my heart I heard my Heavenly Father say, 'I love you no matter your productivity. Let's just hang out. Simply be with Me in each hour.' Reflecting on his greatness and care turned out to be a God-glorifying purpose, even in that condition.

At six in the morning on a cold snowy November day I got another call. I immediately began the ninety minute drive to Denver. As I was navigating along the icy highway my doctor called me again. I was trying to breathe, hold the phone and navigate the roadway. With concern in his voice my doctor said the lungs the hospital had for me were from a former IV drug user who smoked and had spent time in prison. What a dilemma. They would have a low potential, and were definitely high risk. I truly wondered what to do. But I realized I needed to take them as I didn't seem to have many remaining days to live. So I said I wanted to go ahead with it and I was coming in for the operation. After the surgery and extubation it was truly great to breathe freely without oxygen.

However, two months later I learned there had been some complications during the transplant. The clam shell wound was not healing well. They needed to surgically clean out old infected areas from around the new lungs. Doctors said the only medication that would fight the infection was Amikacin, which can cause deafness if the dosage is large. They needed a very large dose. I had to choose between the threat of infection in the new lungs and the likelihood of going deaf. I could not imagine life without my hearing. I work with people daily, and music is a core part of my existence. But I signed off on the harsh antibiotics and began the IV drip.

While trying to recover from this second arm pit to arm pit thoracic grand opening, I depended upon worship music to keep my spirits up. Unable to lie down, and uncomfortable sitting, I spent long nights in our home pacing around the house. The massive IV doses of Amikacin were impacting me. I'd been warned. I'd signed the release of liability. So I was upset that night, but not surprised, when I realized I was losing my hearing. Within hours of my second dose, I could feel myself going deaf. Completely. Permanently. I cried out to God, 'Really?! You grant me new life, then take away my hearing?! Even my ability to hear your praises?' In the ensuing days – starkly alone with my thoughts - I began to realize the unusual opportunity I had been given to better hear God's still small voice. My 'quiet times' in the Word and worship were quieter than ever, and I was more connected with Him as well. And isn't that what life is supposed to be about?

A few months after going deaf, in April I received a cochlear implant on my right ear. It took a lot getting used to. In May we took our victory tour pulling a tent trailer visiting friends and family in six states. It included much celebration, but also camping, hiking biking and kayaking. God is great!

The 24 inch lung transplant incision scar across my chest (which required 100 staples to hold it together post surgery) represents being nearly cut in half. Just think of all the muscles and nerves involved! Getting them reconnected and functional has been a long process. Even after almost seven years, I still have numbness, tingling, and itching, bringing new definition to the term, 'Seven year itch.'"

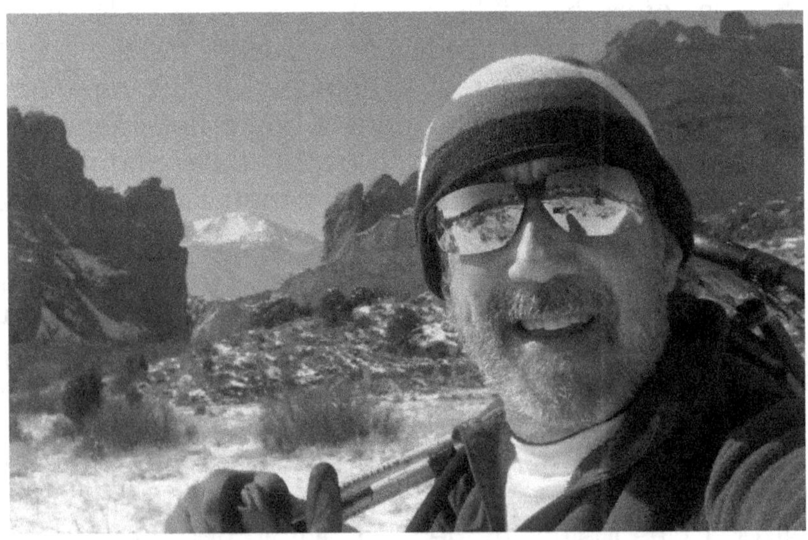

DOUG SNOWSHOEING IN THE COLORADO ROCKIES

Afterword About Our Daughters

Our daughters Shirena and Jessica are both married. Shirena has given us a granddaughter, now age 5. She and her husband have a mobile auto repair business. She is a singer, pianist and songwriter and is an accomplished recording artist. Jessica works full time for a finance investment firm, is learning to play guitar and is a gifted vocalist. Our daughters have been a tremendous joy and support to us through all these trying times.

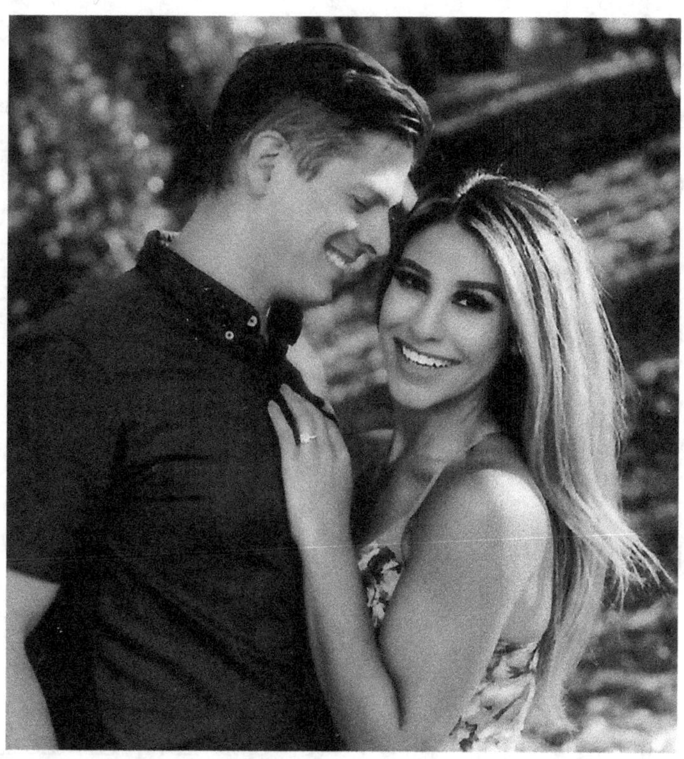

NEWLYWEDS MIKE AND JESSICA

Appendix: Health Record (a partial list)

Surgeries and Procedures

Sinus Surgery (Dr. Nayak)	Oct	2018
Aortic Valve, Tricuspid Valve Replaced, Mitral Repair	Sep	2016
Skin cancers removed surgically (Dr. Honari, Dr. Aasi)	15+	times
Sinus Surgery (Dr Nayak)	Mar	2012
Sinus Surgery (Dr. Nayak)	Mar	2011
Sinus Surgery (Dr. Nayak)	Dec	2009
Aortic valve replacement (stenosis) (Dr. Reitz)	Oct	2008
Thyroidectomy (Dr. Swedenborg)	May	2008
Polypectomy (Dr. Swedenborg)	May	2008
Polypectomy (Dr. Vawter)	Apr	2008
Colonoscopy (Dr. Tu at Kaiser)	Apr	2008
Skin cancer (squamous and basil cell) on head at Kaiser Mar		2008
Sinus surgery (Dr. Vaughn)	June	2007
Endoscopic debridement of sinuses	as	needed
Sinus Surgery (Dr. Gurustan)	Dec	2005
Laparoscopic Repair of Meniscus (Left knee)	July	2003
Aorta root and aortic valve replaced (Dr. Robbins)	Mar	2002
Sinus Surgery (Dr. Vaughn) Aug		2000,
Heart double lung transplant (Dr. Robbins)	Jan	1997
Sinus Surgery (Dr. Moran)	Jan	1996
Gall bladder removal	Nov	1995
Mediport placement in left chest wall (removed in 1997)		1994
Brain abscess removed (left rear hemisphere) (Dr. Huertas)		1978
Tonsillectomy		1962

Other Significant Hospitalizations and Diseases

I was hospitalized for two week periods for lung infections at least 50 times from the years 1976-1996. Sometimes it included some "home care". These occurred in seven different countries. England, Hong Kong, Philippines, Germany, Switzerland, India, and the US. The underlying illness in all of these situations was cystic fibrosis.

Pneumonia	Dec	2019
Blood Infections (six times)		2016
Seizures	1978,	2011
Blood Infection (Pseudomonas)	Sep	2011
Blood Infection (Klebsiella)	Jun	2011
Sepsis (Pseudomonas) heart valve	Apr	2009
Pneumonia (Kaiser, San Jose)	Aug	2008
Lyme Disease	Aug	2007
Shingles	Sep	2007
Urinary Tract Infection	Aug	2006
Blood Infection	Jan	2002
Hepatitis A	Oct	1993
Pancreatitis	1979,	1991
Heat Stroke		1960

Broken Bones

metatarsals r. foot	Feb	2018
Rib, left side	Jun	2011
4th metatarsal r. foot	Nov	2008
2nd, 3rd, 4th, 5th metatarsal r. foot	Jan	2019
5th metatarsal r. foot	Jan	2020
r. forearm	Aug	2006
vertebrae M7, M8, M9 & M11	Aug	2005
5th metatarsal l. foot	Oct	2004

About the Author

Dan Lagasse is a retired pastor, overseas Christian volunteer, teacher, writer and speaker. He has ministered in over forty countries, mostly in the third world. He and his wife, DeAnna, are passionate about sharing the love of Jesus with the lost, especially where Christ is not known. His friends know him as the "miracle man" because of the countless number of times doctors have announced the likelihood of his demise.

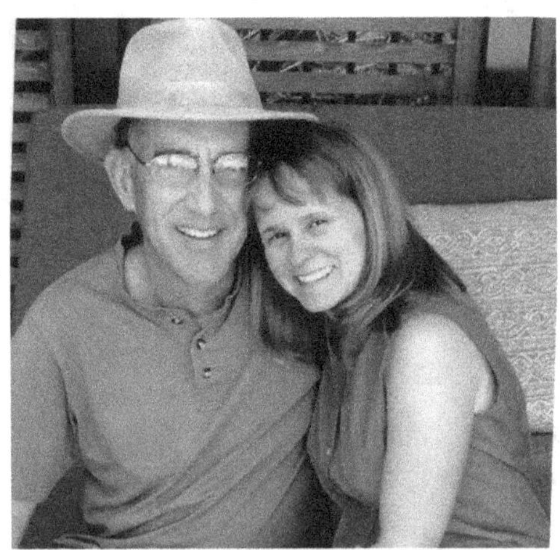

He has been hospitalized over one hundred times (in nine countries). He had a heart-double lung transplant in 1997 and several open-heart surgeries since then. He loves music and plays his trombone in a big band, a jazz band, and a worship band. He loves to learn how to build or fix things. In 2011, he and a friend finished a complete frame-off restoration of a 1936 five-window coupe. You can write Dan at 1936gasser@gmail.com.

Also by Dan Lagasse

Between Iraq and a Hard Place

(Written under the pseudonym Kirk Legacy)

This is the true story of a young couple who leaves Silicon Valley to learn Kurdish in Berlin. They have a passion to share the love of Jesus with the world, particularly those who are oppressed, unloved, and disenfranchised.

As the First Gulf War ends, they are called to lead a team of relief workers into the mountains of eastern Turkey and Iraq to assist the hundreds of thousands of Kurds who have fled for their lives. Their faith is stretched further as they attempt to adopt two starving Kurdish sisters. Finally, their faith in God is stretched to its limits as it becomes clear they will lose their precious children some years after the adoption was finalized.

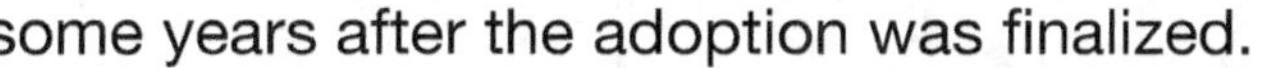

It is a story of two fragile people, facing formidable challenges with scant human resources, and living in extreme conditions. Read about faith when confronted by fear. Witness hope when all seems lost. And see a couple find peace in the midst of life's greatest struggles. Between Iraq and a Hard Place tells the saga of two adults under intense pressure, of two children facing certain death, and of a people facing genocide.

It is available from Amazon at https://smile.amazon.com/Between-Iraq-Hard-Place-Legacy/dp/1098011414/ref=sr_1_1?crid=1BRZ57I2ZWL1B&dchild=1&keywords=between+iraq+and+a+hard+place&qid=1597194006&sprefix=between+Iraq%2Caps%2C351&sr=8-1